MEASURING POVERTY

A New Approach

Constance F. Citro and Robert T. Michael, *Editors*

Panel on Poverty and Family Assistance:
Concepts, Information Needs, and Measurement Methods

Committee on National Statistics

Commission on Behavioral and Social Sciences and Education

National Research Council

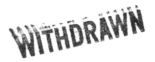

NATIONAL ACADEMY PRESS
Washington, D.C. 1995

NATIONAL ACADEMY PRESS • 2101 Constitution Ave., NW • Washington, DC 20418

NOTICE: The project that is the subject of this report was approved by the Governing Board of the National Research Council, whose members are drawn from the councils of the National Academy of Sciences, the National Academy of Engineering, and the Institute of Medicine. The members of the committee responsible for the report were chosen for their special competences and with regard for appropriate balance.

This report has been reviewed by a group other than the authors according to procedures approved by a Report Review Committee consisting of members of the National Academy of Sciences, the National Academy of Engineering, and the Institute of Medicine.

The project that is the subject of this report was administered under a contract with the Bureau of the Census of the U.S. Department of Commerce, with funding from the Administration for Children and Families of the U.S. Department of Health and Human Services and the Bureau of Labor Statistics of the U.S. Department of Labor. The Food and Nutrition Service of the U.S. Department of Agriculture also provided funding to the Committee on National Statistics for the project.

Library of Congress Cataloging-in-Publication Data

Measuring poverty : a new approach / Panel on Poverty and Family
    Assistance . . . [et al.].
       p. cm.
    Includes bibliographical references and index.
    ISBN 0-309-05128-2
    1. Poverty—United States—Statistical methods. I. Panel on
Poverty and Family Assistance (United States)
    HC110.P6M36   1995
    362.5'2'015195—dc20   95-3901

Printed in the United States of America

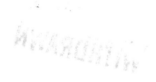

PANEL ON POVERTY AND FAMILY ASSISTANCE: CONCEPTS, INFORMATION NEEDS, AND MEASUREMENT METHODS

ROBERT T. MICHAEL (*Chair*), Harris Graduate School of Public Policy Studies, University of Chicago

ANTHONY B. ATKINSON, Nuffield College, Oxford University

DAVID M. BETSON, Department of Economics, University of Notre Dame

REBECCA M. BLANK, Department of Economics, Northwestern University

LAWRENCE D. BOBO, Department of Sociology, University of California, Los Angeles

JEANNE BROOKS-GUNN, Center for Young Children and Families, Teachers College, Columbia University

JOHN F. COGAN, The Hoover Institution, Stanford University

SHELDON H. DANZIGER, Institute of Public Policy Studies and School of Social Work, University of Michigan

ANGUS S. DEATON, Woodrow Wilson School of Public and International Affairs, Princeton University

*DAVID T. ELLWOOD, Kennedy School of Government, Harvard University

JUDITH M. GUERON, Manpower Demonstration Research Corporation, New York, N.Y.

ROBERT M. HAUSER, Department of Sociology and Institute for Research on Poverty, University of Wisconsin

FRANKLIN D. WILSON, Department of Sociology, University of Wisconsin

CONSTANCE F. CITRO, *Study Director*

NANCY MARITATO, *Research Associate*

ELAINE REARDON, *Research Associate*

AGNES E. GASKIN, *Senior Project Assistant*

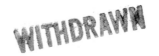

---

*Served until February 1993

Acknowledgments

The Panel on Poverty and Family Assistance wishes to thank the many people who helped make possible the preparation of this report.

An important part of the panel's work was the analysis of implementing the recommended poverty concept and alternative measures on the numbers and characteristics of people in poverty. Panel member David Betson assumed the responsibility for this work and gave unstintingly of his time, energy, and analytical skills in constructing the necessary data files and conducting an extensive series of analyses for the panel's consideration. The panel is greatly in his debt.

The data that Professor Betson analyzed were obtained from many sources, with the gracious help of the following people: Charles Nelson, Bureau of the Census, who provided several March Current Population Survey (CPS) files with the Bureau's estimates of income and payroll taxes and the value of in-kind benefits (he also briefed the panel on the Bureau's tax simulations); Pat Doyle, Agency for Health Care Policy and Research, who provided detailed tabulations of out-of-pocket medical care expenses from the 1987 National Medical Expenditure Survey; and Larry Radbill, Mathematica Policy Research, Inc., who provided analyses of data on child care and other work-related expenses from the Survey of Income and Program Participation (SIPP).

The panel conducted extensive analyses of data from the Consumer Expenditure Survey (CEX) on spending for food, clothing, shelter, and other consumption. This analysis was made possible by the hard work and expertise of staff of the Bureau of Labor Statistics, including Geoffrey Paulin, who, with input from David Johnson, prepared a large of volume of tabulations; and Stephanie Shipp, who saw that the work received priority attention (she also briefed the panel on the CEX). Lynda Carlson and Ivy Harrison of the Energy Information Administration provided useful information on transportation costs from the 1991 Residential Transportation Energy Consumption Survey. An analysis of 1990 census data on geographic variations in housing costs was carried out by Nancy Maritato, research associate for the panel, with a data file provided by Marie Peis of the Census Bureau.

The panel's consideration of using survey responses to derive poverty thresholds benefited from the availability of new data. We thank Donald Clifton, chairman, Gallup Organization, who graciously made space available in the August 1992 Gallup Poll for questions on the poverty line. We also thank Tom Smith of the National Opinion Research Center, who oversaw the addition of questions on the poverty line to the 1993 General Social Survey, and we thank the Wisconsin Letters and Survey Center, which included questions on the poverty line in its ongoing telephone survey.

During the first year of its work, the panel held meetings at which panel members and others presented papers and led discussions on various aspects of poverty measurement. These seminars were always informative and fruitful; they added greatly to the panel's understanding of the issues. We acknowledge particularly the contributions of Marilyn Moon, Urban Institute, who prepared a paper on alternative approaches to the treatment of medical care benefits and costs in a poverty measure; and Harold Watts, Columbia University, who prepared a paper on budget-based concepts of poverty.

We also acknowledge John Coder, Bureau of the Census, who reviewed data quality issues in the March CPS; Greg Duncan, Northwestern University, and Patricia Ruggles, Joint Economic Committee staff, who discussed time periods for measuring poverty; Christopher Jencks, Northwestern University, who discussed consumption and income definitions of family resources; Graham Kalton, Westat, Inc., who reviewed for us the recommendations of the National Research Council Panel to Evaluate SIPP; Brent Moulton, Bureau of Labor Statistics, who reviewed the Bureau's work to develop inter-area price indexes; Kathryn Nelson, U.S. Department of Housing and Urban Development, who briefed the panel on fair market rents and income limits for housing assistance programs; Deborah Phillips, Board on Children and Families, National Research Council, who described research on poverty, child care, and families; Howard Rolston, Administration for Children and Families, U.S. Department of Health and Human Services, who briefed the panel on issues of minimum benefit standards for family assistance programs; Denton Vaughan, Social Security Administration, who described work on estimating poverty levels from Gallup Poll survey data; Daniel Weinberg, Bureau of the Census, who provided an overview of issues in poverty measurement in the United States; and Michael Wolfson, Statistics Canada, who described efforts to revise the Canadian low-income measures. Also, Vee Burke of the Congressional Research Service provided helpful comments on the parts of our report that discuss government assistance programs; and Mary Kokoski of the Bureau of Labor Statistics did the same for our discussion of interarea price indexes.

Regular attendees at our seminars included many of the people listed above, and they and the following people contributed useful insights and perspectives in our public discussions: Richard Bavier and Paul Bugg, U.S. Office of Management and Budget; William Butz, Bureau of the Census; Eva Jacobs, Bureau of Labor Statistics (retired); Bruce Klein, U.S. Department of Agriculture; William Prosser, U.S. Department of Health and Human Services; and Kathleen Scholl, U.S.General Accounting Office. Mollie Orshansky, the originator of the current U.S. poverty measure, gave the panel her unique perspective at our first meeting.

Gordon Fisher, U.S. Department of Health and Human Services (formerly at the U.S. Office of Economic Opportunity), not only attended our seminars but provided the panel with invaluable materials on the history of poverty measurement in the United States. He deserves the thanks of all poverty analysts for assembling and preserving the detailed historical record.

The list of references in our report makes clear the extensive literature on poverty and poverty measurement on which we were fortunate to draw. We acknowledge particularly the useful material for understanding the current U.S. poverty measure and alternative measures in the studies conducted by the 1976 Poverty Studies Task Force, chaired by Bette Mahoney (U.S. Department of Health, Education, and Welfare) and by the Expert Committee on Family Budget Revisions (1980), chaired by Harold Watts. Pat Ruggles' recent book, *Drawing the Line: Alternative Poverty Measures and Their Implications for Public Policy* (1990), is another invaluable review of issues and alternatives. We mention above Gordon Fisher's contributions, which are also cited in the reference list.

Daniel Weinberg and Enrique Lamas, Bureau of the Census; John Holmes, Bureau of Labor Statistics; and Leonard Sternbach, Administration for Children and Families, U.S. Department of Health and Human Services, were the contract monitors and liaisons for the study. They assisted the panel in obtaining needed information and keeping the project on track and by their participation in our public meetings.

An important debt of gratitude is owed to the panel's own staff. Nancy Maritato, who served as research associate, worked closely with the study director on all aspects of the project. She prepared background materials on a wide range of subjects: alternative poverty threshold concepts, subjective measures of poverty obtained from survey responses, geographic variations in living costs, alternative definitions of family resources, poverty indexes, and the incentive effects of government assistance programs. As noted above, she conducted analyses for the panel of interarea housing cost differences, and she worked closely with Bureau of Labor Statistics staff in developing the expenditure information that formed the basis of the panel's recommended threshold concept.

Elaine Reardon, who served as the panel's Chicago-based research associate, provided me with efficient and resourceful assistance. In addition, she prepared background material on alternative equivalence scales for adjusting poverty thresholds by family type and on the effects of poverty and government assistance on children.

Agnes Gaskin served ably as the panel's project assistant. She dealt admirably with the logistics of the panel's numerous meetings and the voluminous materials that the panel generated over the course of the project, culminating in this report. Agnes was assisted at one time or another by virtually all the project assistants of the Committee on National Statistics.

We are very grateful to Eugenia Grohman, Associate Director for Reports of the Commission on Behavioral and Social Sciences and Education, for invaluable assistance in helping the panel organize a large volume of technical material into a coherent and readable report and in shepherding the report through the review and production processes at the National Research Council.

Of course, individual panel members made impressive contributions to the study. Several of them led seminars and prepared background materials and chapter drafts on particular topics; others participated in a working group to explore the relationship of a statistical poverty measure to eligibility standards for government assistance programs; and all contributed a high level of critical thinking and concern for the difficult issues we faced.

Finally, I want to say on behalf of myself and the panel that it has been a joy to work closely with such a fine professional as our study director, Connie Citro. It is she who deserves a disproportionate share of any credit due this panel.

ROBERT T. MICHAEL, *Chair*
Panel on Poverty and Family Assistance

Contents

FIGURES

TABLES

Preface

The concepts and data that underlie the current U.S. measure of poverty are more than 30 years old. Over the past two decades, more and more people have raised questions about the measure and whether it is still appropriate for the end of the twentieth century.

Reflecting these concerns, the Joint Economic Committee of Congress initiated an independent, in-depth review of the U.S. poverty measure, working with the House Subcommittee on Census, Statistics, and Postal Personnel. Funds for a study by the National Research Council (NRC) of the official poverty measure and alternatives to it were appropriated to the Bureau of Labor Statistics (BLS) of the U.S. Department of Labor. The study was to address concepts, measurement methods, and information needs for a poverty measure, but not necessarily to specify a new poverty "line."

Subsequently, the scope of the study was broadened to include consideration of similar conceptual and methodological issues for establishing standards for welfare payments to needy families with children. The Administration for Children and Families (ACF) of the U.S. Department of Health and Human Services provided funding for this second request, which originated from a provision in the 1988 Family Support Act. This provision asked for a study of a national minimum benefit standard for the Aid to Families with Dependent Children program. The NRC said it could not recommend a standard but could consider some of the issues involved. Both ACF and BLS transferred their funding to the Bureau of the Census, U.S. Department of Commerce, for a contract with the Committee on National Statistics at the NRC to establish our panel. The Food and Nutrition Service of the U.S. Department of Agriculture also provided funds to support the study.

Our panel first met in June 1992 and, over two-and-a-half years, worked to come to grips with the range of conceptual and statistical issues involved in defining and measuring poverty and in setting standards for assistance programs. We were very aware of the importance of the poverty measure, which serves as a key social indicator and also determines eligibility for benefits for many government assistance programs. We were also cognizant of the intense interest in the poverty measure among the policy and research communities. Hence, we took steps to educate ourselves as fully as possible about the issues and to ensure that we heard a broad range of views. We held numerous meetings to which we invited staff from many executive and congressional agencies, as well as researchers and analysts with expertise in particular areas. We sent letters to more than 150 researchers and analysts asking for their views on key issues. We reviewed the large body of literature on poverty measurement both in the United States and abroad. Finally, with help from federal agencies, we conducted extensive data analyses of our own.

This report of our work is organized into three distinct parts of disparate lengths. First, a summary highlights key findings and lists all our recommendations. Second, Chapter 1, titled "Introduction and Overview," provides both background on the topic and the arguments for our recommendations; it is designed for a nontechnical audience. Third, Chapters 2-8 (and Appendices B-D) provide detailed reviews and technical analyses of many of the issues related to poverty measurement and the determination of program benefit standards.

On the basis of our deliberations, we recommend a new official poverty measure for the United States. Our recommendation is to retain the basic notion of poverty as material deprivation, but to use a revised concept for setting a threshold and a revised definition of the resources to be compared with the threshold to determine if a family or individual is or is not in poverty. Equally importantly, we recommend procedures for devising an equivalent poverty threshold for families of different sizes and for families in different geographic locations and for updating the poverty threshold over time.

The current poverty measure has weaknesses both in the implementation of the threshold concept and in the definition of family resources. Changing social and economic conditions over the last three decades have made these weaknesses more obvious and more consequential. As a result, the current measure does not accurately reflect differences in poverty across population groups and across time. We conclude that it would be inadvisable to retain the current measure for the future.

In deciding on a new measure to recommend, we used scientific evidence to the extent possible. However, the determination of a particular type of poverty measure and, even more, the determination of a particular poverty threshold are ultimately subjective decisions. "Expertise" can only carry one so far. To help us choose among alternatives, we developed a set of criteria, namely, that the poverty measure should be understandable and broadly acceptable to the public, statistically defensible (e.g., internally consistent), and operationally feasible. Finally, for the most judgmental aspect of a poverty measure, namely, setting the level of the threshold, we recommend a specific *procedure* to follow—but we do not recommend a precise number. We suggest a range that we believe provides reasonable limits for the initial poverty threshold, but we leave the ultimate choice of a specific value to the policy arena.

We also considered the possible relationship of the proposed poverty measure to eligibility and benefit standards for government assistance programs. The issues in this area are complex. For many reasons, there is no necessary relationship between a statistical measure of need and the extent to which programs can or should be devised to alleviate need. We do not offer specific recommendations, but we hope that our discussion of the issues will provide some helpful insights for the ongoing policy debate. We note that our discussion, of necessity, refers to assistance programs as they operated in 1992-1994.

One member of our panel, John F. Cogan, dissents from the panel's decision to recommend a new poverty measure for the United States. He believes that it is inappropriate for a panel of the National Research Council to make such a recommendation, and he questions some of the panel's analysis in his dissent (Appendix A). Although Professor Cogan raises some important issues, we are confident that careful readers of the report will find that we have dealt thoroughly with all of them.

Professor Cogan also questions the scientific basis for our recommendations. There is, indeed, judgment as well as science informing many of the decisions that underlie the recommendations in this report. That is why the panel has taken great care to make clear at each step in the report the character and status of the scientific evidence and the role of judgment. Again, we are confident that careful readers of the report will see clearly how we have dealt with the interplay of science and judgment at every step.

But the panel concluded that it would not serve the public interest for our report simply to lay out the many possible alternatives to the current poverty measure or simply to call for more research on the topics where that might advance our knowledge or reduce the range of possible alternatives. The current U.S. measure of poverty is demonstrably flawed judged by today's knowledge; it needs to be replaced. The panel believes that the measure recommended in our report is a significant improvement over that current measure, and we urge its adoption.

Over time, we know that the nature of scientific evidence will change and the subjective judgments of what seems appropriate today will probably change as well. That was surely one important reason for convening this panel, since the current poverty measure was informed by early 1960s-vintage knowledge and perceptions.   It is also the reason we recommend that a process be established for periodic review of the poverty measure (as is done for other key social indicators, such as the Consumer Price Index).

I know that I speak for all the members of this panel in expressing gratitude for the privilege of serving on it. Its purpose is an important one, and we have each learned much from our work over the past two-and-a-half years.

ROBERT T. MICHAEL, *Chair*
Panel on Poverty and Family Assistance

MEASURING
POVERTY

Summary and Recommendations

$\mathbf{T}$he U.S. measure of poverty is an important social indicator that affects not only public perceptions of well-being in America, but also public policies and programs. The current measure was originally developed in the early 1960s as an indicator of the number and proportion of people with inadequate family incomes for needed consumption of food and other goods and services. At that time, the poverty "line" for a family of four had broad support. Since then, the poverty measure has been widely used for policy formation, program administration, analytical research, and general public understanding.

Like other important indicators, the poverty measure should be evaluated periodically to determine if it is still serving its intended purposes and whether it can be improved. This report of the Panel on Poverty and Family Assistance provides such an evaluation. Our major conclusion is that the current measure needs to be revised: it no longer provides an accurate picture of the differences in the extent of economic poverty among population groups or geographic areas of the country, nor an accurate picture of trends over time. The current measure has remained virtually unchanged over the past 30 years. Yet during that time, there have been marked changes in the nation's economy and society and in public policies that have affected families' economic well-being, which are not reflected in the measure. Improved data, methods, and research knowledge make it possible to improve the current poverty measure.

The panel proposes a new measure that will more accurately identify the poor population today. For example, for 1992, the year for which the panel had data available for analysis, the proposed measure, compared with the current measure, finds a lower poverty rate for people in families on public assistance and a higher poverty rate for people in working families. The

1

differences are largely the result of two factors: first, the proposed measure counts not only cash assistance, but also the value of such in-kind benefits as food stamps; second, the proposed measure counts net earnings, after deductions for taxes and work expenses, instead of gross earnings. Equally important, the proposed measure will more accurately describe changes in the extent of poverty over time that result from new public policies and further social and economic change.

THE CURRENT POVERTY MEASURE: EVALUATION

The current poverty measure has a set of lines, or thresholds, that are compared with families' resources to determine whether or not they are poor. The thresholds differ by the number of adults and children in a family and, for some family types, by the age of the family head. The resources are families' annual before-tax money income.

The current thresholds were originally developed as the cost of a minimum diet times three to allow for expenditures on all other goods and services. The multiplier of three represented the after-tax money income of the average family in 1955 relative to the amount it spent on food. The central threshold for 1963 was about $3,100 for a family of four (two adults and two children). Because the thresholds have been adjusted only for estimated price changes, the 1992 threshold for a two-adult/two-child family of $14,228 represents the same purchasing power as the threshold of $3,100 did 30 years ago.

From the beginning, the poverty measure had weaknesses, and they have become more apparent and consequential because of far-reaching changes in the U.S. society and economy and in government policies.

• First, because of the increased labor force participation of mothers, there are more working families who must pay for child care, but the current measure does not distinguish between the needs of families in which the parents do or do not work outside the home. More generally, the current measure does not distinguish between the needs of workers and nonworkers.

• Second, because of differences in health status and insurance coverage, different population groups face significant variations in medical care costs, but the current measure does not take account of them.

• Third, the thresholds are the same across the nation, although significant price variations across geographic areas exist for such needs as housing.

• Fourth, the family size adjustments in the thresholds are anomalous in many respects, and changing demographic and family characteristics (such as the reduction in average family size) underscore the need to reassess the adjustments.

• Fifth, more broadly, changes in the standard of living call into question the merits of continuing to use the values of the original thresholds updated only for inflation. Historical evidence suggests that poverty thresholds—including those developed according to "expert" notions of minimum needs—follow trends in overall consumption levels. Because of rising living standards in the United States, most approaches for developing poverty thresholds (including the original one) would produce higher thresholds today than the current ones.

• Finally, because the current measure defines family resources as gross money income, it does not reflect the effects of important government policy initiatives that have significantly altered families' disposable income and, hence, their poverty status. Examples are the increase in the Social Security payroll tax, which reduces disposable income for workers, and the growth in the Food Stamp Program, which raises disposable income for beneficiaries. Moreover, the current poverty measure cannot reflect the effects of future policy initiatives that may have consequences for disposable income, such as changes in the financing of health care, further changes in tax policy, and efforts to move welfare recipients into the work force.

The Panel on Poverty and Family Assistance concludes that the poverty measure should be revised to reflect more accurately the trends in poverty over time and the differences in poverty across population groups. Without revision, and in the face of continuing socioeconomic change as well as changes in government policies, the measure will become increasingly unable to inform the public or support research and policy making.

It is not easy to specify an alternative measure. There are several poverty concepts, each with merits and limitations, and there is no scientific basis by which one concept can be indisputably preferred to another. Ultimately, to recommend a particular concept requires judgment as well as science.

Our recommended changes are based on the best scientific evidence available, our best judgment, and three additional criteria. First, a poverty measure should be acceptable and understandable to the public. Second, a poverty measure should be statistically defensible. In this regard, the concepts underlying the thresholds and the definition of resources should be consistent. Third, a poverty measure should be feasible to implement with data that are available or can fairly readily be obtained.

RECOMMENDATION: A NEW POVERTY MEASURE

The official U.S. poverty thresholds should comprise a budget for the three basic categories of food, clothing, shelter (including utilities), and a small additional amount to allow for other needs (e.g., household supplies, personal care, non-work-related transportation). Actual expenditure data should be used to develop a threshold for a reference family of four—two adults and two children. Each year, that threshold should be updated to reflect changes in spending on food, clothing, and shelter over the previous 3 years and then adjusted for different family types and geographic areas of the country. The resources of a family or individual that are compared with the appropriate threshold to determine poverty status should be consistently defined to include money and near-money disposable income: that is, resources should include most in-kind benefits and exclude taxes and certain other nondiscretionary expenses (e.g., work expenses).

The procedure for updating the poverty thresholds over time is an integral part of the proposed measure. Poverty measures tend to reflect their time and place. At issue is whether the thresholds ought to be updated for real changes in living standards only occasionally, or on a regular basis, and by how much. We propose a regular updating procedure to maintain the time series of poverty statistics. We also propose a conservative updating procedure that adjusts the thresholds for changes in consumption that are relevant to a poverty budget, rather than for changes in total consumption.

We recommend that the proposed measure be adopted for official government use. We also urge the Statistical Policy Office in the U.S. Office of Management and Budget (which we presume will oversee the consideration and implementation of our recommendations) to establish a mechanism for regular review of the poverty measure on a 10-year cycle. No measure is without flaws, and it is important to have periodic reviews to identify improvements in concepts, methods, and data that may be needed. Altering a key social indicator is always difficult, but if a measure becomes markedly out of step with societal conditions, its utility as a barometer and guide to policy is greatly reduced.

> RECOMMENDATION 1.1. **The official U.S. measure of poverty should be revised to reflect more nearly the circumstances of the nation's families and changes in them over time. The revised measure should comprise a set of poverty thresholds and a definition of family resources—for comparison with the thresholds to determine who is in or out of poverty—that are consistent with each other and otherwise statistically defensible. The concepts underlying both the thresholds and the definition of family resources should be broadly acceptable and understandable and operationally feasible.**

> RECOMMENDATION 1.2. **On the basis of the criteria in Recommendation 1.1, the poverty measure should have the following characteristics:**

> • **The poverty thresholds should represent a budget for food, clothing, shelter (including utilities), and a small additional amount to allow for other needs (e.g., household supplies, personal care, non-work-related transportation).**

• A threshold for a reference family type should be developed using actual consumer expenditure data and updated annually to reflect changes in expenditures on food, clothing, and shelter over the previous 3 years.

• The reference family threshold should be adjusted to reflect the needs of different family types and to reflect geographic differences in housing costs.

• Family resources should be defined—consistent with the threshold concept—as the sum of money income from all sources together with the value of near-money benefits (e.g., food stamps) that are available to buy goods and services in the budget, minus expenses that cannot be used to buy these goods and services. Such expenses include income and payroll taxes, child care and other work-related expenses, child support payments to another household, and out-of-pocket medical care costs, including health insurance premiums.

RECOMMENDATION 1.3. The U.S. Office of Management and Budget should adopt a revised poverty measure as the official measure for use by the federal government. Appropriate agencies, including the Bureau of the Census and the Bureau of Labor Statistics, should collaborate to produce the new thresholds each year and to implement the revised definition of family resources.

RECOMMENDATION 1.4. The Statistical Policy Office of the U.S. Office of Management and Budget should institute a regular review, on a 10-year cycle, of all aspects of the poverty measure: reassessing the procedure for updating the thresholds, the family resource definition, etc. When changes to the measure are implemented on the basis of such a review, concurrent poverty statistics series should be run under both the old and the new measures to facilitate the transition.

SETTING AND UPDATING THE POVERTY THRESHOLD

We propose that the poverty-level budget for the reference family start with a dollar amount for the sum of three broad categories of basic goods and services—food, clothing, and shelter (including utilities). The amount should be determined from actual Consumer Expenditure Survey (CEX) data as a percentage of median expenditures on food, clothing, and shelter by two-adult/two-child families. This sum should then be increased by a modest additional amount to allow for other necessities. The allowance for "other expenses" is intended to cover such goods and services as personal care, household supplies, and non-work-related transportation. However, it does not include such nondiscretionary expenses as taxes and child care and other costs of working, which are treated as deductions from income (see below).

Once a new reference family threshold is determined, it should be updated each year with more recent expenditure data. The recommended updating procedure will automatically, over time, reflect real changes in the consumption of basic goods and services without the need for a periodic and, inevitably, disruptive readjustment in the level. It represents a middle ground between the approach of simply updating the thresholds for price changes, which ignores changes in living standards over time, and the approach of updating the thresholds for changes in total consumption.

As part of implementing the proposed poverty measure, the current official threshold should be reevaluated in light of the proposed threshold concept, which treats certain expenses as deductions from income rather than as elements of the poverty budget. That evaluation should also consider the real growth in the standard of living that has occurred since the current threshold was first set for 1963.

We do not as a panel recommend a specific threshold with which to initiate the new poverty measure. Ultimately, that decision is a matter of judgment. We do, however, offer our conclusion about a range for that initial threshold. This conclusion represents our own judgment, informed by analysis of thresholds developed from other commonly used concepts, such as expert budgets, relative thresholds expressed as one-half median income or expenditures, and thresholds derived from responses to sample survey questions about the poverty line.

We believe that a reasonable range for the initial threshold for the reference family of two adults and two children is $13,700 to $15,900 (in 1992 dollars). The lower number equals the expenditures for food, clothing, and shelter ($11,950) by families at the 30th percentile of all two-adult/two-children families, with a multiplier of 1.15 for other needed expenditures; the higher number equals the expenditures for food, clothing, and shelter ($12,720) by families at the 35th percentile of all two-adult/two-children families, with a multiplier of 1.25 for other needed expenditures.

> RECOMMENDATION 2.1. **A poverty threshold with which to initiate a new series of official U.S. poverty statistics should be derived from Consumer Expenditure Survey data for a reference family of four persons (two adults and two children). The procedure should be to specify a percentage of median annual expenditures for such families on the sum of three basic goods and services—food, clothing, and shelter (including utilities)—and apply a specified multiplier to the corresponding dollar level so as to add a small amount for other needs.**

RECOMMENDATION 2.2. **The new poverty threshold should be up-dated each year to reflect changes in consumption of the basic goods and services contained in the poverty budget: determine the dollar value that represents the designated percentage of the median level of expenditures on the sum of food, clothing, and shelter for two-adult/two-child families and apply the designated multiplier. To smooth out year-to-year fluctuations and to lag the adjustment to some extent, perform the calculations for each year by averaging the most recent 3 years' worth of data from the Consumer Expenditure Survey, with the data for each of those years brought forward to the current period by using the change in the Consumer Price Index.**

RECOMMENDATION 2.3. **When the new poverty threshold concept is first implemented and for several years thereafter, the Census Bureau should produce a second set of poverty rates for evaluation purposes by using the new thresholds updated only for price changes (rather than for changes in consumption of the basic goods and services in the poverty budget).**

RECOMMENDATION 2.4. **As part of implementing a new official U.S. poverty measure, the current threshold level for the reference family of two adults and two children ($14,228 in 1992 dollars) should be reevaluated and a new threshold level established with which to initiate a new series of poverty statistics. That reevaluation should take account of both the new threshold concept and the real growth in consumption that has occurred since the official threshold was first set 30 years ago.**

ADJUSTING THE THRESHOLD

Given a poverty threshold for a reference family of two adults and two children, the next step is to develop appropriate thresholds for families with more and fewer members and different numbers of adults and children. We recommend that the reference family threshold be adjusted by means of an "equivalence scale" to determine thresholds for other family types. There is no consensus in the scientific literature on the precise form of an appropriate equivalence scale, although there is agreement on some properties of such a scale and that the scale implicit in the official poverty thresholds is flawed.

We recommend that the scale recognize that children under age 18 on average consume less than adults, but that the scale not further distinguish family members by age or other characteristics. We also recommend that the scale add a decreasing amount for each adult (or adult equivalent) family member to reflect economies of scale available to larger families, such as their ability to buy food and other items in bulk and jointly use many durable goods.

Evidence of cost-of-living differences among geographic areas—such as between metropolitan and nonmetropolitan areas—suggests that the poverty thresholds should be adjusted accordingly, but inadequate data make it difficult to determine appropriate adjustments. As a first and partial step, we recommend that the housing component of the poverty thresholds be indexed to reflect variations in housing costs across the country. This adjustment can be made by analyzing decennial census data with the methodology developed by the U.S. Department of Housing and Urban Development (HUD) to estimate rents for comparable apartments in different localities. We believe the available data support reasonable adjustments for several population size groups of metropolitan areas within each of nine regions of the country. The resulting geographic index should be applied to the housing component of the thresholds. It may also be possible to update the index values each year (rather than at 10-year intervals) by applying the updating methods used by HUD.

We do not recommend adjustments for other budget items at this time because good data for such adjustments are lacking and because the available research suggests that variations in the costs of other budget items are not large. However, more research would be very helpful to develop refined methods and data by which to adjust the poverty thresholds more accurately for geographic cost-of-living differences for housing and other goods and services. One source of improved data could be the area price index program of the Bureau of Labor Statistics (BLS).

RECOMMENDATION 3.1. **The four-person (two adult/two child) poverty threshold should be adjusted for other family types by means of an equivalence scale that reflects differences in consumption by adults and children under 18 and economies of scale for larger families. A scale that meets these criteria is the following: children under 18 are treated as consuming 70 percent as much as adults on average; economies of scale are computed by taking the number of adult equivalents in a family (i.e., the number of adults plus 0.70 times the number of children), and then by raising this number to a power of from 0.65 to 0.75.**

RECOMMENDATION 3.2. **The poverty thresholds should be adjusted for differences in the cost of housing across geographic areas of the country. Available data from the decennial census permit the development of a reasonable cost-of-housing index for nine regions and, within each region, for several population size categories of metropolitan areas. The index should be applied to the housing portion of the poverty thresholds.**

RECOMMENDATION 3.3. **Appropriate agencies should conduct research to determine methods that could be used to update the geographic housing cost component of the poverty thresholds between the decennial censuses.**

RECOMMENDATION 3.4. **Appropriate agencies should conduct research to improve the estimation of geographic cost-of-living differences in housing as well as other components of the poverty budget. Agencies should consider improvements to data series, such as the BLS area price indexes, that have the potential to support improved estimates of cost-of-living differences.**

DEFINING FAMILY RESOURCES

It is important that family resources are defined consistently with the threshold concept in any poverty measure. The current measure violates this principle, as has some recent work to investigate alternatives. Examples are measures that add the value of public and private health insurance benefits to families' resources without adjusting the thresholds to account for medical care needs. Such measures should be discontinued.

For consistency, we recommend that family resources be defined as *money and near-money disposable income.* More precisely, the definition should include money income from all sources, as well as the value of such in-kind benefits as food stamps and public housing. It should exclude out-of-pocket medical care expenditures, including health insurance premiums; income and payroll taxes; child care and other work-related expenses; and child support payments to another household. The child care deduction should be capped and apply only to families in which there is no adult at home to provide the care; the deduction for other work expenses should be a flat amount per week worked.

We believe there is widespread agreement among researchers about the appropriateness of such adjustments to income as deducting taxes and work expenses, which are a cost of earning income and cannot be used for consumption, and about adding the value of in-kind benefits that support consumption. The only important area of disagreement concerns medical care benefits.

Trying to account for private and public medical insurance benefits—important as they clearly are—in the same way as in-kind benefits for such items as food and housing would greatly complicate the poverty measure and cloud its interpretation. A chief reason is the wide variation in health care needs among the population: Some people have high medical costs; some have none. Hence, the proposed poverty measure does not include an allowance for medical expenses, either those that might be covered by insurance or paid for out of pocket; for consistency, the proposed resource definition does not add the value of health insurance. Also for consistency, the proposed definition subtracts out-of-pocket medical care expenses from income: even with insurance, many people must pay out of pocket to obtain that insurance or to receive care, and such expenses reduce disposable income.

Although the proposed poverty measure excludes medical care from both the thresholds and resources, it will reflect changes in health care policy that affect disposable income. For example, if changes in health care financing reduce out-of-pocket medical expenditures and thereby free up resources for food, housing, and other consumption, the proposed measure will show a lower poverty rate; the current measure would not show this effect. We also recommend that appropriate agencies develop direct indicators of the extent to which families lack or have inadequate health insurance that puts them at risk of not being able to afford needed treatment. These "medical care risk" measures should be cross-tabulated with but kept separate from the economic poverty measure.

RECOMMENDATION 4.1. In developing poverty statistics, any significant change in the definition of family resources should be accompanied by a consistent adjustment of the poverty thresholds.

RECOMMENDATION 4.2. The definition of family resources for comparison with the appropriate poverty threshold should be disposable money and near-money income. Specifically, resources should be calculated as follows:

• estimate gross money income from all public and private sources for a family or unrelated individual (which is income as defined in the current measure);

• add the value of near-money nonmedical in-kind benefits, such as food stamps, subsidized housing, school lunches, and home energy assistance;

• deduct out-of-pocket medical care expenditures, including health insurance premiums;

• deduct income taxes and Social Security payroll taxes;

• for families in which there is no nonworking parent, deduct actual child care costs, per week worked, not to exceed the earnings of the parent with the lower earnings or a cap that is adjusted annually for inflation;

• for each working adult, deduct a flat amount per week worked (adjusted annually for inflation and not to exceed earnings) to account for work-related transportation and miscellaneous expenses; and

• deduct child support payments from the income of the payer.

RECOMMENDATION 4.3. Appropriate agencies should work to develop one or more "medical care risk" indexes that measure the economic risk to families and individuals of having no or inadequate health insurance coverage. However, such indexes should be kept separate from the measure of economic poverty.

EFFECTS

To consider the effects of our proposed measure, we estimated poverty rates under both the current and the proposed measures with data from the March 1993 Current Population Survey (CPS), supplemented with data from the Survey of Income and Program Participation (SIPP) and other sources.

In one set of comparisons, we kept the overall poverty rate the same for both measures—14.5 percent in 1992. The results show important distributional effects on the makeup of the poverty population under the proposed measure: most strikingly, higher poverty rates for families with one or more workers and for families that lack health insurance coverage and lower rates for families that receive public assistance. The results also show higher poverty rates in the Northeast and West and lower rates in the South and, to a lesser extent, in the Midwest.

In another set of comparisons, we used the midpoint of our suggested range for the two-adult/two-child family threshold—$14,800. With this threshold, a scale economy factor of 0.75, and the other features of our measure, the poverty rate increased from 14.5 percent to 18.1 percent; with a scale economy factor of 0.65, the poverty rate increased to 19.0 percent. The changes in the resource definition increased the rate more than the changes in the thresholds. If we had been able to use SIPP data exclusively, we estimate that the rate would have increased less, from 14.5 percent to 15 or 16 percent (depending on the scale economy factor), because SIPP obtains more complete income reporting for lower income people than does the March CPS.

NEEDED DATA

Full and accurate implementation of the proposed poverty measure will require changes and improvements in data sources. We recommend that SIPP become the source of official poverty statistics in place of the March CPS. SIPP asks more relevant questions than the March CPS and obtains income data of higher quality. Also, because SIPP is an income survey rather than a supplement to a labor force survey, it is better able to satisfy the data requirements for an improved measure of poverty, both now and in the future.

Because analysis with other surveys (including the March CPS) and with the decennial census often requires indicators of poverty status, we encourage research on the estimation of disposable income from these data sources.

Finally, with regard to expenditure data, we support a review of the Consumer Expenditure Survey to identify changes, especially larger sample sizes, that would improve its usefulness for poverty measurement and other important analyses of consumption, income, and savings.

RECOMMENDATION 5.1. **The Survey of Income and Program Participation should become the basis of official U.S. income and poverty statistics in place of the March income supplement to the Current Population Survey. Decisions about the SIPP design and questionnaire should take account of the data requirements for producing reliable time series of poverty statistics using the proposed definition of family resources (money and near-money income minus certain expenditures). Priority should be accorded to methodological research for SIPP that is relevant for improved poverty measurement. A particularly important problem to address is population undercoverage, particularly of low-income minority groups.**

RECOMMENDATION 5.2. **To facilitate the transition to SIPP, the Census Bureau should produce concurrent time series of poverty rates from both SIPP and the March CPS by using the proposed revised threshold concept and updating procedure and the proposed definition of family resources as disposable income. The concurrent series should be developed starting with 1984, when SIPP was first introduced.**

RECOMMENDATION 5.3. **The Census Bureau should routinely issue public-use files from both SIPP and the March CPS that include the Bureau's best estimate of disposable income and its components (taxes, in-kind benefits, child care expenses, etc.) so that researchers can obtain poverty rates consistent with the new threshold concept from either survey.**

RECOMMENDATION 5.4. **Appropriate agencies should conduct research on methods to develop poverty estimates from household surveys with limited income information that are comparable to the estimates that would be obtained from a fully implemented disposable income definition of family resources.**

RECOMMENDATION 5.5. **Appropriate agencies should conduct research on methods to construct small-area poverty estimates from the limited information in the decennial census that are comparable with the estimates that would be obtained under a fully implemented disposable income concept. In addition, serious consideration should be given to adding one or two questions to the decennial census to assist in the development of comparable estimates.**

RECOMMENDATION 5.6. The Bureau of Labor Statistics should undertake a comprehensive review of the Consumer Expenditure Survey to assess the costs and benefits of changes to the survey design, questionnaire, sample size, and other features that could improve the quality and usefulness of the data. The review should consider ways to improve the CEX for the purpose of developing poverty thresholds, for making it possible at a future date to measure poverty on the basis of a consumption or expenditure concept of family resources, and for other analytic purposes related to the measurement of consumption, income, and savings.

OTHER ISSUES IN POVERTY MEASUREMENT

RECOMMENDATION 6.1. The official poverty measure should continue to be derived on an annual basis. Appropriate agencies should develop poverty measures for periods that are shorter and longer than a year, with data from SIPP and the Panel Study of Income Dynamics, for such purposes as program evaluation. Such measures may require the inclusion of asset values in the family resource definition.

RECOMMENDATION 6.2. The official measure of poverty should continue to use families and unrelated individuals as the units of analysis for which thresholds are defined and resources aggregated. The definition of "family" should be broadened for purposes of poverty measurement to include cohabiting couples.

RECOMMENDATION 6.3. Appropriate agencies should conduct research on the extent of resource sharing among roommates and other household and family members to determine if the definition of the unit of analysis for the poverty measure should be modified in the future.

RECOMMENDATION 6.4. In addition to the basic poverty counts and ratios for the total population and groups—the number and proportion of poor people—the official poverty series should provide statistics on the average income and distribution of income for the poor. The count and other statistics should also be published for poverty measures in which family resources are defined net of government taxes and transfers, such as a measure that defines income in before-tax terms, a measure that excludes means-tested government benefits from income, and a measure that excludes all government benefits from income. Such measures can help assess the effects of government taxes and transfers on poverty.

RELATING THE POVERTY MEASURE
TO ASSISTANCE PROGRAMS

More than 25 government programs that provided benefits and services to low-income families in 1994—such as food stamps, Head Start, Legal Services, Medicaid—linked their need standard for determining eligibility for some or all applicants to the U.S. Department of Health and Human Services poverty guidelines, which are derived from the official poverty thresholds. The use of the proposed measure would improve the targeting of benefits to needy families, and we encourage program agencies to consider adopting it as an eligibility criterion in place of the current measure. In doing so, program agencies should consider whether the proposed measure may need to be modified to better serve program objectives. For example, the proposed definition of family resources may add administrative burdens in programs that currently obtain crude measures of applicants' gross money income to assess eligibility because more information is needed to determine applicants' disposable income. In these instances, it may be preferable to implement a less detailed definition.

Program agencies should also consider the implications of the recommended method for updating the poverty thresholds. There may be consequences for program caseloads or waiting lines and costs if, over time, thresholds developed under that method rise at a faster rate than thresholds that are simply adjusted for inflation. With constrained budgets, the relationship of program need standards to the poverty thresholds may need periodic adjustment.

In the Aid to Families with Dependent Children (AFDC) program, for which we were asked to consider issues of a national minimum benefit standard, federal law currently defines "countable income." The definition is similar in concept, if not in specifics, to the proposed disposable income definition of family resources. However, a unique feature of AFDC is that the states establish need standards for eligibility but are allowed to and often do pay benefits below that standard. Most state need standards and, even more so, most state benefit standards are considerably below the poverty thresholds, and the level varies widely across states—more widely than can be explained by differences in living costs.

Currently, more than a dozen states link their need standard in some way to the current poverty guidelines. Again, the proposed measure would be an improvement for this purpose. We encourage the states to consider the use of the proposed measure, which includes an adjustment to the thresholds for geographic differences in housing costs, in setting their need standard for AFDC.

It would also seem reasonable to consider the thresholds that are developed under the proposed measure as a goal or benchmark in any debate about state or federal AFDC benefit standards. However, many factors properly enter into a determination of program benefit levels, and the result may well be standards that differ from those that make sense for a statistical measure of poverty. Such factors include constraints on available funding, the desire to target benefits to particular population groups, interactions among programs, and the desire to provide incentives to participants and potential participants, such as incentives to prefer work over welfare. Ultimately, the determination of appropriate assistance program benefit standards involves political judgments about the appropriate balance of competing program objectives within the constraints of scarce resources. We hope, by reviewing the issues, to help clarify the policy debate.

> RECOMMENDATION 7.1. Agencies responsible for federal assistance programs that use the poverty guidelines derived from the official poverty thresholds (or a multiple) to determine eligibility for benefits and services should consider the use of the panel's proposed measure. In their assessment, agencies should determine whether it may be necessary to modify the measure—for example, through a simpler definition of family resources or by linking eligibility less closely to the poverty thresholds because of possible budgetary constraints—to better serve program objectives.

> RECOMMENDATION 8.1. The states should consider linking their need standard for the Aid to Families with Dependent Children program to the panel's proposed poverty measure and whether it may be necessary to modify this measure to better serve program objectives.

Introduction and Overview

1

The Social Security Administration (SSA) began publishing poverty statistics in the early 1960s, using a poverty measure developed by staff economist Mollie Orshansky (1963, 1965a). This measure had a set of poverty thresholds for different types of families that consisted of the cost of a minimum adequate diet multiplied by three to allow for other expenses. The threshold value for the base year 1963 for a family of two adults and two children was about $3,100. To determine a family's poverty status, its resources, defined as before-tax money income, were compared with the appropriate threshold.

In 1965 the Office of Economic Opportunity (OEO) adopted the SSA thresholds for statistical and program planning purposes; in 1969 the U.S. Bureau of the Budget (now the U.S. Office of Management and Budget) issued a statistical policy directive that gave the thresholds official status throughout the federal government. The Census Bureau took over the job of publishing the official annual statistics on the number and proportion poor (the poverty rate) by comparing the SSA thresholds to estimates of families' before-tax money income from the March Current Population Survey (it first issued poverty statistics in August 1967).[1] For these comparisons, the SSA thresholds are updated annually for price inflation and so are not changed in real dollar terms: in other words, the 1992 threshold value of $14,228 for a family of four (two adults and two children) represents the same purchasing power as the 1963 threshold value of about $3,100 for this type family.[2]

---

[1] See Fisher (1992b, summarized in 1992a) for a detailed history of the origins and development of the official U.S. poverty measure.

[2] We cite the 1992 threshold here and elsewhere because the latest data available to us were for that year.

The official poverty measure has important effects—direct and indirect—on government policies and programs. Some government assistance programs for low-income people determine eligibility for benefits or services by comparing families' resources to the poverty thresholds or a multiple of them.[3] Also, some formulas for allocating federal funds include state or local poverty rates as a factor.

The poverty measure influences policy making more broadly as an indicator of economic well-being to which policy makers, advocates, analysts, and the general public are sensitive. Trends in poverty rates over time and differences in poverty rates across population groups are often cited as reasons that a particular policy (or set of policies) is, or is not, needed. For example, the recent expansion of the Earned Income Tax Credit (EITC) was prompted by statistics on poverty among working families.

The poverty measure also plays a role in evaluating government programs for low-income people and, more generally, the effects of government policies and economic growth on the distribution of income. In academia, there is a large literature on the characteristics of the poor, factors leading to poverty and other kinds of deprivation, and the effects of poverty on other behaviors and outcomes.

Consequently, each year's poverty figures are sought by policy makers, researchers, and the media, who look to see if the rate has changed for the nation as a whole and for specific population groups and to understand the causes and consequences of changes in the rate and their implications for public policy. For all of these users, it is critical that the measure provide an accurate picture of trends over time and of differences among groups, such as children, the elderly, minorities, working people, people receiving government assistance, people in cities, and people in rural areas.

Poverty statistics regularly make the headlines, but, increasingly over the past decade, so do stories that question the soundness of the concepts and methodology from which the official numbers derive. In response to a request of the U.S. Congress, the Committee on National Statistics of the National Research Council established a study panel to address the concerns about the poverty measure and also to consider related conceptual and methodological issues in establishing standards for welfare payments to needy families.

Our panel—the Panel on Poverty and Family Assistance: Concepts, Information Needs, and Measurement Methods—has concluded that revisions to the current poverty measure are long overdue. We have developed a new measure, embracing both the concept of the poverty standard or threshold

---

[3] Most of the programs that relate eligibility to the poverty measure actually use the poverty guidelines, which were originally developed by OEO and are issued annually by the U.S. Department of Health and Human Services. The poverty guidelines are constructed by smoothing the official thresholds for different size families (see Fisher, 1992c). For historical reasons, the guidelines are higher than the thresholds for Alaska (by 25%) and Hawaii (by 15%).

itself (i.e., the standard of need), how it is updated over time, and the definition of families' resources that are available to meet this poverty standard. We considered the relevance of our proposed poverty measure—and other factors—for setting standards for government assistance programs. Although we offer few recommendations in this latter area, we try to illuminate and clarify the issues.

This overview presents the panel's findings, conclusions, and recommendations in a nontechnical way, for the general reader. The other chapters of this report discuss the issues involved in poverty measurement in detail: alternative concepts for developing and updating poverty thresholds (Chapter 2); alternative adjustments of the thresholds for different family circumstances, such as family size and geographic location (Chapter 3); alternative definitions of family resources (Chapter 4); data requirements for implementing the panel's proposed poverty measure and the effects on the distribution of poverty (Chapter 5); other issues in poverty measurement, such as the time period and unit of economic analysis covered (Chapter 6); and the potential relationship of the poverty measure to government assistance programs, both generally (Chapter 7) and, specifically, to the program for Aid to Families with Dependent Children (Chapter 8). Appendices provide additional information on specific topics.

In this overview we first explain what we mean by economic poverty, in contrast to other types of deprivation. We then describe the current official U.S. poverty measure and assess its adequacy. We also review alternative poverty measures, summarizing their merits and limitations. We base our choice of a measure on scientific evidence to the extent possible; however, we stress that the decision to recommend a particular measure (and the specific features of a measure) ultimately cannot rest on science alone, but also involves judgment. We describe the criteria that we used to guide our judgments. We then present our recommendations for the poverty measure. Finally, we present our findings and views regarding the applicability of our revised poverty measure for eligibility standards and payment levels in assistance programs for low-income families.

WHAT IS POVERTY?

We define poverty as economic deprivation. A way of expressing this concept is that it pertains to people's lack of economic resources (e.g., money or near-money income) for consumption of economic goods and services (e.g., food, housing, clothing, transportation). Thus, a poverty standard is based on a level of family resources (or, alternatively, of families' actual consumption) deemed necessary to obtain a minimally adequate standard of living, defined appropriately for the United States today.[4]

---

[4] We refer to "family resources" throughout this report, as distinguished from the country's economic resources, more broadly defined. Properly, the term should be "family or unrelated individual resources" (or needs) to accord with the units for which poverty is currently measured.

There are many other forms of deprivation. One can be deprived of psychological or social well-being (e.g., one can have impaired self-esteem or heightened anxiety and stress or be socially isolated), and one can lack physical well-being (e.g., one can have a chronic disease or disabling condition or be subjected to a high risk of violence in one's neighborhood). There are also many conditions that can lead to deprivation on one or more of these dimensions. For example, people who live with a family member who abuses drugs or alcohol likely suffer deprivation in terms of their psychological health, and perhaps their physical health and economic standard of living as well. People who live in a crime-ridden neighborhood may be deprived in a number of ways—through the psychological fear they are likely to harbor, the actual physical harm or property loss that they may experience, and the adverse social and economic effects (e.g., declining property values) that may result because the broader society shuns their neighborhood. People who are illiterate may experience many deprivations to full participation in society: they may have great difficulty in finding and keeping a good job; they may have problems in traveling around their area or in negotiating a good price for the products they buy; they may avoid voting for public office; and they may experience social shame. People who are without health insurance may be at risk of psychological and economic, as well as physical, deprivation. People who lose their job or who have never been successful in finding one may suffer a deprivation of both income and psychic esteem. Finally, people who, for one or another reason, lack sufficient resources to provide for an adequate standard of living may suffer not only economic hardship, but psychological stress and physical problems as well.

We encourage the development of indicators for monitoring trends over time and among population groups on all of these different dimensions of deprivation. Also, we encourage work on the relationships among them. For example, one element of economic or material deprivation may be inadequate housing, which, in turn, can imply exposure to risks that go well beyond income inadequacy (e.g., fire hazard, lead poisoning). For fuller understanding and to inform policy, a breadth of information and analysis is needed on the well-being of the population, including and going beyond the economic dimension.

But the focus of our work is on economic deprivation, narrowly defined. We are concerned with the concept, definition, and measurement of economic poverty, or what many call material poverty. We contend that this relatively narrow conceptualization of poverty is appropriate for an official poverty measure for several reasons. First, it is a familiar concept that, in a broad sense, has formed the basis of official poverty measurement in the United States for the past several decades. It is a notion of poverty that accords with political rhetoric as least as far back as Franklin D. Roosevelt's concern for Americans who were ill-housed, ill-clad, and ill-nourished.

Second, while it is surely not easy to arrive at a specific concept or measurement of economic deprivation (see below), the same problem applies to other kinds of deprivation, and the notion of economic deprivation has the advantage that policy makers and the public have experience with its measurement and intuition about its interpretation and movement over time. Third, since many public programs and debates pertain to the economic sphere of life, it is important to have a time-series measure of economic deprivation. If a broader concept for the official "poverty" measure were adopted, there would still be a need for a measure to track the effects of programs and policies on the economic domain.

The nation's understanding about and commitment to the alleviation of poverty has been informed for many years by the official measure of economic deprivation. We think the function of that measure should be retained much as it is now. If the current measure were internally consistent and not flawed, in ways we describe below, we would be inclined to recommend its continuation. But we do find it unacceptably flawed for its important uses with respect to government policies and programs, academic research, and public understanding; thus, we recommend a new measure, but one that retains the concept of economic deprivation as the core notion of poverty.

This concept of poverty must be distinguished from "welfare" and "well-being." Poverty is a circumstance, defined by a set of specific conditions that are considered to reflect economic deprivation. One is said to be "in poverty" if those conditions are met (i.e., if one's resources are below a threshold level for needed economic consumption) and "not in poverty" if those conditions are not met. Welfare is a term for certain government assistance programs or the resources that are transferred by those programs, such as Aid to Families with Dependent Children. More generally, the term welfare is sometimes used to mean well-being, which is a much broader term capturing the overall condition of a person. In contrast, "economic poverty" refers to a circumstance defined by a low level of material goods and services or a low level of resources to obtain those goods and services. This distinction is maintained by the concept of poverty that we use here.

While we use economic deprivation as the underlying concept of poverty and devote most of this report to its definition and measurement, we acknowledge that it is not easy to specify in a precise manner what it means to be economically deprived, even in a narrow sense. The general idea certainly seems intuitive and transparent. For instance, Adam Smith as far back as 1776 linked economic poverty to the want of "necessaries," which he defined as "not only the commodities which are indispensably necessary for the support of life, but whatever the custom of the country renders it indecent for creditable people, even of the lowest order, to be without." Commonly, such a concept is translated into a dollar level that is deemed adequate to obtain necessary goods and services. The official U.S. poverty measure was developed along these lines, although only one "necessity"—a minimum diet—was specified; other necessary consumption was subsumed in the multiplier of three applied to the costs of the minimum diet.

More recently, Townsend (1979, 1992:5, 10) has given a social dimension to economic deprivation. Townsend observes that people are "social beings expected to perform socially demanding roles as workers, citizens, parents, partners, neighbors, and friends." He argues that economic poverty should be defined as the lack of sufficient income for people to "play the roles, participate in the relationships, and follow the customary behavior which is expected of them by virtue of their membership of society." As an example, one could argue that having a telephone is essential in a developed country for everything from job seeking to having relationships with family and friends.

Given a concept such as Smith's or Townsend's or, indeed, virtually any concept of economic deprivation, the issue is how to define the key terms— "necessaries," "indecent . . . to be without," "customary behavior." Although there may be a general sense in a society of what are "necessities" or what is "customary behavior," the attempt to be specific inevitably raises questions and leads to debate about the very meaning of economic poverty.

Throughout this report, our approach is pragmatic. We first assess how well the official U.S. poverty measure is serving as a barometer and benchmark for policy, research, and general public understanding about an important aspect of deprivation. We conclude that, given socioeconomic and public policy changes since the measure was developed, it is no longer satisfactory for those purposes. We then review the properties of some common alternative measures to determine which of them could represent an improvement. Our goal is not to develop the ideal poverty measure on which everyone would agree (which surely does not exist), but to propose a measure that is a marked improvement over the current one—just as the official measure, when first developed by Mollie Orshansky, was regarded as a marked improvement over competing measures at that time.

Our measure includes a specific concept of economic poverty by which to develop a new poverty threshold for a reference family type: inadequate resources to obtain basic living needs. We define those basic needs as food, clothing, and shelter. There are other needs as well (e.g., personal care, transportation), but there is less agreement about them, and so our approach provides a small amount for other needed spending by means of a multiplier that is applied to the amounts for food, clothing, and shelter.

This concept of poverty as insufficient resources for basic living needs accords with traditional public concerns for the needy, whether expressed in provisions for homeless shelters, soup kitchens, and clothing drives, or the provision of cash or in-kind benefits for basic consumption. It is also not inconsistent with and, in our view, improves on, the concept that was originally used to derive the current thresholds, namely, the application of a multiplier for other needed spending to a minimum allowance for food.

Yet general agreement about basic needs does not mean that everyone agrees about the level of consumption that distinguishes a state of poverty from a state of adequacy. Thus, there is a question about how much food, shelter, and clothing distinguish a person in poverty from one who is not in poverty. This question cannot be answered in the abstract. No concept of economic poverty, whether ours or another, will of itself determine a level for a poverty threshold. That determination necessarily involves judgment. Moreover, as we show below and in Chapter 2, no matter what the particular concept, the determination of a poverty threshold invariably considers people's actual spending patterns and hence, inevitably, has a relative aspect.

Under our threshold concept, we propose that the values for food, shelter, and clothing—the basic bundle—and for a small amount of other needed spending—the multiplier—be developed by direct reference to spending patterns of American families below the median expenditure level. More important, we propose that real changes in spending on food, clothing, and shelter be used to update the poverty thresholds each year. By so doing, the thresholds will maintain a relationship to real changes in living standards, but only to the extent that these changes affect consumption of basic goods and services that pertain to a concept of poverty, not all goods and services. In this sense, our concept is quasi-relative in nature.

Because the most judgmental aspects of any poverty measure concern the reference family threshold, there is a danger that the need to improve the official measure may founder on debates about the "right" concept and level of that threshold. (We do not recommend a particular value for that threshold; rather, we suggest a range within which we believe it could reasonably fall.) It is important that a threshold concept satisfy the criteria we outline below and that the level chosen for the threshold is credible, but other characteristics of a poverty measure are equally or more important. Significant improvements will result in the accuracy of official U.S. poverty statistics by implementing our recommendations for adjusting the threshold along the three dimensions of family composition, geographic location, and time period and by implementing our recommended definition of family resources. It is in these recommendations that we are confident that the new measure of poverty is a considerable improvement over the current official measure.

Finally, by focusing on and recommending a specific measure of economic poverty, as we do, we do not advocate the idea that there is but a single measure of economic deprivation that should be featured as sacrosanct in policy evaluations. Rather, we urge the Census Bureau to develop reports on a range of poverty statistics, just as the Bureau of Labor Statistics (BLS) publishes a range of unemployment statistics in addition to the official unemployment rate. Examples of such useful poverty indicators, in addition to the poverty rate itself, would include measures of the intensity of poverty in terms of the average income and distribution of income of the poor.

THE OFFICIAL U.S. POVERTY MEASURE

Development of the Measure

The poverty thresholds that are used in estimating the official U.S. poverty statistics were originally developed by SSA staff economist Mollie Orshansky as the cost of a minimum diet times a "multiplier" (or factor) of three to allow for other needed expenses, such as housing and clothing. The diet was constructed by the U.S. Department of Agriculture (USDA), by examining data on the food-buying patterns of lower income households from a 1955 Household Food Consumption Survey, modifying the patterns to develop a nutritionally balanced food plan, and costing out the items included in the plan. The USDA developed several food plans at varying cost levels; the one used as the basis of the poverty thresholds was the "Economy Food Plan," the lowest cost plan designed for "temporary or emergency use when funds are low."[5] The plan allowed for no eating at restaurants, called for careful management of food storage and food preparation, and was acknowledged by its developers to provide a nutritious but monotonous diet. The multiplier of three was derived from the same 1955 survey, which showed that the average family of three or more persons—the average of all such families, not the average of low-income families—spent about one-third of its after-tax money income on food.

The poverty thresholds were varied to account for the differing food needs of children under age 18 and of adults under and over age 65 and to account for economies of scale for larger households. Originally, the thresholds also varied by the gender of the family head and whether or not the family resided on a farm and could be expected to grow some of its own food. The thresholds are the same across the nation; there are no allowances for differences in cost of living in different geographic areas. Each year the thresholds are updated for price inflation by the Census Bureau.

In 1969 the Bureau of the Budget gave official status to the following two changes in the poverty thresholds, which were adopted by an interagency committee: to use the overall Consumer Price Index (CPI) to update the thresholds for price changes instead of the Economy Food Plan cost index and to raise the farm thresholds from 70 to 85 percent of the nonfarm thresholds. (Turned down was an SSA proposal to revise the thresholds to reflect newer data from the 1965-1966 Nationwide Food Consumption Survey; see Fisher, 1992b:38-49.) In 1979 Carol Fendler of the Census Bureau wrote a paper with Orshansky describing various possible changes that could be made in the poverty thresholds, including a revision of the thresholds using a multiplier of

---

[5] Orshansky also developed a set of poverty thresholds on the basis of the Low Cost Food Plan, the second lowest cost of four USDA plans, but these thresholds were never adopted for official use.

3.4 derived from the 1965-1966 survey. In 1979-1980, an interagency committee was asked to consider possible small changes in the thresholds (not including the use of a higher multiplier) and recommended the following minor changes discussed by Fendler and Orshansky, which were adopted in 1981: the nonfarm thresholds were applied to all families; the thresholds for families headed by women and men were averaged; and the largest family size category for the thresholds was raised from families of seven or more to families of nine or more persons (Fisher, 1992b:64-68).

Overall, except for the minor changes in the number of different thresholds and the change in the price index for updating them, the poverty line has not been altered since it was first adopted in 1965. In the language of poverty measurement, the United States has an "absolute" poverty threshold that is updated for price changes but not for real growth in consumption. Thus, the poverty line no longer represents the concept on which it was originally based—namely, food times a food share multiplier—because that share will change (and has changed) with rising living standards. Rather, the poverty threshold reflects in today's dollars the line that was set some 30 years ago.

Each year, the official thresholds are compared with an estimate of resources for each family (or individual) in the March Current Population Survey (CPS), which includes about 60,000 households, to determine the number and proportion poor (the poverty rate). Resources are defined as before-tax money income from all sources—for example, earnings, pensions, interest, rental income, other income from assets, cash welfare. Although the multiplier of three used in constructing the poverty thresholds was based on after-tax income, there was no methodology for calculating taxes from the March CPS, so income is defined on a before-tax basis. No valuations for in-kind benefits, such as food stamps, are included in income, nor are asset holdings accounted for in any way. Since 1982 the Census Bureau has published poverty estimates that do exclude most taxes from income and do include the value of major in-kind benefits, but these estimates are labeled "experimental" and do not represent the official statistics (see, e.g., Bureau of the Census, 1993a, 1995). The official poverty statistics for the United States, based on the March CPS, are currently published each fall as a Current Population Report in the P-60 Series (for the latest such report, see Bureau of the Census, 1995).

Adequacy of the Current Measure

There are several different approaches to developing a measure of poverty, both for the thresholds and for the definition of family resources, each of which has some merit and none of which is without difficulties. So one might ask why the United States should consider replacing a measure that has served for many years. Moreover, it will undoubtedly be disruptive to an important statistical time series if a different measure is adopted.

Yet, historically, poverty measures have tended to reflect their time and place. When it was adopted by OEO for official use, the SSA measure was viewed as a distinct improvement over a widely cited measure developed by the Council of Economic Advisers (CEA) for 1962. The SSA thresholds were based on an explicit concept of need and were adjusted for family size and other characteristics; the CEA measure had just one threshold for families of all sizes with a second, lower threshold for single individuals. The SSA measure also had the advantage that its central threshold for a family of four in 1963 was about the same as the CEA family threshold of $3,000. In turn, the CEA family threshold had been based on considering such factors as the minimum wage and public assistance levels; see Fisher (1992b:30). Gallup Poll data from the early 1960s, as analyzed by Vaughan (1993), suggest that public opinion would also have agreed with a four-person family poverty threshold of about $3,000. Also, such a level represented about one-half median after-tax four-person family income, which is a standard often used in comparative analyses of poverty across nations. In other words, the SSA thresholds accorded well with other views about what it meant to be poor in America in the mid-1960s.

Yet if the SSA approach of developing the thresholds as food costs times a food share multiplier were to be used today, it would produce a different result from the current thresholds—which represent the original 1963 thresholds adjusted for inflation—because changes in consumption patterns have increased the multiplier. Similarly, the use of the SSA approach for a period earlier than 1960 would have given a different result from the official thresholds extended back in time in real dollars because the multiplier would have been lower.

Two questions in evaluating the current poverty measure are whether it makes sense to continue to use the real value of the original 1963 thresholds and, if not, whether the original SSA approach or some other procedure should be used to update them. From the perspective of providing accurate comparisons of poverty status across population groups and across time, there is also the important question of whether other aspects of the current measure—namely, the adjustments to the thresholds for family size and type and the definition of family resources—remain relevant at the end of the twentieth century. Given the important role that the poverty measure and poverty statistics play in contemporary U.S. society, it seems imperative to make the most careful assessment possible of the current measure to determine its adequacy.

We find that the current official poverty measure has a number of weaknesses, involving both the thresholds and the definition of family resources. (Some of these problems were pointed out in the 1960s by Orshansky herself.) Although they were not necessarily important or obvious at the time the measure was adopted, these problems have become more evident and more consequential because of far-reaching social and economic changes, as well as changes in public policy, that have occurred since the 1950s and 1960s. These changes involve labor force participation, family composition, geographic price differences, growth in medical care costs and benefits, government taxation, the provision of in-kind benefits to families and individuals, and the overall increase in the standard of living.

Work Patterns of Families with Children

Over the period from 1955 (the date of the survey underlying the original poverty thresholds) to 1993, the percentage of women with a child under age 6 who were in the labor force more than tripled, increasing from 18 to 58 percent. During that same time, the labor force participation rate of women whose youngest child was age 6 or older almost doubled, increasing from 38 to 75 percent (U.S. House of Representatives, 1994:Table 12-1). As a consequence of these changes, there are many more families who must make arrangements for child care in order to earn at least some of their income.

Child care expenditures were a negligible component of consumer expenditures in the 1950s; at that time, one could readily assume that in most U.S. families a parent was available at home. Today, one can no longer make that assumption, and many families face high out-of-pocket child care expenses. Estimates from the 1991 National Child Care Survey are that 57 percent of families with working mothers of pre-school-aged children paid cash for child care and that child care expenses for the average family with such expenses amounted to 10 percent of total family income (U.S. House of Representatives, 1994:Table 12-8). The current poverty measure does not distinguish between families with and without these expenses, either by having separate thresholds for working and nonworking families or by deducting child care costs from earnings; hence, the current measure does not accurately portray the relative poverty status of these two groups.

Composition of Families and Households

Among families with children, one of the most dramatic changes over the past few decades has been the rise in the number that are headed by a single parent, most often a woman: such families increased from 11 to 26 percent of all families with children over the period 1970-1992. As a proportion of all households, single-parent families increased from 5 to 8 percent over the same period (see Bureau of the Census, 1993d:Tables 65, 75). In order to work, such single parents face the problem noted above of finding—and, in many instances, paying for—child care.

Concurrent with the rise in the number of single-parent families is the growth in the number of people who live apart from their children. Many noncustodial parents pay child support, which means that they have fewer resources with which to support their own households. One study of men aged 18-54 estimated that about 16 percent were noncustodial parents, of whom 44 percent paid child support. On average, these payments accounted for 9 percent of their family income (Sorenson, 1993). Again, the current poverty measure does not distinguish between families with and without these expenses, so that it does not accurately reflect the relative economic status of the two groups.

Among all households, a striking change has been the growth in nonfamily households, which increased from 15 to 30 percent from 1960 to 1992 (Bureau of the Census, 1993d:Table 65). Most nonfamily households consist of persons living alone (84% in 1992). One of the concerns that has been raised about the current poverty measure is the nature of the adjustment to the thresholds for single persons relative to families—an application of what is termed the "equivalence scale." A change in the scale value for persons living alone would likely affect the total poverty rate as well as the rate for that group, given the large and growing proportion that single adults represent of all households.

Multiperson nonfamily households (including cohabitors and roommates), although smaller in numbers, exhibited even higher growth rates over the 1960-1992 period, increasing from 2 to 5 percent of all households (Bureau of the Census, 1993d:Table 65). The current poverty measure treats each member of such a household as a separate economic unit, but to the extent that cohabitors and roommates share resources and hence benefit from economies of scale, the current measure likely overstates the poverty rate for such people.

Finally, households headed by someone aged 65 or over increased from 18 to 22 percent of all households between 1960 and 1992 (Bureau of the Census, 1967:Table 18; 1993d:Table 67). Most such households are comprised of a single person or a married couple. One of the most widely criticized aspects of the official measure is that the thresholds for one- and two-person units headed by someone aged 65 or over are lower than the thresholds for other such units. This difference resulted from the USDA diets, which assumed lower caloric requirements for older people. A change in the threshold values for older household heads relative to younger heads might affect both the total poverty rate and the distribution of poverty across groups.

Geographic Differences in Prices

Measuring differences in consumer prices across geographic areas of the country is a difficult task, yet there is evidence suggesting that such differences exist to a significant extent. In 1981, the last year for which BLS published family budgets for various locales, the relative cost of the lower level budget was higher in metropolitan areas than in nonmetropolitan areas and in the West and (to a lesser extent) the Northeast than in the South (Bureau of Labor

Statistics, 1982:Table 4).[6] Furthermore, over the period 1982-1992, prices have increased at a faster rate in the Northeast and West than in the Midwest and South (Bureau of the Census, 1993d:Table 761). Interarea price differences appear to be especially large for shelter; housing costs ranged from 52 to 183 percent of the national average in one study of metropolitan areas for 1989 (Kokoski, Cardiff, and Moulton, 1992). Yet the current poverty measure has the same poverty threshold for all regions and types of areas.

Increases in Medical Care Costs and Benefits

Per capita medical care spending has increased dramatically over the past few decades, rising from $1,166 to $2,566 over the period 1970-1990 (in 1990 dollars) (Moon, 1993). Health insurance coverage—including Medicare, Medicaid, and employer-provided insurance—has increased substantially as well. As a consequence, individuals' out-of-pocket costs for medical care (including insurance premiums) have declined as a share of total costs. However, their out-of-pocket costs in real dollar terms have actually increased somewhat—from $478 in 1963 to $597 in 1990 (Moon, 1993:23). One reason is that not everyone has insurance; another reason is that people with insurance coverage often contribute to the premiums and pay for a part of covered expenses. Also, there is wide variation in both total and out-of-pocket medical care costs by such characteristics as age, health status, and type of insurance coverage. Yet the current poverty measure does not distinguish among the health care needs of different kinds of families, nor does it reflect the role of insurance coverage in reducing families' medical care expenditures.

Taxes

When the U.S. poverty measure was first developed in the 1960s, the burden of income and payroll taxes on the low-income population was relatively light. Hence, the use of a before-tax definition of income to compare with thresholds that were developed on an after-tax basis was not problematic. However, there have been periods when the tax burden on low-income people has been relatively high. One estimate is that the effective federal individual income tax rate on the poorest 10 percent of the population increased from about 1 percent in 1966 to about 4 percent by 1985, and the effective Social Security payroll tax rate for this group increased from about 3-5 percent in 1966 to about 9-11 percent in 1985 (Pechman, 1985). Because

---

[6] There are problems in using the BLS family budget data to infer differences in the cost of living across geographic areas (e.g., the composition of the budgets differed across areas). However, Sherwood (1975) continued to find such differences in an analysis that made the budgets more comparable (see Chapter 3).

the official poverty measure uses a before-tax definition of family resources, it did not capture the adverse effects of these tax policy changes for low-income working families. Subsequently, expansion of the Earned Income Tax Credit reduced the tax burden on low-income working families, but the official measure similarly could not capture the ameliorative effects of this policy change.

Provision of In-Kind Benefits

When the U.S. poverty measure was first developed, there was relatively little provision of public or private benefits to the low-income population in the form of goods or services; since then, such benefits have expanded dramatically. As just one example, the Food Stamp Program did not operate nationwide in 1970; in 1993 it provided benefits to 10 percent of the population (U.S. House of Representatives, 1994:Table 18-9).

There are difficult problems of assigning monetary values to many in-kind benefits: for example, valuing a benefit like public housing at the full cost to the government may overstate the value to recipients, who might accept less money than the cost of the housing. Particularly difficult is the treatment of medical care benefits, whether public benefits (such as Medicaid and Medicare), benefits from employer-provided insurance, or uncompensated services provided by emergency rooms. It is easy to make sick people look like rich people by assigning monetary values to their medical care benefits, even when they have little or no other income with which to obtain such essentials as food and housing. Nonetheless, if in-kind benefits that are largely equivalent to money and that support consumption are not counted as income, the extent of poverty among the recipients is overstated. Such an approach also understates the efficacy of government income-support measures, which have increasingly favored in-kind benefit programs.

Increase in the Standard of Living

When the official poverty measure was first developed for 1963, the threshold of about $3,100 for a four-person family represented about one-half median after-tax four-person family income (see Vaughan, 1993). Between 1963 and 1992, median after-tax four-person family income increased by 28 percent in real terms, but the thresholds remained constant. Families' total expenditures also increased in real terms, and spending on nonfood items rose more rapidly than spending on food: expenditures on food accounted for one-third of the total in the 1950s but less than one-sixth of the total in the 1990s (see Bureau of the Census, 1993d:Table 708). Hence, if the original approach were used to develop the poverty thresholds today, their value would be significantly higher. One may question whether a poverty threshold should be updated for changes in total consumption, which includes spending on luxuries as well as necessities. One may also question whether a poverty threshold should remain fixed in real terms, so that it progressively declines in relation to the standard of living, not only overall but for such necessities as food and housing.

ALTERNATIVE POVERTY MEASURES
AND CRITERIA FOR A MEASURE

In this section we first consider different approaches to constructing poverty thresholds. We then consider the definition of family resources, which is the other side of the calculation needed to determine if a given person or family is poor. Establishing a poverty measure also requires that several other issues be addressed, particularly the time period, the unit of analysis, and how information about those in poverty is presented; these are treated below (see "Other Issues in Poverty Measurement"). Last, we present three criteria that we believe are critical in assessing any measure of poverty for consideration as the official U.S. measure.

Types of Poverty Thresholds

Absolute and Relative Thresholds

The literature often distinguishes between "absolute" and "relative" poverty thresholds. Absolute thresholds are fixed at a point in time and updated solely for price changes; relative thresholds are updated regularly (usually annually) for changes in real consumption. In this sense, the U.S. measure is an absolute one.

Absolute thresholds generally carry the connotation that they are developed by "experts" with reference to basic physiological needs (e.g., nutritional needs). In contrast, relative thresholds, as commonly defined, are developed by reference to the actual expenditures (or income) of the population. A typical approach is to select a cutoff point in the distribution of total family expenditures or income adjusted for family composition—say, one-half the median—and designate that dollar amount as the poverty threshold for a reference family, with thresholds for other family types developed by use of an equivalence scale. The European Community often uses relative thresholds to facilitate cross-national comparisons (see, e.g., O'Higgins and Jenkins, 1990).[7]

One criticism of relative thresholds is that the choice of the expenditure or income cutoff is arbitrary or subjective, rather than reflecting an objective

---

[7] Most developed countries do not have official poverty measures (see Will, 1986). However, studies of poverty have been carried out in most countries using various measures developed by researchers or social welfare policy analysts.

standard of economic deprivation. It is also argued that relative poverty thresholds do not provide a stable target against which to measure the effects of government programs because they change each year in response to increases or decreases in real consumption levels instead of remaining fixed in real terms. However, it is important to stress that relative poverty thresholds are not so distinct as one might imagine from thresholds developed according to expert standards of need: the latter also embody a great deal of relativity and subjectivity (see below). Moreover, it is rare for expert (or other) standards to be maintained in absolute terms over long periods of time. The more common experience is that an old standard is replaced after some period of time by a new standard that is higher in real terms (in this regard, see Fisher, 1993, for the history of unofficial poverty budgets in the United States prior to Orshansky). In other words, updating for real growth in consumption occurs, but at occasional intervals rather than on a regular basis.

Expert Budgets: The U.S. Experience

Expert budgets typically involve the development of standards for a large number of goods and services (e.g., food, clothing, shelter, utilities, transportation, personal care) with perhaps a small "other" or "miscellaneous" category. Although not an expert budget in this sense, the original U.S. poverty thresholds were based on expert standards for a key commodity, food. The experts were USDA home economists, and the poverty budget developed by Orshansky at SSA was based on the USDA estimates of the cost of the Economy Food Plan with a multiplier to account for other consumption items.

Relativity and subjectivity entered into the determination of both the food component and the multiplier for the original poverty thresholds. The Economy Food Plan was developed by considering the food-buying patterns of lower income families, as well as nutritional requirements. The USDA experts could have developed the Economy Food Plan at an even lower cost level and still provided for nutritional balance if they had been willing to ignore the eating patterns of Americans, who, even at lower income levels, showed a preference for meat as well as rice and beans. They could also have developed the Economy Food Plan at a higher cost level to allow for somewhat greater variety of diet and an occasional restaurant meal. That is, they had to make judgments that cannot be supported by nutritional science alone; they were guided in these judgments by data on Americans' actual food choices. Orshansky then explicitly introduced another element of relativity into the thresholds by choosing to use a multiplier that was based on the spending patterns of the average American family rather than on expert standards for other needed budget items.

Subjective judgment and relativity cannot be avoided by developing a detailed budget that eschews the use of a multiplier. The Family Budgets

Program of the BLS is a case in point. For the mid-1940s, 1959, and 1966, BLS developed detailed budgets for particular family types at an "intermediate" standard of living (earlier termed a "modest but adequate" or "moderate" standard). For 1967, BLS developed "higher" and "lower" budgets by scaling the intermediate budget up and down. In time intervals between budget revisions, the budgets were updated by repricing the budget, or, after 1966, by adjusting its cost by the change in the CPI.[8]

To develop the budgets, BLS used expert standards when they existed, including the USDA food plans (for the at-home component of food) and housing standards developed by the predecessors to the U.S. Department of Housing and Urban Development (HUD). For other budget items (e.g., clothing, transportation), BLS analysts used econometric methods to determine the spending levels that demarcated "necessary" from "excess" spending. These methods proved quite problematic in concept and application: they often produced unclear results, which, just as for the expert standards, necessitated choices that could only be guided by considering actual spending preferences (see Expert Committee on Family Budget Revisions, 1980). Overall, on each occasion when BLS revised its family budgets, the baseline intermediate-level budget typically approximated median spending levels of American families at the time. In other words, the budget reflected changes in the standard of living, but on a periodic basis rather than every year as would occur with a conventional relative measure.

Poverty standards developed by experts have historically been conditioned by their time and place. Thus, the modern Economy Food Plan and its successor, the Thrifty Food Plan, are much more generous in terms of allowed quantities than the food components of minimum budgets that were developed in major American cities between 1906 and 1929; similarly, the implicit allowance for nonfood items in the original SSA poverty thresholds is considerably more generous than the allowance in the pre-1929 budgets, when incomes were lower and the percentage spent on food was, consequently, higher (Appelbaum, 1977).

Although budget-based poverty thresholds are essentially relative in their development, and hence not as different as one might suppose from thresholds that are explicitly relative, they do have some distinctive features. By incorporating one or more explicitly named commodities, budget-based thresholds convey some type of paternalistic or normative concept of "needs," which may be more appealing to policy makers and the general public than a purely relative concept, such as one-half median family income. Of course, people will argue about which commodities should be part of the budget and which should be left out: obtaining consensus may be easier to the extent that broad

---

[8] The BLS Family Budgets Program was discontinued in the early 1980s for lack of adequate funds to improve it.

budget categories are used (e.g., clothing) rather than specific budget items (e.g., a raincoat). There still remains the problem of setting the specific dollar value for each named commodity and for the multiplier (if there is one) and determining how (and how often) to update those values: most expert budgets rely heavily on people's actual spending patterns.

Other Approaches

There are still other ways of determining poverty thresholds. One approach, which has been the subject of considerable research, particularly in Europe, is to ask a representative sample of the population to specify a minimum necessary income or to evaluate the adequacy of various income levels. There are various methods to calculate these "subjective" poverty thresholds from survey data of this type, each of which has positive and negative features. Generally, subjective poverty thresholds are sensitive to question wording and the particular method used in their derivation. Also, there tends to be wide variation in respondents' answers.

Despite their problems, subjective poverty thresholds—particularly a time series derived from consistent questions and procedures—can provide information that helps determine the extent to which other kinds of thresholds are more or less in agreement with broad public perceptions. One such series has been developed for the United States on the basis of responses to questions in the Gallup Poll over the period 1947-1989 (Vaughan, 1993), and there is similar information available from 1992 and 1993 polls.[9] This series suggests that people, on average, would have perceived about the same poverty level for a four-person family as the official threshold when it was first developed in the early 1960s. However, for the period prior to 1957, the data suggest that people, on average, would have perceived the poverty level in real terms to be below the official threshold. In contrast, since 1966, the data suggest that people, on average, would have perceived the poverty level to be higher than the official threshold.

Overall, there is a marked consistency from the late 1940s to the early 1990s between these subjective estimates of the poverty threshold and a time series of relative estimates based on median family income. For close to half a century these two quite distinct concepts have moved in similar ways and at similar levels. Figure 1-1 shows the official poverty threshold for a two-adult/

---

[9] The Gallup Poll asked: "What is the smallest amount of money a family of four (husband, wife and two children) needs each week to get along in this community?" In 1989 the Gallup Poll also included a question specifically about the poverty line. Vaughan (1993) used the relationship of the average amounts for the poverty and get-along questions in 1989 to construct a time series of subjective poverty thresholds from 1947 to 1989. A poverty line question in the 1992 Gallup Poll and the 1993 General Social Survey gave results similar to the 1989 Gallup Poll (see Chapter 2).

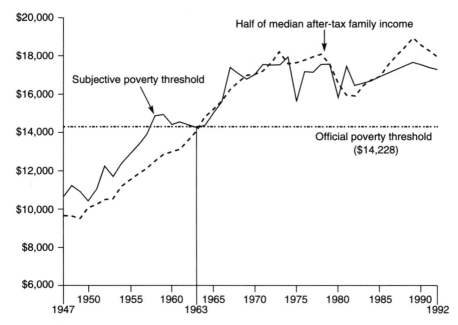

FIGURE 1-1 Alternative poverty thresholds for four-person families, in constant 1992 dollars.

two-child family, the subjective estimate of that threshold based on Vaughan's (1993) work, and a relative estimate of that threshold, defined as one-half after-tax median income of four-person families. In 1963, the base year for the official poverty threshold, the subjective and relative estimates are in close agreement, which surely helps explain why the official threshold was so generally acceptable at that time.

Researchers abroad have proposed yet another method of establishing poverty standards, namely, identifying a list of specific activities, items of ownership, and types of consumption that are believed to be essential for people to be able to participate normally in their society. In the United Kingdom, Townsend (1979) developed a "deprivation index" that included 12 components, including such items as not having taken a vacation in the past year and having gone through one or more days in the past fortnight without a cooked meal. He used the scores on this index to attempt to determine income levels (poverty thresholds) below which the deprivation index scores rose markedly. Other researchers refined the Townsend index by including only those elements that at least one-half of the respondents to a national survey claimed to be "necessary" for a minimal standard of living in the United Kingdom and by asking those lacking a given item whether they lacked it because they could not afford it or because they did not want it

(Mack and Lansley, 1985). The resulting deprivation index was used directly as a measure of poverty: those experiencing "enforced lack" due to budget constraints of 3 or more of the 22 items in their list were deemed poor.[10]

A conceptual underpinning for a deprivation index approach has been proposed that posits a normative standard, in terms of a fixed set of needed capabilities—for example, the ability to obtain a job, literacy, good health (Sen, 1983, 1989, 1992; see also Atkinson, 1989). The standard is then made operational in a relative manner by determining items that are necessary to achieve these capabilities in a particular time and place: for example, it can be argued that one needs a telephone to be able to obtain a job in modern U.S. society.

Deprivation indexes have their advantages and disadvantages. Like poverty thresholds expressed in monetary terms, they, too, involve difficult questions of choice—How many and which items to include in the list?—and inevitably embody a large element of subjectivity and relativity. Deprivation indexes appear less useful than monetary thresholds as an official measure of poverty for such purposes as determining eligibility for government assistance, but they can broaden understanding of what it means to have less resources than the official thresholds.

Definitions of Family Resources

Given a set of poverty thresholds, one must then define the resources that are to be counted to determine if each family and individual is above or below the appropriate threshold. Common resource definitions pertain to family income, which is the definition used in the United States and Canada, or to family expenditures (or consumption), which is the definition often used in Europe.

Conceptually, an income definition is more appropriate to the view that what matters is a family's *ability* to attain a living standard above the poverty level by means of its own resources. Thus, an income definition will not count as poor anyone who had an income above the threshold for the period of measurement, even if he or she consumed less than the poverty level, for whatever reason—pure choice or perhaps because of anticipating a drop in future income. Conversely, an income definition will count as poor anyone who had inadequate income, even if he or she was able to maintain consumption above the poverty level by such actions as borrowing, carrying a credit card balance, or depleting savings. In contrast to an income definition, an expenditure (or consumption) definition is more appropriate to the view that what matters is someone's *actual* standard of living, regardless of how it is

---

[10] In the United States, Mayer and Jencks (1993) have looked at items of ownership and types of consumption as indicators of material more than social deprivation, analyzing the proportion of low-income people who do not own a home or a car, who do not have air conditioning, etc.

attained. In practice, the availability of high-quality data is often a prime determinant of whether an income- or expenditure-based family resource definition is used.

Whichever type of family resource definition is used, decisions must be made about its precise components. In the case of an income definition, one must decide whether to include or exclude taxes or in-kind income and whether to take account of expenses involved in earning income (e.g., commuting or child care expenses). One must also decide whether to include any value for asset holdings that could be used to provide cash income. For the definition of expenditures, one must decide which types of expenditures to include.

A basic principle for a poverty measure, but one that has not always been followed, is that the threshold concept and the family resource definition should be consistent. Relative measures, such as one-half median family income, achieve consistency because the thresholds are defined from the same data that are used to estimate resources. Other types of thresholds are typically defined on the basis of different data from those used to estimate resources. Hence, explicit attention must be paid to achieving consistency between the two components: for example, if child care expenses are treated as a deduction from income on the grounds that the money so spent is a cost of earning income and is not available for consumption, such expenses should not be part of the poverty-level budget. In general, income is used for consumption, savings, and taxes, and it does not make sense to base the threshold and family resource concepts on different components of these elements.

Criteria for a Poverty Measure

Science alone cannot determine whether a person is or is not poor. Thus, there is no scientific basis on which one might unequivocally accept or reject a budget-based, or a purely relative, or a subjective concept for developing an official poverty measure. Each has some merit, and each has limitations; one concept may be more useful for one purpose and another for some other purpose. Although there are options that are clearly incorrect or internally inconsistent and there are better and worse ways of determining needs or resources, there is no way to reach a judgment solely on scientific grounds. Even if there were such a basis for an underlying concept, there is no purely scientific basis for specifying the level that should be defined as the threshold for poverty. This is at its essence a matter of judgment.

Given the limits of science, other criteria must be brought to bear in weighing alternatives and reaching decisions about an appropriate concept to underlie an official poverty indicator. We, as a panel that has deliberated about these matters at considerable length and benefited from the counsel of many experts, believe that three criteria are important in considering a concept and level for the official U.S. poverty measure, in addition to what can be learned from science: public acceptability; statistical defensibility; and operational feasibility. We have been guided by these three in our deliberations and in the formation of our recommendations.

Public Acceptability

Public acceptability is both a demanding and a lenient criterion. One of the key reasons that the SSA measure of poverty became quickly and broadly acceptable as the "official" measure in the early 1960s was that there was, for whatever reason, broad consensus that a level of income of about $3,000 was then a sensible cutoff for the threshold for poverty in the United States. A concept—then or now—that varies greatly from a generally accepted intuitive notion of what constitutes poverty would probably fail to gain political acceptance.

But this criterion demands that there be some rationale that has face validity. Just proclaiming a number—for example, the income level $10,000 as the benchmark for poverty—is not useful and would not become influential as a benchmark or policy guide. There should be some underlying sense to the concept, some reasonable explanation that is persuasive. The measure should be understandable and broadly acceptable. The general public may not care to understand details about the calculation of components of the measure (e.g., the equivalence scale computations), but the basic notion that the poverty measure reflects should accord with common sense.

Statistical Defensibility

Statistical defensibility, or statistical integrity, is an important criterion partly because the measure will be used by analysts and policy makers, and the technical details of its computation must meet the accepted standards of those analysts and of the many scholars who conduct research on the issue of poverty. Any newly proposed concept or method will be scrutinized and assessed before it becomes widely accepted, and it must withstand this demanding test.

The measure must be logically consistent. One of the central complaints against the current measure, as we note throughout this report, is that the poverty threshold is an after-tax concept, but the annual computation of the proportion and characteristics of people in poverty uses a before-tax family resource definition; this does not make sense.

More subtly, a poverty measure must allow for reasonable comparative analyses (within the limits of available data) across time, across places, across types of families, and across population groups. Analysts and policy makers want to be able to say something about the incidence of poverty compared with 10 years ago; about its incidence in the Northeast or Southwest; about its prevalence among minority groups, among female-headed families, among children, or among employed householders. The concept and measurement of poverty must apply as well to these various groups and over time and space as it does to the population as a whole for a given year.

Operational Feasibility

Operational feasibility implies that data can be collected that will in fact measure the prevalence of the conditions underlying the concept of poverty. Income and expenditures are concepts that are generally understood and can be measured and so these should be the core of the concept and measure of poverty.

As the capacity to measure and to survey improves, the measures of poverty that are used may well also improve. One rationale for a new measure now is that, indeed, knowledge of and capacity to collect accurate data on income and expenditures is far superior to that which informed the construction of the poverty thresholds in the early 1960s. Another 30 (or fewer) years, one hopes, will again provide far superior data, theory, and technical capacity to gather and analyze relevant information.

A NEW APPROACH TO POVERTY MEASUREMENT: RECOMMENDATIONS

A New Poverty Measure

We conclude that it is time to revise the official U.S. measure of poverty, even though a revision will affect the time series of poverty statistics. This section presents our recommendations for a new poverty measure and its implementation. We describe and explain the type of measure that we propose with regard to the threshold for a reference family, the updating procedure, adjustments to the threshold for differing family circumstances, and the family resource definition. We then summarize the results of an empirical analysis of the likely effects of the proposed poverty measure on the distribution of poverty and the overall rate. Finally, we summarize our recommendations for the kinds of data that are needed to fully implement the recommended new measure and other issues in poverty measurement (e.g., the time period and economic unit).

RECOMMENDATION 1.1. The official U.S. measure of poverty should be revised to reflect more nearly the circumstances of the nation's families and changes in them over time. The revised measure should comprise a set of poverty thresholds and a definition of family resources—for comparison with the thresholds to determine who is in or out of poverty—that are consistent with each other and otherwise statistically defensible. The concepts underlying both the thresholds and the definition of family resources should be broadly acceptable and understandable and operationally feasible.

RECOMMENDATION 1.2. On the basis of the criteria in Recommendation 1.1, the poverty measure should have the following characteristics:

• The poverty thresholds should represent a budget for food, clothing, shelter (including utilities), and a small additional amount to allow for other needs (e.g., household supplies, personal care, non-work-related transportation).

• A threshold for a reference family type should be developed using actual consumer expenditure data and updated annually to reflect changes in expenditures on food, clothing, and shelter over the previous 3 years.

• The reference family threshold should be adjusted to reflect the needs of different family types and to reflect geographic differences in housing costs.

• Family resources should be defined—consistent with the threshold concept—as the sum of money income from all sources together with the value of near-money benefits (e.g., food stamps) that are available to buy goods and services in the budget, minus expenses that cannot be used to buy these goods and services. Such expenses include income and payroll taxes, child care and other work-related expenses, child support payments to another household, and out-of-pocket medical care costs, including health insurance premiums.

Table 1-1 contrasts the elements of the proposed measure and the current measure. Not only do we propose a different concept for the reference family threshold (and suggest a realignment of the level of that threshold), but we also propose different ways of adjusting the threshold by family type, by geographic area, and over time, as well as a different definition of family resources. The current definition is gross money income; the proposed definition is disposable money and near-money income, which recognizes the value of near-money in-kind benefits and the unavailability for consumption of taxes and other nondiscretionary expenses. We also recommend using a different data source with which to measure disposable money and near-money income, namely, the Survey of Income and Program Participation (SIPP).

These other elements of a poverty measure—that is, the elements besides the concept and level of the threshold on which attention so often focuses—have important implications for differences in poverty rates for groups and areas and over time. In contrast to poverty statistics that are produced with the

TABLE 1-1 Elements of the Current and Proposed Poverty Measures

Element	Current Measure	Proposed Measure
Threshold Concept	Food times a large multiplier for all other expenses	Food, clothing, and shelter, plus a little more
1992 level (two-adult/ two-child family)	$14,228	Suggest within range of $13,700-$15,900
Updating method	Update 1963 level each year for price changes	Update each year by change in spending on food, clothing, and shelter over previous 3 years by two-adult/two-child families
Threshold Adjustments By family type	Separately developed thresholds by family type; lower thresholds for elderly singles and couples	Reference family threshold adjusted by use of equivalence scale, which assumes children need less than adults and economies of scale for larger families
By geographic area	No adjustments	Adjust for housing cost differences by region and size of metropolitan area
Family Resource Definition (to compare with threshold to determine poverty status)	Gross (before-tax) money income from all sources	Gross money income, plus value of near-money in-kind benefits (e.g., food stamps), minus income and payroll taxes and other nondiscretionary expenses (e.g., child care and other work-related expenses; child support payments to another household; out-of-pocket medical care expenses, including health insurance premiums)
Data Source (for estimating income)	March Current Population Survey	Survey of Income and Program Participation
Time Period of Measurement	Annual	Annual, supplemented by shorter term and longer term measures
Economic Unit of Analysis	Families and unrelated individuals	Families (including cohabiting couples) and unrelated individuals

TABLE 1-2 Policy and Other Changes Affecting Poverty Statistics

Type of Change	Reflected in	
	Current Measure	Proposed Measure
Increase/decrease in federal or state income taxes	No	Yes
Increase/decrease in Social Security payroll taxes	No	Yes
Increase/decrease in Social Security benefits	Yes	Yes
Increase/decrease in receipt or benefits under Aid to Families with Dependent Children Program	Yes	Yes
Increase/decrease in food stamp receipt or benefits	No	Yes
Increase/decrease in public or private health insurance coverage	No	Yes
Increase/decrease in child care or commuting subsidies	No	Yes
Increase/decrease in child support awards and enforcement	Partly[a]	Yes
Economic recession/recovery	Yes	Yes

[a]Gross money income includes child support *received* by families, but does not deduct child support *paid* by families to other households.

current measure, the proposed measure will capture more fully the effects of government policy initiatives, as well as social and economic changes, on the disposable money and near-money income that different types of families have available to meet their basic needs; see Table 1-2. We believe that the proposed poverty measure represents a marked improvement over the current measure, particularly for comparing the extent of poverty across population groups and geographic areas and across time.

Periodic Reviews

The procedure we propose for updating the poverty thresholds should link them more closely to societal norms about the appropriate level for a poverty line. Our proposal is to update the thresholds for real changes in the consumption of food, clothing, and shelter (see below). In contrast, the current measure simply updates the thresholds for price changes. The proposed measure, thus, is a type of relative measure, but it is not the same as a fully relative measure, such as one-half median income or expenditures, that would update the thresholds for changes in total consumption, including luxuries as well as basic goods and services.

However, adopting the proposed updating procedure does not obviate the need for periodic reviews of the poverty measure to determine whether, conceptually, it remains useful and appropriate and to identify and effect improvements on the basis of new data collection or research knowledge. No measure is without flaws, and a continuing process of review and improvement is needed. Thus, we also recommend periodic reassessments of all aspects of the poverty measure to determine what further improvements could be made. Indeed, it is dismaying that such a process has not been followed for the current poverty measure.

Although we do not fully understand the reasons, it seems that the "official" standing of the U.S. measure and the fact that it is used to determine eligibility for a number of government assistance programs have made it almost impervious to change. Other statistical measures with equally great political and budgetary consequences, such as the CPI, are regularly reviewed and revised, but even obvious changes—such as defining income in after-tax terms once the Census Bureau had developed reasonably good procedures for estimating income and payroll taxes—have not been made to the poverty measure. Although maintaining a concept over time is desirable to facilitate analysis of trends, it is dangerous to let a key social indicator become so frozen in place that, when societal conditions change, it can no longer adequately reflect what it was designed to measure.

We believe it makes sense to conduct a comprehensive review of the poverty measure on a 10-year cycle, as is done with other important statistical indicators, such as the CPI. The review should address all aspects of the poverty measure, including the concepts underlying the thresholds and the family resource definition, the performance of the updating procedure, and whether better data are available with which to derive the thresholds and estimate resources.

Should changes to the measure result from one of these periodic reviews, it will be important for policy makers, researchers, and other users to understand the implications for the time series of poverty statistics. To facilitate the transition for users, two poverty rate series should be produced for a period of several years—the official series that is based on the new measure and a second series that is based on the old measure.

There is a question of who should implement the proposed revised poverty measure and carry out the 10-year reviews. The poverty measure, unlike the CPI or unemployment rate, does not have a clear "home" within the federal government. The Census Bureau publishes the official poverty statistics, but it has never been empowered to change the measure. The U.S. Office of Management and Budget (OMB) issued directives implementing the minor changes to the thresholds that were adopted in 1969 and 1981, but it has not played an active role in the debate about the underlying concepts and does not have research or operational capabilities.

Based on past practice, it seems likely that the Statistical Policy Office of OMB will convene an interagency group representing program and statistical agencies to review this report and determine the response to our recommendations. On the assumption that OMB will play this role, we believe the Statistical Policy Office is the appropriate office to oversee implementation of our recommendations if they are accepted and to manage the 10-year review process. Obviously, the Census Bureau will have a major role to play, not only in publishing statistics under the new measure, but also in implementing needed data improvements and conducting research on various aspects of the measure. The Bureau of Labor Statistics will also have an important role in light of our recommendations for deriving and updating the reference family poverty threshold from consumer expenditure data (see below). Other agencies can also make important contributions to the continued improvement of the measure, as can researchers at academic institutions. In this regard, we urge OMB to seek the involvement of all appropriate agencies in the implementation and continued improvement of the poverty measure.

> **RECOMMENDATION 1.3. The U.S. Office of Management and Budget should adopt a revised poverty measure as the official measure for use by the federal government. Appropriate agencies, including the Bureau of the Census and the Bureau of Labor Statistics, should collaborate to produce the new thresholds each year and to implement the revised definition of family resources.**

> **RECOMMENDATION 1.4. The Statistical Policy Office of the U.S. Office of Management and Budget should institute a regular review, on a 10-year cycle, of all aspects of the poverty measure: reassessing the procedure for updating the thresholds, the family resource definition, etc. When changes to the measure are implemented on the basis of such a review, concurrent poverty statistics series should be run under both the old and the new measures to facilitate the transition.**

The Poverty Threshold

To understand fully the concept we recommend for developing and updating the poverty threshold and why we recommend it, the reader should keep several things in mind. First, the proposed threshold concept applies to a reference family, which we recommend be a family of two adults and two children.[11] It is possible with some concepts to develop thresholds indepen-

---

[11] It is important for technical reasons relating to the equivalence scale for the reference family to fall in the middle of the size distribution. Of course, the four-person family is not the

dently for each family type (as the official thresholds were originally constructed). However, we believe that it makes more sense to develop a threshold for a reference family and then use a formal equivalence scale to adjust that threshold for different numbers of adults and children. We also recommend that the thresholds be further adjusted by an index of differences in the cost of housing across geographic areas as a feasible way of implementing a cost-of-living adjustment (see below).

Second, we believe that in addition to accounting for different needs of families by number of adults and children and geographic area of residence, it is critical to account for different needs due to the fact that some families incur nondiscretionary expenses that are not available for consumption. For example, some families pay for child care in order to earn income, whereas other families (and individuals) make no such payments, yet the official thresholds are the same for both situations. One way to recognize these different circumstances is to develop additional thresholds, such as thresholds for nonworking families, working families with children who pay for child care, and other working families. We recommend instead that nondiscretionary expenses—which we define as taxes, child care and other work-related expenses, child support payments to another household, and out-of-pocket medical care expenditures (including health insurance premiums)—be deducted from the income of families with such expenses. This approach will more accurately capture the poverty status of families in different circumstances than would the approach of trying to develop a range of different thresholds. However, our approach has implications for comparing poverty thresholds across concepts: a reference family threshold developed as we propose will necessarily exclude some expenses that are typically averaged in for all such families.

Third, we consider that the decision about whether (and to what extent) to update the official poverty line for real growth in consumption has important implications for the choice of a poverty threshold concept and, indeed, for how much attention one needs to give to the threshold concept as opposed to other aspects of the poverty measure. We briefly discuss the updating issue before turning to our recommended threshold concept.

---

predominant living arrangement in American society. Of all households (including family households and those headed by unrelated individuals), the single largest type consists of adults living alone (25% in 1992), followed by married couples with no other family member (22%). Four-person families, comprising a married couple and two other family members, are the next largest group (13%). However, such four-person families are the modal type in terms of how many people they represent: in 1992, they accounted for 20 percent of all people, compared with 17 percent for married couples living alone, and 10 percent for single-adult households (Rawlings, 1993:Table 16).

Updating the Thresholds

Although developed in a largely relative fashion with reference to actual spending patterns, the official U.S. poverty thresholds are absolute in that they are updated each year solely for price changes. If one believes it appropriate to continue to maintain the current official poverty standard in absolute terms, then there is little need to debate the underlying threshold concept. One would want to review other aspects of the measure, including adjustments to the threshold for different family circumstances and the family resource definition. One would also want to consider the appropriate price index for updating: some have argued, for example, that it is preferable to use an index based on a market basket that reflects the spending patterns of low-income people rather than the overall CPI. But it would not be necessary to reconsider the level or concept of the reference family threshold itself.

(We note that whatever the merits of continuing with an absolute poverty standard, the argument that is sometimes made for it—namely, that only with an absolute standard is it possible to reduce poverty—is incorrect. In fact, the only way in which the poverty rate cannot go down is if the poverty level is defined each year as that income value not exceeded by, say, the lowest 20% of families—by definition, 20% of families are always below that level. In contrast, with such relative concepts as one-half median family income, changes in the distribution of income below the median can lower the poverty rate even when median income—and hence the dollar value of the poverty threshold—rises in real terms.)

An alternative approach would be to conclude from the historical evidence—as we do—that poverty thresholds, when they are set, are inherently relative to time and place but argue that it is important to maintain a set of thresholds, once chosen, in absolute terms for reasonably long periods of time. This approach would reject the notion of maintaining a poverty level unchanged for longer than, say, a generation (or, perhaps, a decade), but, between realignments, would maintain a stable target in real terms for such purposes as evaluating the effects of economic growth and government assistance programs on the extent of poverty.

The question then becomes whether now is the time for a realignment of the official thresholds and, if so, what is a reasonable level to adopt. (Other aspects of the poverty measure, such as the adjustments to the reference family threshold and the family resource definition, would also need to be considered, as would the appropriate price index for updating.)

A pragmatic first step is to look at the reference family threshold level produced by several concepts (e.g., the original SSA concept, other budget approaches, one-half median income or expenditures, subjective survey responses) in comparison with the official threshold. To the extent that the various levels from other concepts both differ from the official threshold and are reasonably congruent with each other, it may be possible to reach a consensus as to an appropriate realignment—just as the original SSA threshold for a family with two adults and two children commanded broad support in 1963.

It turns out that recently calculated thresholds for a two-adult/two-child family (or, in some cases, a four-person family) range from $17,200 to $21,800 (in 1992 dollars); see Table 1-3. By comparison, the official 1992 two-adult/two-child threshold is $14,228. (All the thresholds in Table 1-3 are after taxes; however, they average the needs of families with and without other types of

TABLE 1-3   Poverty Thresholds for Two-Adult/Two-Child (or Four-Person) Families Set by Various Methods for 1989-1993, in 1992 Dollars (Rounded)

Type and Source of Threshold	Amount
Absolute Threshold	
Official Orshansky, 1963: Economy Food Plan times 3.0, updated by the change in the CPI	14,228
Expert Budget Thresholds	
Adaptation by the panel of Orshansky (1963, 1965a): food times a multiplier of 4.4	20,700
Adaptation by the panel of Ruggles (1990): housing times a multiplier of 3.3	21,600
Weinberg and Lamas (1993), version A: food plus housing times a multiplier of 2.0	20,300
Weinberg and Lamas (1993), version B: (food plus a higher housing standard times a multiplier of 2.0	21,800
Adaptation by the panel of Renwick and Bergmann (1993): budget for food, housing and household operations, transportation, health care, clothing, child care, and personal care	17,600
Schwarz and Volgy (1992): detailed budget for single-earner family	19,000
Relative Thresholds	
One-half median after-tax four-person family income: extension of series developed by Vaughan (1993)	18,000
Adaptation by the panel of Expert Committee on Family Budget Revisions (1980): one-half average expenditures of four-person consumer units	20,000
Subjective Thresholds	
1989 Gallup Poll "poverty" line: from Vaughn (1993)	17,700
1993 General Social Survey "poverty" line	17,200

SOURCE: See Chapter 2, especially Table 2-5.

NOTE: All thresholds are after taxes except that survey respondents to the Gallup Poll and General Social Survey may not have answered the question on the poverty line in after-tax terms.

nondiscretionary expenses, such as child care.) These numbers indicate both that it would be appropriate to revise the level of the official thresholds and that there is room for debate about the extent of the realignment. For that debate, it would be important to consider the comparative merits of different concepts and the quality of the data underlying them, for two reasons: first, in order to reach consensus on a new reference family poverty threshold, and, second, to recommend improvements to the data and methods for various concepts so as to provide a sounder basis for repeating the realignment in the future.

There is yet a third alternative: an automatic mechanism for updating the thresholds on an annual basis for real changes in living standards. (The question of the price index is then irrelevant, except to account for lags in data availability.) In our view, this approach has several advantages over the approach of realigning the thresholds every so often. First, it avoids major breaks in the time series of poverty statistics that will inevitably occur with periodic realignments. Second, it ensures that an adjustment is in fact carried out and is not delayed or negated for political or other considerations. Third, it obviates the controversy that is likely to occur with periodic readjustments.

With a decision to update the poverty thresholds annually for changes in living standards, it becomes quite important to look at alternative concepts. Each of the concepts we reviewed, in our view, can contribute to the process of reaching consensus on a new threshold with which to initiate a new time series of poverty statistics. However, each concept has somewhat different implications for updating the poverty thresholds, particularly for the extent of the updating—that is, whether the thresholds are updated for real changes in all consumption or only in basic consumption. We believe it will be more acceptable to update the poverty thresholds in a "conservative" manner, that is, to update them for growth in consumption of basic goods and services that pertain to a notion of poverty, rather than to update them for growth in consumption of all goods and services.

Threshold Concepts: Assessment

Having reviewed the many possible concepts for deriving and updating the official reference family threshold in light of our criteria (see above), we acknowledge the strong attraction of the original SSA concept in terms of public acceptability and understandability. After all, food—more precisely, what is deemed a "minimally adequate" diet—is undeniably a necessary item of consumption. And developing a threshold that is food times a multiplier to allow for such other economic necessities as housing is a simple concept to understand. Also, the concept is easy to implement with available consumer expenditure data.

However, we question the use of expert-based standards of need even for

an item, such as food, that seems relatively well grounded in human physiol-
ogy. It may be feasible for experts to develop "minimum" standards for food
on the basis of nutrition needs alone, but because tastiness and some variety are
part of the notion of a minimally adequate diet, even experts will rely on
actual consumption patterns and not just nutritional need. In this way, judgment inevitably enters any calculation. We believe it best if these judgments
are introduced and explained explicitly.

Even more we question the use of a large multiplier applied to a single
commodity, particularly a multiplier that reflects the total expenditures of the
average family. With this approach, if applied regularly, the thresholds will be
updated to reflect increased spending on most goods and services, not just
basic goods and services. In other words, it is more akin to a completely
relative concept, like one-half median family income or expenditures (see
Table 1-3).

An expert budget approach in which standards are set for a number of
goods and services, with perhaps only a small "other" or "miscellaneous"
category, avoids the problem of a large multiplier. However, this approach
necessitates making a large number of specific judgments about approved
expenditures for the poor, each of which must be reexamined for updating
purposes. It is true that any approach involves judgments, and the poverty
thresholds that result from expert budgets may prove no less acceptable than
other thresholds (just as the original SSA thresholds found wide acceptability).
However, we believe it best for deriving the official U.S. poverty thresholds to
minimize the number of judgments required and, further, to link the thresholds directly, rather than indirectly, to actual spending patterns.

A relative concept for the reference family poverty threshold, such as one-
half the median level of family income or expenditures (adjusted for family
composition), makes explicit the judgment that is involved in setting a poverty
level. Although one-half the median is the commonly used standard, it could
just as well be some other percentage of median income. Also, as usually
implemented, a relative concept provides for an automatic, regular updating of
the poverty thresholds for real changes in living standards, as new data on
income or expenditures become available.

In spite of these attractive characteristics, we believe that a completely
relative concept would find little public support. First, it makes no reference
at all to a budget and, hence, gives no sense of what a poverty standard entails,
except that it is some fraction of median income or expenditures. Second, a
relative concept, applied regularly, will update the poverty thresholds for real
changes in total consumption, including luxuries as well as necessities. Moreover, the thresholds will reflect short-term changes in the business cycle—
both up and down—as well as longer term changes. In an economic downturn, the thresholds will likely decline in real terms, with the possibly
counterintuitive result that the poverty rate falls as well. It certainly seems

plausible that, if there is a serious depression or even a long-running recession, people will change their views about an appropriate poverty threshold, setting it at a lower dollar figure than previously. Also, a decline in the threshold does not necessarily mean a lower proportion of people in poverty (nor does an increase in the threshold necessarily mean a higher proportion of people in poverty). However, it seems undesirable to have the thresholds fluctuate with yearly ups and downs in the business cycle.

From the perspective of public acceptability and also from the view that the poverty level is inherently relative to a particular society, one could argue for using the responses of a representative sample of the population to set the level. In support of this approach, evidence from the Gallup Poll series and other studies show that subjective poverty thresholds tend to track changes in living standards, although on a less than one-to-one basis (i.e., they tend to change in a quasi-relative fashion). However, we believe that methodological problems—such as sensitivity of the results to question wording, large variance in responses—make this approach unsuitable for determining the official U.S. poverty thresholds. There is also the possibility with a public opinion survey that the results could be biased if people realize that their answers could affect the poverty line and thus respond differently than they otherwise would.

Recommended Threshold Concept and Updating

We propose that a new poverty threshold for the United States be developed as a hybrid of the budget-based and relative approaches. In our view, the poverty-level budget should start with a dollar amount for the sum of three broad categories of necessary goods—food, clothing, and shelter (including utilities). This sum should then be increased by a modest additional amount to allow for other necessary expenditures, such as personal care, household supplies, non-work-related transportation. We selected food, clothing, and shelter because they represent basic living needs with which no one would quarrel. That is, people may quarrel about the need for specific kinds of food, housing, and clothing—such as whether air conditioning is essential—but not about the need for food, housing, and clothing in broad terms. Indeed, the United States has major assistance programs to provide food and housing; there is no clothing program, but clothing allowances historically were separately identified grants under Aid to Families with Dependent Children (AFDC). There are other needs besides these three, of course, but there will be debate about which other goods and services represent necessities (e.g., whether to include reading materials). We believe that the use of a multiplier is a better way to provide an allowance for other needs without having to designate particular goods and services as necessary or unnecessary.

A difference in our approach is that we propose to obtain dollar amounts for the budget categories directly from tabulations of actual expenditures, rather than from expert judgments about standards of need. Specifically, we recommend that a new poverty threshold for the reference family be derived by specifying a percentage of median expenditures on the sum of food, clothing, and shelter by two-adult/two-child families in the Consumer Expenditure Survey (CEX), and applying a multiplier to that dollar value so as to add a small amount for other needed expenditures. (CEX data can also inform the selection of the multiplier.)

Having specified a percentage of the median and a multiplier, these values would then be used to update the poverty threshold for the reference family each year on the basis of more recent CEX data. To smooth out year-to-year fluctuations and to lag the adjustment to some extent, we propose to perform the calculations for each year by averaging the most recent 3 years' worth of CEX data, with the data for each of those years brought forward to the current period by using the change in the CPI. Once the threshold is updated for the reference family, the thresholds for other family types can be calculated (see below).

An important advantage of our proposed threshold concept is its implications for updating over time. Historically, spending on food, clothing, and shelter has increased at a slower rate in real terms than has total spending. We have estimated the elasticity with respect to real total expenditures of real spending on food, clothing, and shelter (including utilities) for the period 1960-1991 at about 0.65: in other words, for each 1 percent increase in real expenditures for all items, we estimate that expenditures on food, clothing, and shelter increased by about two-thirds of 1 percent (see Council of Economic Advisers, 1992:Table B-12). Hence, tying the poverty thresholds to spending levels for these three necessary commodities is a conservative way of updating; it adjusts the thresholds for real increases in consumption of basic goods and services, rather than for all goods and services.[12] Supporting the reasonableness of this degree of updating is the evidence that subjective poverty thresholds have an elasticity in the range of 0.65-0.80 with respect to median income: when people are asked in successive years to set a value for a minimum income, their answers reflect changes in living standards but on less than a one-for-one basis (see Figure 1-1).

RECOMMENDATION 2.1. A poverty threshold with which to initiate a new series of official U.S. poverty statistics should be derived from

---

[12] One could argue that a completely relative updating procedure is preferable to a "conservative" procedure on the grounds that, over time, "luxuries" become "necessities" (e.g., as in the case of radios and televisions). However, we argue that it is appropriate for a *poverty* measure to reflect such changes with a lag. An example is modern-day computing technology. Our proposed updating procedure will not immediately reflect the spread of such technology to consumers; however, when the technology becomes so integrated into the American life-style that housing and utilities are reconfigured to accommodate it, our measure will likely pick up that change.

Consumer Expenditure Survey data for a reference family of four persons (two adults and two children). The procedure should be to specify a percentage of median annual expenditures for such families on the sum of three basic goods and services—food, clothing, and shelter (including utilities)—and apply a specified multiplier to the corresponding dollar level so as to add a small amount for other needs.

RECOMMENDATION 2.2. The new poverty threshold should be updated each year to reflect changes in consumption of the basic goods and services contained in the poverty budget: determine the dollar value that represents the designated percentage of the median level of expenditures on the sum of food, clothing, and shelter for two-adult/two-child families and apply the designated multiplier. To smooth out year-to-year fluctuations and to lag the adjustment to some extent, perform the calculations for each year by averaging the most recent 3 years' worth of data from the Consumer Expenditure Survey, with the data for each of those years brought forward to the current period by using the change in the Consumer Price Index.

A concern with an updating procedure that adjusts for real increases in consumption is that the poverty thresholds will be too closely tied to changes in the business cycle. Our proposed updating procedure should moderate such fluctuations, both because of the use of 3 years' worth of expenditure data to calculate the reference family threshold each year and because the updating is tied to the basic necessities of food, clothing, and shelter.

The lack of a consistent historical time series of CEX data limited our ability to assess the performance of our updating procedure over the past 30 years. With data available beginning in 1980, however, we were able to determine that our procedure is less sensitive to the business cycle than a completely relative updating procedure (e.g., one-half median income or expenditures). Also, our procedure in fact performed conservatively over this period, in that the thresholds increased in real terms but not as much as thresholds derived in a completely relative manner (see Chapter 2).

Nonetheless, for evaluation purposes, we believe it would be useful to produce a second set of poverty rates from the proposed measure in which the thresholds are updated only for price changes. This second set of rates will permit evaluating changes in the official rates, based on updating the thresholds according to our recommended procedure, relative to changes in the business cycle.

RECOMMENDATION 2.3. When the new poverty threshold concept is first implemented and for several years thereafter, the Census Bureau should produce a second set of poverty rates for evaluation

purposes by using the new thresholds updated only for price changes (rather than for changes in consumption of the basic goods and services in the poverty budget).

In summary, we see the following advantages to our proposed concept for the poverty threshold. First, the concept is readily described as "food, clothing, and shelter, plus a little more." Although it is an oversimplification, as is a description of the original official concept as "food times a multiplier," it represents a clear and understandable level of need. Second, by relying on observed expenditure data, the concept avoids the difficulties of trying to develop and justify expert-based standards for a number of budget categories. Our approach explicitly links the measure of poverty to actual expenditures on basic goods and services. Finally, our proposed updating procedure has properties that we believe are desirable for the official U.S. poverty measure—namely, that the thresholds be updated on an automatic, regular basis, and that the updating be linked to spending on basic goods and services instead of total consumption.

Setting the Initial Threshold

In our empirical analysis (see below), we determined a two-adult/two-child reference family poverty threshold that, together with all of the other changes we recommend to the thresholds and family resource definition, produced the same overall poverty rate as the official rate for 1992. The purpose of this exercise was to illustrate the effects of the proposed measure, compared with the current measure, on the distribution of poverty among population groups and areas of the country.

The threshold for this exercise, however, is simply an artifact of the analysis. Thus, there remains the question of where to set the reference family threshold to serve as the starting point for a new series of poverty statistics with a new measure. Since we propose a new concept for the threshold, in which work and certain other expenses are subtracted from income rather than included in the poverty budget, one must allow for that concept in considering values for the reference family threshold. Data limitations make it difficult to convert threshold values developed on the basis of other concepts to the proposed concept with any exactitude, but it is possible to make rough estimates. Thus, a rough estimate is that the official 1992 threshold of $14,228 for a two-adult/two-child family is about $12,000 in terms of the proposed concept; see Table 1-4.[13] This adjustment only transforms the one budget con-

---

[13] The value of $12,000 is lower than the value of $13,175 that, together with the proposed changes to the poverty measure, produces the same overall poverty rate as the official rate for 1992 (see section below on "Effects"). The reason is that the threshold value for this exercise has to exactly offset the effects of all the other changes, not just the new threshold concept.

TABLE 1-4 Poverty Thresholds for Two-Adult/Two-Child (or Four-Person) Families Set by Various Methods for 1989-1993, as Developed and as Converted, in 1992 Dollars (Rounded)

Type and Source of Threshold	Amount as Developed	Amount as Converted[a]
Absolute Threshold		
Official Orshansky, 1963:	14,228	12,000
Economy Food Plan times 3.0		
updated by the change in the CPI		
Expert Budget Thresholds		
Adaptation by the panel of Orshansky	20,700	17,400
(1963, 1965a): food times 4.4		
Adaptation by the panel of Ruggles (1990):	21,600	18,100
housing times 3.3		
Weinberg and Lamas (1993), version A:	20,300	17,100
food plus housing times 2.0		
Weinberg and Lamas (1993), version B:	21,800	18,300
food plus a somewhat higher housing		
standard times 2.0		
Adaptation by the panel of Renwick	17,600	13,100
and Bergmann (1993): budget for food,		
housing and household operations,		
transportation, health care, clothing,		
child care, and personal care		
Schwarz and Volgy (1992): detailed budget	19,000	15,600
for single-earner family		
Relative Thresholds		
One-half median after-tax income for	18,000	15,100
four-person families: extension of		
series developed by Vaughan (1993)		
Adaptation by the panel of Expert	20,000	16,800
Committee on Family Budget Revisions		
(1980): one-half average expenditures		
of four-person consumer units		
Subjective Thresholds		
Gallup Poll "poverty" line: from Vaughan (1993)	17,700	14,900
General Social Survey "poverty" line	17,200	14,400
Suggested Threshold Range		
Recommended concept developed by panel:	13,700–	13,700–
percentage of median expenditures	15,900	15,900
on food, clothing, and shelter,		
plus a little more		

NOTE: All thresholds are after taxes (except that survey respondents to the Gallup Poll and General Social Survey may not have answered the question on the poverty line in after-tax terms). See Chapter 2 (especially Table 2-5) for more information on each threshold.

[a]"As converted" amounts for Renwick and Bergmann and Schwarz and Volgy are from inspection of their budgets, which gives ratios of "as converted" to "as developed" amounts of 0.74 and 0.82, respectively. These ratios are low because the budgets assume that every family spends the maximum allowance for such items as work expenses. "As converted" amounts for other thresholds are based on a ratio of 0.84, which is the ratio of "as converted" and "as developed" amounts for one-half median after-tax income of two-adult/two-child families. The "as converted" amount was obtained by subtracting one-half average work-related, child care, and out-of-pocket-medical care expenditures as imputed by the panel to the March 1993 CPS for two-adult/two-child families with after-tax income around the median.

cept into the other; we believe that the adoption of a new measure should also occasion a reevaluation of the appropriate level of the threshold.

We have recommended that, once adopted, the new reference family threshold be updated on an annual basis for real growth in the consumption of three categories of basic goods and services—food, clothing, and shelter. Consistent with this recommendation, we conclude that it is appropriate in setting the initial threshold to consider the real growth in the standard of living since 1963 when the current threshold was fixed in real terms.

RECOMMENDATION 2.4. As part of implementing a new official U.S. poverty measure, the current threshold level for the reference family of two adults and two children ($14,228 in 1992 dollars) should be reevaluated and a new threshold level established with which to initiate a new series of poverty statistics. That reevaluation should take account of both the new threshold concept and the real growth in consumption that has occurred since the official threshold was first set 30 years ago.

Over the period 1963-1992, median before-tax money income of four-person families increased by 36 percent in real terms (the real increase in median after-tax income was 28%; the real increase in average expenditures was 45%; see Chapter 2), but the poverty threshold did not change. There is, of course, a judgment to be made about how much to adjust the current poverty threshold. An adjustment that is somewhat less than the real increase in total consumption would be consistent with the proposed updating procedure, given our earlier observation that real growth in spending on food, clothing, and shelter has been less than real growth in total spending.

Because of the limitations of historical data on family expenditure patterns, one cannot readily apply the proposed updating procedure over time to determine a value for the threshold today (see Chapter 2). Even if the data were adequate for this purpose, however, the decision about the appropriate level for the reference family threshold for a particular time and place would remain inherently a matter of judgment.

For this reason, we concluded that we would not make a formal recommendation about the initial threshold for the two-adult/two-child reference family. However, we do offer our conclusion about what we believe is a reasonable range for that initial threshold. This conclusion is informed by our analysis of thresholds that result from a variety of approaches and concepts in the published literature, as well as our judgment.

We conclude that reasonable values for the starting threshold for a two-adult/two-child family lie in the range of about $13,700 to $15,900 (in 1992 dollars). Compared with the range of threshold values of $17,200 to $21,800 shown in Table 1-3, the values we suggest appear to represent little or no updating in real terms of the official 1992 threshold of $14,228 for a two-adult/two–child family. However, when other threshold values are converted (as best as can be done) to *our budget concept*, their range is $13,100 to $18,300, or 9 to 53 percent above the comparable value of $12,000 for the official level; see Table 1-4. Our suggested range of $13,700 to $15,900 is 14 to 33 percent higher than the comparable current level. This range falls within but toward the lower end of the estimated range of other thresholds. Thus, it represents a conservative updating in real terms of the current threshold, consistent with our recommendation.

In terms of our proposed budget concept, the lower end of our suggested range, $13,700, equals 1.15 times (or 15% more than) the spending on food, clothing, and shelter by two–adult/two–child families at the 30th percentile of the distribution estimated from the 1989-1991 CEX (expressed in 1992 dollars). That is, if one sets aside 15 percent for all other spending items, then that threshold level permits a family to spend as much on food, clothing, and shelter as families that ranked at the 30th percentile of all two–adult/two–child families, which was $11,950. Similarly, one can characterize the upper end of our suggested range, $15,900, as equal to 1.25 times (or 25% more than) the spending on food, clothing, and shelter by two–adult/two–child families at the 35th percentile of the distribution, which was $12,720.[14]

What could these amounts buy? Illustratively, a family at the 30th percentile might spend $355 per month or $4,260 annually for food (the value of the Thrifty Food Plan for a four-person family); $545 per month or about $6,550 per year for rent and utilities (including telephone) for a two-bedroom apartment (the fair market rent in 1992 for such units that is the basis for federal housing assistance); and $95 per month ($24 per family member) or $1,140 per year for clothing. A family at the 35th percentile could spend another $64 per month, or $770 per year, on food, clothing, and shelter. The multiplier adds another $1,750-$3,180, or about $145-$265 per month, for all other needed expenditures.

Values of the multiplier of 1.15 to 1.25 are below the values of the multiplier in other approaches (see Table 1-4). However, the multiplier in the proposed concept applies to a larger bundle of basic goods and services (food, clothing, and shelter) than is true for other approaches; also, it excludes such expenses as child care and out-of-pocket medical care costs, which are treated as deductions from income.

Analysis that we conducted with CEX data supports the range for the multiplier of 1.15 to 1.25. (In this analysis, we examined the amounts spent on such items as personal care and non–work-related transportation relative to the amounts spent on food, clothing, and shelter by two–adult/two–child

---

[14] Both the lower and the upper ends of our suggested range for the initial reference family threshold could be expressed in terms of some other combination of values for food, clothing, and shelter and a multiplier for other expenditures.

families spending below the median level on these three categories—see Chapter 2.) Multipliers in recently published expert budgets (Renwick, 1993a; Schwarz and Volgy, 1992), after adjustment to the proposed concept, fall in the range of 1.14 to 1.30 for the reference family type.

The ranges that we suggest for food, clothing, and shelter and the multiplier produce a reasonable threshold, even though the range for food, clothing, and shelter is 78-83 percent of the median level of spending on these categories by two-adult/two-child families; in 1992 that median was $15,344. The reason that the threshold is reasonable is because the average family (*not* the average low-income family) spends only about 45 percent of its budget on food, clothing, and shelter (Bureau of the Census, 1993d:Table 708). Hence, taking a relatively large proportion of median expenditures on food, clothing, and shelter, which represent less than half the typical budget, and applying a multiplier in the range of 1.15 to 1.25 will produce a threshold that is lower than a relative threshold of one-half median total expenditures (or after-tax income).

Whatever level is selected for the initial threshold, the key point of our procedure is how that level is updated over time. Each year, the updating procedure will use the same percentage of median expenditures on food, clothing, and shelter and the multiplier that were determined for the initial threshold and use them to update the threshold with newer expenditure data.[15] Consequently, the updating over time will be pegged to the level of spending on food, clothing, and shelter, not to the spending on all goods or to the growth in income overall. This difference is quite important because food, clothing, and shelter expenditures are likely to increase proportionately less than total expenditures (or income). Hence, a threshold that is updated as we recommend is likely to increase less than would a purely relative threshold.

Finally, we want to make clear that building a poverty threshold on food, clothing, and shelter plus a little more—and linking changes in the thresholds to changes in consumption of these items—do not imply that families must spend their income accordingly. For example, families that spend less on food, clothing, and shelter than implied in the poverty threshold are not necessarily poor—perhaps they grow some of their own food or make some of their own clothing in order to increase their income for other spending (e.g., on books, haircuts, or a vacation). Such families are poor if their total income (net of nondiscretionary expenses) is below the poverty line, but not otherwise. Conversely, families that spend more on food, clothing, and shelter than

---

[15] It is convenient in setting the initial threshold to look at percentiles of the expenditure distribution on food, clothing, and shelter (i.e., the dollar values that include the lowest 20%, 25%, 30%, 35%, 40%, and so on of two-adult/two-child families). However, for updating purposes, the dollar level for food, clothing, and shelter must be expressed as a percentage of median expenditures on these categories; see Chapter 2.

implied in the poverty threshold may (or may not) be poor, depending on their net income compared with the poverty threshold.

Just as we have urged the development of indicators of other kinds of deprivation (e.g., physical, social) in addition to the economic poverty measure, it would be useful to have indicators that directly measure inadequate food consumption (including hunger) and inadequate housing (including homelessness). It would also be useful to have tabulations of how people below the poverty threshold spend their income. For this to be possible, improvements must be made in both the expenditure and the income data in the CEX (see below).

Adjusting the Thresholds—Equivalence Scale

A poverty threshold that is appropriate for one type of family is not necessarily appropriate for another. One difference is that the level of consumption needed for a child is not the same as that for an adult. Also, a larger family enjoys some economies of scale: it can make bulk purchases and use hand-me-down clothing, and although it may need more bedrooms, it does not need more kitchens or living rooms than a smaller family. Adjustments to the reference family poverty threshold to reflect differences in family size and composition are made by applying an "equivalence scale." Unfortunately, there is no research-based consensus about how large the scale economies are for larger families, nor about how much children consume, on average, relative to adults. Hence, there are no clear guidelines for adjusting the poverty threshold for families of different sizes and structures.

For family size, if one starts with some benchmark family of a specific size and with some specific expenditure level, there is no completely objective way to determine what level of expenditure by a family of some other size is in fact equivalent in terms of well-being or satisfaction. Thus, there is no way to specify the "scale economy factor" by which the poverty threshold for a reference family should be adjusted for different size families. Yet the magnitude of this factor can have a very large influence on the composition and magnitude of the poverty population.[16]

At one extreme, no adjustment for family size (i.e., a scale economy factor of 0.0) would give the same poverty threshold for an unrelated individual and for a family of five or more. The implication is that all additional family members beyond the first are completely costless, and the result would surely be to underestimate the extent of poverty for larger families relative to smaller families. At the other extreme, a "full" adjustment (i.e., a scale economy

---

[16] The reader needs to keep in mind that a lower value of the scale economy factor (i.e., closer to zero) means greater scale economies, and a higher value of the factor (i.e., closer to 1.0) means lesser scale economies.

factor of 1.0) would result in a poverty threshold for a family of five that is five times as much as the threshold for a single individual. The implication is that there are no economies of scale whatsoever—that each added member costs the family as much as the first member—and the result would be to overestimate the extent of poverty for larger families relative to smaller families. Neither extreme is defensible, and the debate in the research literature can be understood as a debate about the correct level for this factor, somewhere between the two extremes.

There is growing consensus, however, that the equivalence scale implicit in the official poverty thresholds is not internally consistent and exhibits an irregular pattern. The inconsistency comes from the fact that the scale is based on the dietary needs of family members even though the economies of scale appear to be different for food and for other goods, like housing or transportation. In addition, the current measure reflects ad hoc adjustments for single people living alone or without other relatives and for two-person families. Finally, the current measure has lower thresholds for single people and couples who are aged 65 or older than for younger single people and couples.

We conclude that the equivalence scale that is embedded in the official poverty thresholds should not be retained. We recommend that the scale for the poverty thresholds account for differences between the needs of adults and children under 18 but not further distinguish family members (adults or children) by age or other characteristics. We also recommend that the scale incorporate a scale economy factor to reflect economies for larger families.

The equivalence scale should take the following general form:

$$(A + PK)^F.$$

The quantity A is the number of adults in a family; the quantity K is the number of children, each of whom is treated as a proportion P of an adult. Thus, $(A + PK)$ reflects the size of the family in adult equivalents, and F is the scale economy factor that converts these adult equivalents into comparable units in terms of their efficient use of the family's resources. We recommend values for both P and F near 0.70; to be specific, we recommend setting P at 0.70 (i.e., each child is treated as 70% of an adult) and F in the range of 0.65 to 0.75.

The result of implementing the formula for the reference family of two adults and two children, with P equal to 0.70 and F equal to 0.75, is an equivalence scale value of 2.5 (3.4 adult equivalents raised to a power of 0.75). To calculate the poverty threshold for any other combination of adults and children, the ratio of the scale value from the formula for that family type to the scale value of 2.5 is applied to the reference family threshold. For example, the scale value for a one-adult/one-child family, with P equal to 0.70 and F equal to 0.75, is 1.49 (the result of raising 1.7 adult equivalents to a power of 0.75). Hence, the poverty threshold for a one-adult/one-child family is 60 percent (1.49/2.5) of the threshold for the two-adult/two-child family.

We are confident that this equivalence scale has an appropriate form; however, the selection of the two key parameters—for the proportionate needs of children and the scale economy factor—involves judgment. In selecting the values for these parameters, it is important to recognize the interaction between them. For example, several studies and advisers to the panel have suggested the use of a scale economy factor of 0.50 (implying greater economies than our suggested range of 0.65-0.75), but coupled with the assumption that children cost the same as adults. Given a scale, such as we propose, in which children are assumed to need less than adults, it is appropriate to raise the scale economy factor closer to a value of 1, although how much closer is, to repeat, a matter of judgment.

> **RECOMMENDATION 3.1.   The four-person (two adult/two child) poverty threshold should be adjusted for other family types by means of an equivalence scale that reflects differences in consumption by adults and children under 18 and economies of scale for larger families. A scale that meets these criteria is the following: children under 18 are treated as consuming 70 percent as much as adults on average; economies of scale are computed by taking the number of adult equivalents in a family (i.e., the number of adults plus 0.70 times the number of children), and then by raising this number to a power of from 0.65 to 0.75.**

Figure 1-2 portrays the equivalence scale for selected family types under our proposal compared with the scale implicit in the current poverty thresholds. The graph indicates the percentage by which a single person's poverty threshold is increased when that person acquires a spouse and when the couple subsequently has a first, second, third, and fourth child. The figure makes clear the irregularities and anomalies in the current scale. For example, under the current scale, a spouse adds only 29 percent to family costs; the first child adds almost as much (26%), and the second child adds a yet greater amount (40%). These patterns are not consistent with the view that adults need more than children nor with economies of scale for larger families. In contrast, our proposed scale adds 57-68 percent for a spouse (depending on whether the scale economy factor is 0.65 or 0.75), 34-42 percent for the first child, and a decreasing percentage for each additional child.

Adjusting the Thresholds—Geographic Variations

A frequently voiced criticism of the current poverty thresholds is that they take no account of variations in the cost of living in different geographic areas of the country. Such variations—for example, large differences in housing

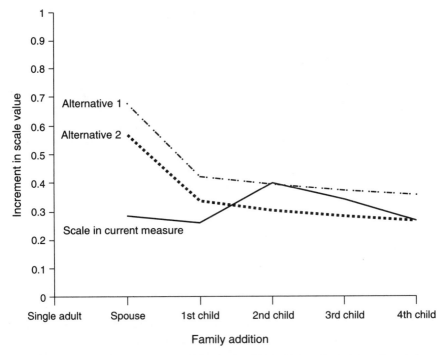

FIGURE 1-2 Alternative equivalence scales. NOTES: Alternatives 1 and 2 use scale economy factors of 0.75 and 0.65, respectively; both alternatives assume children need 70 percent as much as adults. The increments are relative to a scale value of 1.0 for a single adult.

costs between coastal metropolitan areas and the heartland—seem obvious to the public, and, indeed, are often the subject of media attention. Poverty thresholds that recognize such differences seem clearly preferable to those that do not. Unfortunately, this is a topic for which limitations in data greatly constrain one's options. For example, although BLS publishes price indexes for a number of metropolitan areas, no indexes are published for nonmetropolitan areas. Moreover, the BLS price indexes are not designed to permit comparisons of cost-of-living differences across areas; rather, they compare rates of change in price inflation: one can determine whether prices are rising faster in Los Angeles than in New York City, for example, but not whether the cost of living is higher in one or the other area.

Despite data limitations, we believe that some adjustment to the poverty thresholds should be made for geographic cost-of-living variations. Research conducted by BLS analysts suggests that variations are minor for some items, such as food (Kokoski, Cardiff, and Moulton, 1994), but that they are large for housing (including utilities), which is a large component of the proposed poverty-level budget. Also, data are available from the 1990 census with which to estimate differences in rental housing costs across the entire country, making possible at least a partial adjustment of the poverty thresholds for geographic cost-of-living differences.

We analyzed the census data to determine adjustments that, in light of other studies, seem reasonable to apply to the housing component of the proposed poverty thresholds. We believe that at this stage of knowledge the adjustments should be made for relatively large geographic areas. Our analysis examined census-based housing cost adjustments by region and state and by several population size categories of metropolitan areas.[17] On balance, it appears that size of place is a more important correlate of housing costs than is state of residence; most states include urban and rural areas that vary widely in population density and housing costs. Hence, we recommend that adjustments for housing cost differences—calibrated to reflect the share of housing in the proposed poverty budget—be implemented for nine regions of the country and, within each region, by several population size categories of metropolitan areas. The adjustments that we developed from our analysis and used in estimating the effects of the proposed measure are provided in Table 1–5.[18]

RECOMMENDATION 3.2. **The poverty thresholds should be adjusted for differences in the cost of housing across geographic areas of the country. Available data from the decennial census permit the development of a reasonable cost-of-housing index for nine regions and, within each region, for several population size categories of metropolitan areas. The index should be applied to the housing portion of the poverty thresholds.**

It would be desirable to update the adjustment factors that are applied to the housing component of the poverty thresholds more frequently than once every 10 years. We encourage research to determine reasonable updating methods. For example, it may be that HUD's methods for updating fair market rents could be adapted for this purpose.

RECOMMENDATION 3.3. **Appropriate agencies should conduct research to determine methods that could be used to update the geographic housing cost component of the poverty thresholds between the decennial censuses.**

---

[17] We adapted the HUD methodology for constructing fair market rents by locality.

[18] We did not address the special circumstances of Alaska and Hawaii, for which a housing cost adjustment based on the Pacific states region as a whole may not be sufficient to reflect the high cost of living in these states. Also, although we do not recommend state-by-state adjustments for the statistical measure of poverty, such adjustments may make sense for the AFDC program (see Chapter 8).

TABLE 1-5   Poverty Thresholds Adjusted for Differences in Cost of Housing, Expressed as Percentages Above or Below a National Poverty Threshold

Region and Area	Percentage Difference
North	
New England (Connecticut, Maine, Massachusetts, New Hampshire, Rhode Island, Vermont)	
Nonmetropolitan areas and metropolitan areas under 250,000 population	+12.8
Metropolitan areas 250,000–500,000 pop.	+12.8
Metropolitan areas 500,000–1,000,000 pop.	+14.8
Metropolitan areas 1,000,000–2,500,000 pop.	+14.1
Metropolitan areas 2,500,000 or more pop.	+20.9
Middle Atlantic (New Jersey, New York, Pennsylvania)	
Nonmetropolitan areas and metropolitan areas under 250,000 population	−9.2
Metropolitan areas 250,000–500,000 pop.	−0.3
Metropolitan areas 500,000–1,000,000 pop.	+2.0
Metropolitan areas 1,000,000–2,500,000 pop.	−2.5
Metropolitan areas 2,500,000 or more pop.	+18.7
Midwest	
East North Central (Illinois, Indiana, Michigan, Ohio, Wisconsin)	
Nonmetropolitan areas and metropolitan areas under 250,000 population	−10.4
Metropolitan areas 250,000–500,000 pop.	−4.1
Metropolitan areas 500,000–1,000,000 pop.	−1.3
Metropolitan areas 1,000,000–2,500,000 pop.	−0.5
Metropolitan areas 2,500,000 or more pop.	+5.9
West North Central (Iowa, Kansas, Minnesota, Missouri, Nebraska, North Dakota, South Dakota)	
Nonmetropolitan areas and metropolitan areas under 250,000 population	−13.9
Metropolitan areas 250,000–500,000 pop.	−3.8
Metropolitan areas 500,000–1,000,000 pop.	−1.9
Metropolitan areas 1,000,000–2,500,000 pop.	+2.8
Metropolitan areas 2,500,000 or more pop.	N.A.
South	
South Atlantic (Delaware, District of Columbia, Florida, Georgia, Maryland, North Carolina, South Carolina, Virginia, West Virginia)	
Nonmetropolitan areas and metropolitan areas under 250,000 population	−10.1
Metropolitan areas 250,000–500,000 pop.	−3.9

continued on next page

TABLE 1-5 *Continued*

Region and Area	Percentage Difference
South Atlantic—*continued*	
Metropolitan areas 500,000–1,000,000 pop.	+0.7
Metropolitan areas 1,000,000–2,500,000 pop.	+4.3
Metropolitan areas 2,500,000 or more pop.	+11.9
East South Central (Alabama, Kentucky, Mississippi, Tennessee)	
Nonmetropolitan areas and metropolitan areas under 250,000 population	−17.3
Metropolitan areas 250,000–500,000 pop.	−6.5
Metropolitan areas 500,000–1,000,000 pop.	−5.3
Metropolitan areas 1,000,000–2,500,000 pop.	N.A.
Metropolitan areas 2,500,000 or more pop.	N.A.
West South Central (Arkansas, Louisiana, Oklahoma, Texas)	
Nonmetropolitan areas and metropolitan areas under 250,000 population	−14.2
Metropolitan areas 250,000–500,000 pop.	−8.9
Metropolitan areas 500,000–1,000,000 pop.	−5.8
Metropolitan areas 1,000,000–2,500,000 pop.	−3.8
Metropolitan areas 2,500,000 or more pop.	+0.5
West	
Mountain (Arizona, Colorado, Idaho, Montana, Nevada, New Mexico, Utah, Wyoming)	
Nonmetropolitan areas and metropolitan areas under 250,000 population	−11.2
Metropolitan areas 250,000–500,000 pop.	−2.4
Metropolitan areas 500,000–1,000,000 pop.	+3.9
Metropolitan areas 1,000,000–2,500,000 pop.	+0.3
Metropolitan areas 2,500,000 or more pop.	N.A.
Pacific (Alaska, California, Hawaii, Oregon, Washington)	
Nonmetropolitan areas and metropolitan areas under 250,000 population	−3.1
Metropolitan areas 250,000–500,000 pop.	+1.8
Metropolitan areas 500,000–1,000,000 pop.	+2.8
Metropolitan areas 1,000,000–2,500,000 pop.	+10.4
Metropolitan areas 2,500,000 or more pop.	+21.7

NOTES: Housing cost indexes are calculated from 1990 census data on gross rent for apartments with specified characteristics, adjusted to reflect the share of housing in the proposed poverty budget (see Chapter 3). Nonmetropolitan areas are combined with metropolitan areas of less than 250,000 population because of restrictions on geographic area coding in the Current Population Survey and Survey of Income and Program Participation.

N.A., not applicable.

Finally, further research and perhaps additional data collection are needed on adjustments to the poverty thresholds for geographic cost-of-living differences. We encourage research that could lead to more sophisticated adjustments for differences in housing costs and, ultimately, to adjustments that reflect cost differences for other goods and services.

RECOMMENDATION 3.4. **Appropriate agencies should conduct research to improve the estimation of geographic cost-of-living differences in housing as well as other components of the poverty budget. Agencies should consider improvements to data series, such as the BLS area price indexes, that have the potential to support improved estimates of cost-of-living differences.**

Defining Family Resources

Under the official U.S. poverty measure, a family's poverty status is determined by comparing its gross money income to the appropriate threshold. A number of researchers have argued that a preferable comparison is between a family's consumption (or expenditures) and the appropriate poverty threshold. One can make arguments for either approach, depending in part on one's view as to whether poverty is more appropriately assessed as the actual or the potential attainment of a minimally adequate standard of living. Whatever one's view, the United States does not have adequate data sources with which to develop a consumption or expenditure-based poverty measure: the sample size of the CEX is too small to provide reliable poverty measures for population groups or by geographic area. To make the CEX adequate for purposes of poverty measurement would require an expensive expansion of the sample size and a redesign of the survey, which is focused on providing information needed to revise the market basket for the CPI.

In contrast, the United States has large, well-developed surveys for measuring income. Thus, we conclude that the measurement of poverty in the United States must continue, at least for some years, to be based on an income-based definition of family resources. However, we believe that the current concept of gross money income is inadequate in many respects and needs to be modified in order to be consistent with the proposed threshold concept.

We stressed earlier the importance of consistency between the concept underlying the poverty thresholds and the definition of resources. The current measure violates this principle, as has some recent work to investigate alternatives. For example, estimates by the Census Bureau (see, e.g., Bureau of the Census, 1993a) and others in which the value of public and private health insurance benefits is added to families' resources are inconsistent with the thresholds. The reason is that, since the official thresholds were first developed, medical care costs have escalated greatly, so that the effect of including insurance values without also raising the thresholds is to ignore the added costs of staying out of poverty.

RECOMMENDATION 4.1.   **In developing poverty statistics, any signifi-cant change in the definition of family resources should be accom-panied by a consistent adjustment of the poverty thresholds.**

To achieve consistency with the proposed poverty budget, the definition of family resources (or income) must represent disposable money and near-money resources: it should include the value of in-kind resources that are available for consumption, and, conversely, it should deduct from income required expenditures that are not available for consumption. We note that the major public assistance programs, such as food stamps and AFDC, cur-rently use a similar definition of disposable or "countable" income to deter-mine eligibility and benefits.

RECOMMENDATION 4.2.   **The definition of family resources for com-parison with the appropriate poverty threshold should be disposable money and near-money income. Specifically, resources should be calculated as follows:**

- **estimate gross money income from all public and private sources for a family or unrelated individual (which is income as defined in the current measure);**
- **add the value of near-money nonmedical in-kind benefits, such as food stamps, subsidized housing, school lunches, and home en-ergy assistance;**
- **deduct out-of-pocket medical care expenditures, including health insurance premiums;**
- **deduct income taxes and Social Security payroll taxes;**
- **for families in which there is no nonworking parent, deduct actual child care costs, per week worked, not to exceed the earnings of the parent with the lower earnings or a cap that is adjusted annually for inflation;**
- **for each working adult, deduct a flat amount per week worked (adjusted annually for inflation and not to exceed earnings) to ac-count for work-related transportation and miscellaneous expenses; and**
- **deduct child support payments from the income of the payer.**

In-Kind Benefits—Nonmedical

The official poverty thresholds, as originally conceived, and the panel's pro-posed thresholds, although developed in somewhat different ways, reflect the concept of a budget for consumption needs. Hence, it is clear that the definition of family resources should add to money income the value of near-money in-kind benefits that are intended to support consumption. Thirty years ago, assistance programs that provided in-kind benefits rather than money were small in number and scope. Subsequently, such programs—which include food stamps, subsidized housing, school lunches, meal programs for the elderly, and home energy assistance—have expanded greatly, and the poverty measure should take account of their effects.

Some in-kind benefits are harder to value than others because they are less fungible (i.e., less interchangeable with other resources) and of less value to the recipient than the same amount of money income: public housing raises the most problems in this regard. Also, for some types of benefits (e.g., employer-provided housing or meals), there is little information or experience with how to value them. However, we believe that the Census Bureau has sufficient experience with valuing the major types of in-kind benefits so that reasonable estimates can be added to money income without waiting for further research. Of course, research should continue on improved methods for valuing in-kind benefits, and changes in methodology should be made as appropriate. (Employer-provided benefits that are necessary for work, such as subsidized child care, parking, or free uniforms or tools, should not be valued as part of income because the proposed definition of disposable income subtracts out-of-pocket costs for child care and other work-related expenses, net of any employer subsidy.)

Medical Care Costs

Perhaps the most striking omission from the list of in-kind benefit programs that we propose to count as family resources for purposes of measuring poverty is medical care benefits. Certainly, Medicare, Medicaid, and employer-provided health insurance have helped many millions of Americans over the past three decades. It seems odd that the proposed poverty measure does not explicitly reflect this achievement of public policy and also does not explicitly reflect the gaps in health insurance coverage of the population that still exist. In fact, the proposed measure does take account of health insurance benefits, but indirectly—in terms of the extent to which they reduce out-of-pocket medical care expenses and thereby increase disposable income for other consumption. Also, we recommend that separate measures be developed of the economic risk from inadequate or no health insurance coverage to accompany the measure of economic poverty.

Researchers have wrestled with the valuation of health care benefits for purposes of poverty measurement for over a decade, without providing satisfactory solutions. One reason is that, in contrast to such benefits as food stamps, health care benefits are not very fungible. Food stamps are fungible for two reasons: essentially all households spend at least some money for food, so the receipt of food stamps frees up money income for consumption of other goods; also, the maximum food stamp allowance is low enough that it is unlikely households would receive more benefits than the amount they would otherwise choose to spend on food. Neither of these conditions holds for medical care benefits. First, not all households have medical care needs during the year. Second, although medical care benefits for, say, a low-cost prescription or for a doctor's visit may free up money income for other consumption, the "extra" benefits received from insurance (or free care) to cover, say, expensive surgery are not likely to free up money income commensurately. Hence, it is misleading to add medical care benefits to resources without also acknowledging the costs of medical care in the poverty budget. But the development of appropriate adjustments to the thresholds is a difficult task because of the great variation in health care needs across the population.

One proposal is to have a "two-index" poverty measure, in which people must satisfy two tests to be considered not poor: they must have adequate resources to obtain nonmedical necessities (e.g., food), *and* they must have adequate medical insurance coverage or sufficient resources with which to buy such coverage. Such an approach is appealing, but it poses considerable operational difficulties, for example, determining what is "adequate" health insurance coverage, in general, and for different groups. Also, the two components of the measure are not consistent, in that the medical component measures a risk (e.g., an expensive illness) that may or may not have materialized for a family or individual over the time span for which poverty is determined, while the nonmedical component measures the actual ability of the family or individual to obtain such universally required items as food.

Further complicating the whole issue is that, despite widespread medical care coverage, many people still face high out-of-pocket costs, such as the employee share of health insurance premiums, payments for deductibles, copayments, and payments for noncovered services. Very little consideration has been given to the appropriate treatment of such costs in a poverty measure. The original thresholds implicitly allowed for some out-of-pocket medical care expenditures in the multiplier, but not for the fact that such costs differ substantially by people's health status and other characteristics. Because the official thresholds do not reflect such differences, the poverty rate for some groups is underestimated, and for other groups it is overestimated.

We argue for an approach that separates the measurement of economic poverty from the measurement of medical care needs and the adequacy of resources to meet those needs. Hence, the proposed threshold concept includes such goods and services as food and housing but not medical care. For consistency, we do not propose to add the value of medical care benefits to income, and, further, we propose to subtract out-of-pocket medical care expenses from income. The result is a consistent measure of economic poverty.[19]

Although the proposed measure excludes medical care from both the poverty thresholds and family resources, it does not ignore the effect of changes in health care policy on economic poverty. Thus, the proposed measure will capture the effects of policy changes (e.g., extension of health insurance coverage) that reduce the need for out-of-pocket expenditures for medical care and thereby increase disposable income to spend on food, housing, and other goods and services. It will also capture the effects of policy changes (e.g., tax increases to pay for health insurance) that reduce disposable income. The proposed measure will not, however, directly assess the extent to which people have access to an adequate package of health insurance benefits that protects them against risk. Hence, we believe it would be highly desirable to publish regularly a "medically needy" index (more properly, an index of the risk of not being able to afford needed care) and to cross-tabulate it with the poverty measure. However, we do not believe such a medically needy index should be a part of the poverty measure because it would inordinately complicate the measure.

Finally, as changes are made to the U.S. system of health care, it will be important to reevaluate the treatment of medical care expenses in the definition of family resources. As an example, if relatively generous health insurance coverage is made available to everyone, the amount of out-of-pocket costs that is subtracted from income should likely be subject to an upper limit or cap.

RECOMMENDATION 4.3. **Appropriate agencies should work to develop one or more "medical care risk" indexes that measure the economic risk to families and individuals of having no or inadequate health insurance coverage. However, such indexes should be kept separate from the measure of economic poverty.**

Taxes

The appropriate definition of family resources for comparison with a poverty threshold that does not include income or payroll taxes is an after-tax definition. Income and payroll tax dollars are assuredly not available for consumption. Also, it is misleading for the poverty measure not to reflect changes in tax laws when such changes affect the amount of disposable income that is available for consumption. The alternative would be to include taxes in the

---

[19] Canada and Western European countries do not take account of medical care benefits in their poverty measures. Because they have some type of national health insurance, they treat medical care benefits as they do public education or the police force, namely, as government services that are universally available and whose effects would simply cancel out in a poverty measure (i.e., a benefit would be added to resources that matched whatever expenditure might be deemed "necessary" in the poverty budget).

poverty thresholds, but this approach would unnecessarily complicate them: for example, at a minimum, there would have to be different thresholds for workers and nonworkers. The Census Bureau has considerable experience with developing after-tax estimates of income so that subtracting income taxes and payroll taxes from gross family income for calculating poverty rates will not be difficult. Sales and property taxes do not need to be subtracted since they are included in the CEX expenditure data and hence accounted for in the poverty thresholds.

Work-Related Expenses

To earn money from a job almost always requires a worker to use some of that money on work expenses. Just as income used for taxes is not available for consumption, neither is the amount of earnings devoted to work expenses; hence, such expenses should not be counted as family resources. Specifically, child care costs that are necessary for a parent to hold down a job should be deducted from earnings, as should an allowance for other work-related expenses (e.g., commuting costs).

We propose that actual child care expenses be deducted per week worked for families in which there is no nonworking parent, up to the earnings of the parent with the lower earnings or a cap that is adjusted annually for inflation (whichever value is lower). The cap could initially be based on the maximum employment-related child care expenses—$2,400 for one child and $4,800 for two or more children—that are allowed in computing the federal dependent care income tax credit.

Alternatively, the cap could be developed as a percentage of median child care expenditures by families with one or two or more children, similar to the proposal for developing the food, clothing, and shelter component of the poverty threshold. In the 1990 SIPP, the annualized value of median weekly expenditures (in 1992 dollars) for families who paid for child care was about $2,300 for families with one child and $2,700 for families with two or more children. The issue of an appropriate cap is complicated by the age of a family's children: a more generous cap seems appropriate for pre-school-aged children than for older children. Indeed, the relatively low median child care expenses by families with two or more children relative to families with one child, as measured in SIPP, is undoubtedly because more families in the former group have older children.

In the case of other work-related expenses, such as commuting, we propose that a flat allowance per week worked, updated annually for inflation, be deducted from the earnings of each adult worker in the family. The reason to deduct a flat amount, rather than actual expenses, is because of the tradeoff that people often make between housing and commuting costs, by choosing a more expensive home closer to work or a less expensive one farther away. As each family in an area will have the same adjustment to the poverty threshold for housing costs, so each worker needs to have the same work expense deduction.

For a family with child care expenses, the total of child care costs plus other work-related expenses for the parent with the lower earnings should not exceed that parent's earnings. The amount of the flat deduction for other work-related expenses could be developed as a percentage of the median. Data from the 1987 SIPP indicate that median weekly expenditures of adult workers for commuting and other work expenses (e.g., tools and uniforms) are about $17.00 (in 1992 dollars).

Instead of deducting child care and other work-related expenses from earnings, an alternative approach would be to include them in the poverty budget. However, this approach would require separate thresholds for working families with and without children and by number of earners, as well as for nonworking families.

Child Support Payments

The argument for excluding child support payments from the family income of the payer is the same argument of consistency that we have made throughout this discussion. At present, child support payments are counted as part of gross money income of the families that receive them, which is appropriate, because the payments are available for consumption by these families. However, the amounts are not deducted from the income of the families that pay them, which is inappropriate, because the payments are not available for consumption by those families. Thus, we propose that child support payments be deducted from the income of families that pay them.

Services from Home Ownership

Estimates of families' economic resources, to be comparable for renters and homeowners, should take account of the flow of services that owners obtain from their homes. Thus, people with low or no mortgage payments or other ownership costs do not face the same housing costs as renters or other homeowners and so should have a rental equivalence value (a type of in-kind benefit) added to their income. Alternatively, one could lower the threshold for such families to recognize that they do not have the same budgetary requirements for shelter as other families. However, it does not seem feasible with available data to develop adequate rental imputations. Hence, valuation of home ownership services is a priority area for further research and consideration for implementation in the poverty measure at a later date.

Assets

Some researchers have argued that families' asset holdings should be considered in some way in determining their poverty status. Financial assets, such as savings accounts and stocks, can often be converted to cash to tide families over a period of low income. Property assets (e.g., houses, land, cars, household furnishings) can also be converted to cash, although often not as readily. Assistance programs such as AFDC and food stamps allow families to have their own home, furnishings, and a cheap car, but otherwise place a low limit on the assets they can hold and still be eligible for benefits. The reason for the asset limit is the programs' short accounting periods: they allow families to qualify for benefits on the basis of having low income for a period as short as 1 or 2 months, provided that the families have few or no financial assets on which they can draw.

For purposes of poverty measurement, however, for which the accounting period is a year, it does not seem sensible to add asset values to nonasset income. In most cases, asset values will only raise income-poor people above the poverty line for short periods, after which they are still poor. It is more appropriate, instead, to define resources as disposable income from all sources, including any income from assets, such as interest or rents (although very few income-poor people have financial assets in any case; see Chapter 4). However, we recognize that for some purposes it may be desirable to have companion measures that take account of some types of assets. Thus, measures for shorter periods (e.g., 4 months) may be more useful than annual measures to evaluate how effectively assistance programs with short accounting periods target benefits to needy people. For consistency with program rules, short-term poverty measures will need to include financial asset values.

Effects

What difference would it make to poverty statistics to adopt the proposed measure in place of the current measure? Developing a few concrete examples of prototypical families and their poverty status under the two measures can help illustrate the differences between them. Figure 1-3 shows four examples of single-parent families with two children who, under our proposal, have different poverty thresholds—relative to the official threshold—depending on where they live. These examples are somewhat contrived, but they illustrate the potential effects of adopting the proposed measure for families with different sources of income in different areas of the country.

The family on welfare in a big New England city, Case 1, is poor under the current measure and is also poor under the proposed measure: adding the value of in-kind benefits to the family's cash welfare income does not raise that income above either the official threshold or the adjusted threshold (which is higher due to the cost of housing). In contrast, the family on welfare in a rural area of the upper Midwest, Case 2, is poor under the current measure but is not poor under the proposed measure: in this case, adding the value of in-

CASE 1: Three-person family in big New England city

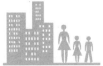

Official threshold:	$11,304
Revised threshold:	$13,522

Gross regular money income: $ 6,662—from AFDC; maximum benefit
Disposable income: $ 9,583—from AFDC; food stamps, school lunch and breakfast

Poverty status, current: Poor
Poverty status, proposed: Poor

CASE 2: Three-person family in rural area of upper Midwest

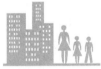

Official threshold:	$11,304
Revised threshold:	$ 9,322

Gross regular money income: $ 6,390—from AFDC; maximum benefit
Disposable income: $ 9,385—from AFDC; food stamps, school lunch and breakfast

Poverty status, current: Poor
Poverty status, proposed: Not poor

CASE 3: Three-person family in big New England city

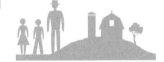

Official threshold:	$11,304
Revised threshold:	$13,522

Gross regular money income: $13,000—wages from full-time job paying $6.50 per hour
Disposable income: $ 9,798—wages plus EITC minus payroll taxes, child care, work expenses, out-of-pocket medical expenses

Poverty status, current: Not poor
Poverty status, proposed: Poor

CASE 4: Three-person family in rural area of upper Midwest

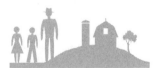

Official threshold:	$11,304
Revised threshold:	$ 9,322

Gross regular money income: $10,000—wages from full-time job paying $5.00 per hour
Disposable income: $ 7,969—wages plus EITC minus payroll taxes, child care, work expenses, out-of-pocket medical expenses

Poverty status, current: Poor
Poverty status, proposed: Poor

FIGURE 1-3 Poverty status of hypothetical three-person (one-adult/two-child) families under current and proposed poverty measures, 1992. NOTE: Revised thresholds are based on the 0.75 scale economy factor and the relevant housing cost adjustment factor.

kind benefits raises the family's income above the adjusted poverty threshold (which is lower than the official threshold because of the housing cost adjustment).

The family with a working parent in a big New England city, Case 3, is not poor under the current measure but is poor under the proposed measure: subtracting such expenses as child care reduces the family's income below both the official threshold and the adjusted threshold. In contrast, the family in the rural upper Midwest, with a parent who works at a lower pay rate, Case 4, is poor under both the current measure and the proposed measure.

We also conducted an extensive analysis with the March 1993 Current Population Survey data files of poverty rates under the current measure and the proposed measure (see Chapter 5). To implement the proposed family resource definition with the March 1993 CPS, we performed imputations for such components as child care and out-of-pocket medical care expenses by using data from SIPP and the National Medical Expenditure Survey. We were able to take advantage of the Census Bureau's research and development program for other components, such as income and payroll taxes and non-medical in-kind benefits.[20] Although our data adjustments and imputations are not without problems, we believe the comparisons we obtained between gross money income and disposable money and near-money income for 1992 are reasonably accurate.[21]

Distributional Effects

We carried out one set of comparisons to illustrate the effects of the current and proposed measures on the characteristics of people who are poor, holding constant the poverty rate for the total population. For this exercise, we determined the two-adult/two-child family threshold that, together with the proposed threshold adjustments (including the use of a 0.75 scale economy factor) and the proposed family resource definition, gave the same 1992 poverty rate as the official rate, 14.5 percent. The total number of poor people was about the same as the official number of 36.9 million. (The official reference family threshold for 1992 was $14,228; the threshold that gave the same result with the proposed measure turned out to be $13,175, a number that is purely an artifact of the analysis.)

In this exercise, the proposed measure produces about the same number

---

[20] The only income component that we did not implement was an adjustment for child support payments. The March CPS lacks any information with which to determine who would most likely make such payments; this lack could be easily remedied by adding a question to the survey.

[21] We are grateful for the help we received from many agencies in obtaining the data with which to implement our proposed family resource definition with the March CPS (see Acknowledgments).

of poor people as the current measure, but they are not all the same people. Under the proposed measure, 7.4 million people are moved out of poverty, and 7.4 million are moved into poverty. That is, the proposed measure has significant effects on the composition of the poor population, changing about 20 percent of that population. Table 1-6 shows these changes for groups categorized by age, race, ethnicity, receipt of cash welfare, work status, health insurance status, and region of residence. This table also shows the poverty *rates* for each group under the current and proposed measures.

The greatest effect of the proposed measure is to decrease the percentage

TABLE 1-6 Poverty Statistics, 1992: Current Measure and Proposed Measure, Keeping the Overall Poverty Rate Constant

Population Group	Percent of Total Population	Percent of Poor Population		Poverty Rate for Population Group (%)	
		Current Measure	Proposed Measure	Current Measure	Proposed Measure
Age					
Children under 18	26.3	39.6	39.2	21.9	21.7
Adults 18–64	61.5	49.6	51.8	11.7	12.2
Adults 65 and older	12.2	10.8	9.0	12.9	10.8
Race					
White	83.6	66.8	69.3	11.6	12.0
Black	12.5	28.6	25.7	33.2	29.8
Other	3.9	4.6	5.1	17.4	19.1
Ethnicity					
Hispanic	8.9	18.1	20.9	29.4	34.0
Non-Hispanic	91.1	81.9	79.1	13.1	12.6
Welfare Status of Family					
Receiving cash welfare	9.9	40.4	29.9	59.4	44.0
Not receiving welfare	90.1	59.6	70.1	9.6	11.3
Work Status of Family					
One or more workers	81.1	50.8	58.9	9.1	10.6
No workers	18.9	49.2	41.1	37.9	31.7
Health Insurance Status of Family					
No health insurance	13.7	30.1	35.7	32.0	37.9
Some health insurance	86.3	69.9	64.3	11.8	10.8
Region of Residence					
Northeast	20.0	16.9	18.9	12.3	13.8
Midwest	24.0	21.7	20.2	13.1	12.2
South	34.4	40.0	36.4	16.9	15.4
West	21.6	21.4	24.5	14.4	16.5

NOTE: In the first, second, and third columns, the percentages for the categories within each characteristic (age, race, etc.) add to 100; in the last two columns, the percentages (rates) apply to each category individually. See text for thresholds used.

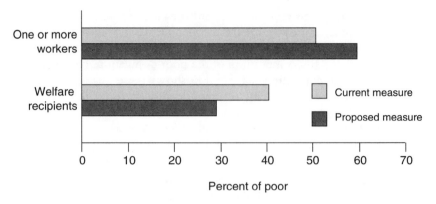

FIGURE 1-4 Effects of the proposed measure on the percentage of poor people in working families and families receiving cash welfare.

of poor people who are in families receiving cash welfare, AFDC and Supplemental Security Income (SSI), and to increase the percentage who are in working families; Figure 1-4.[22] Largely because of the additions to income of the value of in-kind benefits, people in families receiving cash welfare account for just 30 percent of poor people under the proposed measure, compared with 40 percent under the current measure. In contrast, largely because of deductions from income of taxes, work expenses, and out-of-pocket medical care expenses, people in families with one or more earners account for 59 percent of poor people under the proposed measure, compared with 51 percent under the current measure. People in families receiving cash welfare still have a much higher poverty rate than the people in working families, but the difference is not as large under the proposed measure: the poverty rate for people in welfare families is 44 percent under the proposed measure and 59 percent under the current measure; the rate for people in working families is 11 percent under the proposed measure and 9 percent under the current measure.

Another effect of the proposed measure is to increase the poverty rate for people in families lacking health insurance coverage. They make up 36 percent of the poor under the proposed measure, compared with 30 percent under the current measure.

By age, children make up about the same percentage of poor people (39–40%) and have about the same, higher-than-average poverty rate (22%) under both the current and the proposed measures—because poor children live both in families receiving cash welfare and in families with one or more earners.

---

[22] Families receiving cash welfare and those with one or more earners overlap to some extent; people not in either group include some retirees, students, and others.

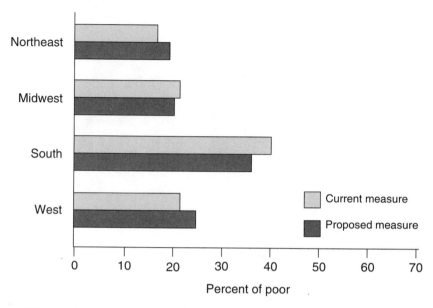

FIGURE 1-5 Effects of the proposed poverty measure on the geographic distribution of poor people.

However, the poverty rate for the elderly and their share of the poverty population are somewhat lower under the proposed measure, compared with the current measure, while the poverty rate for working-age adults and their share of poor people are somewhat higher.

By region of the country, the poverty rates for residents of the Northeast and West are higher, and they make up larger percentages of poor people under the proposed measure, compared with the current measure. In contrast, the poverty rates for residents of the South and Midwest are lower, and they make up smaller percentages of poor people under the proposed measure; see Figure 1-5. These shifts occur because of adjustments to the thresholds for geographic differences in the cost of housing.[23]

Effects of Selected Components

We next considered the effects of specific components of the proposed measure on the overall poverty rate of 14.5 percent; see Figure 1-6. Adjusting the thresholds for geographic differences in the cost of housing, while having significant distributional effects, has little effect on the poverty rate for the total population. However, the use of a scale economy factor of 0.75 for determin-

---

[23] For the areas and states included in each region, see Table 1-5, above.

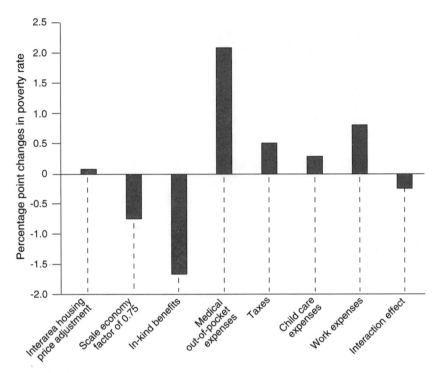

FIGURE 1-6 Effects of selected components of the proposed measure on the poverty rate. NOTE: The official poverty rate in 1992 was 14.5 percent; see text for a discussion of the interaction effect.

ing equivalent thresholds for other family types decreases the rate somewhat (by 0.7 of a percentage point).

The addition to income of nonmedical in-kind benefits (e.g., food stamps) has a sizable effect, decreasing the rate by 1.7 percentage points. The subtraction of out-of-pocket medical care expenditures increases the rate by 2.1 percentage points. The subtraction of taxes, work expenses, and child care expenses increases the rate by 0.5, 0.8, and 0.3 of a percentage point, respectively.[24] In addition, there is an interaction effect that decreases the rate by 0.2 of a percentage point: this effect occurs because a combination of changes may move a family above (or below) the poverty line when a single change does not.[25]

---

[24] From tabulations with SIPP, we estimate that the subtraction of child support payments would also increase the poverty rate by a small fraction of a percentage point.

[25] The interaction effect would be positive if our analysis did not use a reference family threshold of $13,175 in order to maintain the official 1992 poverty rate of 14.5 percent; this threshold value reduces the overall poverty rate by 1.2 percentage points.

Effects on the Poverty Rate

We carried out another set of comparisons to illustrate the effects on the overall poverty rate of raising the poverty threshold in real terms, as well as implementing the recommended adjustments to the threshold and family resource definition. For this exercise, we used a two-adult/two-child family threshold of $14,800, representing the midpoint of our suggested range for that threshold of $13,700 to $15,900.

Under the proposed measure—with a $14,800 reference family threshold and a 0.75 scale economy factor—46.0 million people would have been classified as poor in 1992, for a poverty rate of 18.1 percent, compared with the official count of 36.9 million and the official poverty rate of 14.5 percent. Figure 1-7 shows the effects for both a 0.75 and a 0.65 scale economy factor,

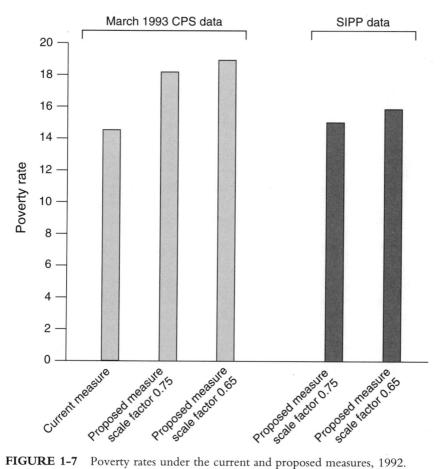

FIGURE 1-7 Poverty rates under the current and proposed measures, 1992.

using both CPS and SIPP data.[26] The reason for the lower rates with SIPP data is that SIPP achieves more complete income reporting for lower income people.[27]

A higher reference family threshold explains part of the increase in the poverty rate, but the proposed changes to the resource definition (including the interaction of such changes as subtracting taxes and work expenses) account for the larger portion of the increase. Although the use of a $14,800 reference family threshold and the proposed changes to the resource definition increase the number of poor, not all of the movement is in the same direction. For example, with a 0.75 scale economy factor, 4.2 million people are moved out of poverty, and 13.3 million people are moved into poverty.

Time Trends

It is clear that the proposed poverty measure has important distributional and cross-sectional effects on estimates of poverty. What is less clear is the effect on time trends. We attempted to conduct the same kinds of analyses summarized above for 1992 with the March 1990, 1984, and 1980 CPS files, using the official thresholds for 1989, 1983, and 1979 and thresholds developed under the proposed concept for earlier years. However, we were not able to develop adequate imputations for 1979 or 1983 for such important components of the proposed resource definition as out-of-pocket medical care expenditures. Hence, the time-series results we obtained are not strictly comparable with our cross-sectional analyses for 1992. The results do show, however, the effects with the proposed poverty measure of changes in tax laws and changes in the provision of in-kind benefits, such as the curtailment of eligibility and benefits in the early 1980s—effects that are not evident with the current measure. (Both measures show the effects of changes in the business cycle over the 1980s.)

In looking to the future, it is likely that trends under the proposed measure will diverge from trends under the current measure. Certainly, the proposed measure will provide a more accurate picture of the effects of important government policy initiatives. For example, changes in the health care financing system that affect out-of-pocket medical care costs or changes in tax provisions that affect disposable income would be reflected in the proposed measure; they cannot affect the poverty rate under the current measure. We estimated the effects of the expansion of the Earned Income

---

[26] The estimate for SIPP is based on the average difference of 3.2 percentage points between the overall poverty rates from SIPP and the March CPS for the period 1984-1991 (see Chapter 5). We could not use SIPP for our analysis because the Census Bureau had not yet completed work on procedures to estimate taxes and value in-kind benefits for this survey; however, we did use SIPP for some of our imputations to the March CPS.

[27] See Chapter 5 on the reason for higher poverty rates with a 0.65 scale economy factor.

Tax Credit that is scheduled to take full effect in 1996: adjusted to 1992, the result would be to reduce the poverty rate under the proposed measure from 18.1 to 17.2 percent (using a $14,800 reference family threshold and 0.75 scale economy factor).

The proposed measure will also more accurately reflect the effects of any welfare reform that puts a time limit on the receipt of benefits and thereafter requires recipients to work. If the jobs obtained by former welfare recipients include child care and health insurance benefits, the proposed measure would likely show a different poverty rate than if the jobs do not provide such benefits; the current measure would not distinguish between those situations.

Needed Data

Clearly, the availability of relevant, high-quality, and timely data is critical for determining the poverty rate, in order to estimate resources for a representative sample of families and individuals to compare with the appropriate poverty thresholds. The survey that has supplied the United States with its income and poverty statistics is the March income supplement to the CPS. The March CPS has served the nation well, but it is inherently limited in the extent and quality of data that it can provide because it is a supplement to a continuing survey of the labor force that is the basis of the official monthly unemployment rate. Its major focus is on unemployment, not poverty.

The March CPS currently obtains information on a family's previous year's income from a large number of sources, and it also asks about receipt of benefits from the major in-kind programs. However, it does not ask about taxes, medical care costs, child support, work expenses, or assets. It also does not provide information for constructing poverty measures for periods other than a calendar year.

To remedy these deficiencies in the March CPS and to improve the quality of income reporting, SIPP was begun in 1983. Although SIPP had start-up problems, including cuts in sample size, it has largely achieved the goal of providing a richer set of higher quality data on income and related topics than the March CPS. One of the criticisms of using income rather than actual expenditures as the measure of resources is that income reporting errors in surveys lead to an overestimate of the poverty rate. However, poverty estimates calculated from SIPP, with more complete income reporting for lower income families than in the March CPS, are comparable to estimates developed from the CEX that use a consumption or expenditure concept of resources (see Chapter 5). Also, a number of improvements will be made to SIPP, beginning in 1996—including an expansion of the overall sample to about that of the March CPS—that will further strengthen it.

The proposed changes to the family resource definition, and continued research on various aspects of the resource definition (e.g., valuation of home ownership services), will increase the data needed for measuring poverty. SIPP, with its focus on income data, is in a position to respond to these needs; the March CPS, which must always be geared primarily to the requirements of the nation's main labor force survey, is not. Hence, we recommend that SIPP become the basis of the nation's official income and poverty statistics in place of the March CPS. This change should take effect when the slated improvements to SIPP are introduced in 1996.

A decision to use SIPP to produce the official poverty rates means that the SIPP design and questionnaire must be reviewed to determine if modifications are needed to enhance the survey's ability to provide accurate statistics under the proposed measure. (A panel that recently evaluated SIPP made a similar recommendation about using SIPP for income and poverty statistics [Citro and Kalton, 1993:85-87], and many of its recommendations on the SIPP design and questionnaire are relevant.)

In regard to the overall SIPP design, we are concerned that the Census Bureau's decision for 1996 to have new samples ("panels") introduced every 4 years, each of which is followed for a 4-year period, may be problematic for providing a reliable time series of annual poverty statistics because of biases that result from attrition from the samples over time. Every 4 years there may be a break in the time series because of the introduction of a new sample; in addition, because there is no overlap between the samples, it will be difficult to evaluate whether the changes in the poverty rate are real or not.

Such a nonoverlapping design also limits the usefulness of SIPP to analyze important policy changes, such as changes in welfare programs or health care financing: if policy changes take effect near the beginning or end of a 4-year sample, there is limited information available either before or after the change to adequately evaluate its effects. The SIPP evaluation panel recommended that SIPP samples be followed for 4 years but that a new sample be introduced every 2 years. Poverty rates under this design may also be affected by attrition and other biases, but, with the sample overlap, it will be possible to evaluate and, one hopes, adjust for the effects. Also, under this design, a new sample is in the field every 2 years, which should facilitate analysis of policy changes.[28]

It is important to carry out methodological research that can lead to yet further improvements in SIPP data quality for purposes of poverty measurement. A high priority is research to improve the population coverage in SIPP (and other household surveys), especially among lower income minority groups, particularly young black men (the Census Bureau has such research

---

[28] The disadvantage for longitudinal analysis of the overlap design recommended by the SIPP panel is that the sample size is half that of the design of 4-year samples with no overlap; however, for the estimation of annual poverty statistics, the total sample size of the overlap design, added across the two samples in the field each year, is the same as that of the nonoverlap design.

under way). These groups are missed at high rates in surveys relative to estimates derived from the decennial census because they are not reported as household residents. We note, however, that SIPP (and other household surveys) will necessarily overlook some population groups who may be particularly at risk of poverty, including the homeless and people in institutions. The decennial population census (see below) includes these groups, although coverage is far from complete.

> RECOMMENDATION 5.1. **The Survey of Income and Program Participation should become the basis of official U.S. income and poverty statistics in place of the March income supplement to the Current Population Survey. Decisions about the SIPP design and questionnaire should take account of the data requirements for producing reliable time series of poverty statistics using the proposed definition of family resources (money and near-money income minus certain expenditures). Priority should be accorded to methodological research for SIPP that is relevant for improved poverty measurement. A particularly important problem to address is population undercoverage, particularly of low-income minority groups.**

To aid in making the transition to a SIPP-based series of official poverty statistics and to help evaluate that new series, it would be helpful for the Census Bureau to produce a concurrent time series of poverty rates from the March CPS on the basis of the proposed measure. Both the SIPP and the March CPS series should be extended backward to 1984, when SIPP was first introduced. Also for the foreseeable future, the Census Bureau should issue public-use files from both SIPP and the March CPS that include values for the thresholds under the new concept and estimates of disposable income (and its components) under the new resource definition. The availability of such files will enable researchers to conduct poverty analyses with either survey.

> RECOMMENDATION 5.2. **To facilitate the transition to SIPP, the Census Bureau should produce concurrent time series of poverty rates from both SIPP and the March CPS by using the proposed revised threshold concept and updating procedure and the proposed definition of family resources as disposable income. The concurrent series should be developed starting with 1984, when SIPP was first introduced.**

> RECOMMENDATION 5.3. **The Census Bureau should routinely issue public-use files from both SIPP and the March CPS that include the Bureau's best estimate of disposable income and its components (taxes, in-kind benefits, child care expenses, etc.) so that researchers can obtain poverty rates consistent with the new threshold concept from either survey.**

Many other federally sponsored surveys besides SIPP and the March CPS provide income and poverty variables for analysis purposes: examples include the American Housing Survey, Consumer Expenditure Survey, National Health Interview Survey, National Medical Expenditure Survey. However, these surveys, which are focused on other topics, cannot usually afford the questionnaire space needed to collect all of the information needed for an accurate estimate of disposable money and near-money income. Research on the most appropriate set of income questions to include in such surveys would be useful. With limited space, it may be preferable to ask questions about expenses that need to be deducted from gross income, rather than to ask detailed questions about the sources of that income. Even more important is research on methods to develop poverty estimates from limited income information that approximate the estimates that would be obtained under a disposable income definition from a detailed survey like SIPP.

> **RECOMMENDATION 5.4. Appropriate agencies should conduct research on methods to develop poverty estimates from household surveys with limited income information that are comparable to the estimates that would be obtained from a fully implemented disposable income definition of family resources.**

Another source of income and poverty statistics is the U.S. decennial census. It provides data every 10 years for small geographic areas for which reliable estimates cannot be obtained in household surveys. Small-area poverty estimates serve many important purposes, for example, to allocate federal funds to local school districts. Questionnaire space in the decennial census is even more limited than in most surveys: the 1990 census asked about 8 types of income, compared with more than 30 in the March CPS and more than 50 in SIPP. No information was obtained about taxes, in-kind benefits, medical costs, child support, work expenses, or assets. We encourage research on methods to adjust census small-area poverty estimates to more closely approximate the estimates that would result from using our proposed family resource definition. Also, while recognizing the constraints on the census questionnaire, we urge serious consideration of adding perhaps one or two simple yes-no questions—for example, whether a family received food stamps or paid for child care in the past year—that would facilitate such adjustments.

> **RECOMMENDATION 5.5. Appropriate agencies should conduct research on methods to construct small-area poverty estimates from the limited information in the decennial census that are comparable with the estimates that would be obtained under a fully implemented disposable income concept. In addition, serious consideration should be given to adding one or two questions to the decennial census to assist in the development of comparable estimates.**

Finally, with regard to data sources, we believe it is vitally important to improve the available data on consumer expenditures, an area in which the United States lags behind other developed countries. Our evaluation of alternative methods for updating poverty thresholds was hampered by the fact that the United States did not have a continuing consumer expenditure survey until 1980. Moreover, small sample sizes in the present CEX impair its usefulness for developing poverty budgets and completely preclude its use for measuring family resources. The CEX also has data quality problems, such as high nonresponse rates by sample households, high rates of recall error, and underreporting of expenditures and income. We urge BLS to conduct (or commission) a study that evaluates the CEX and assesses the costs and benefits of changes to the survey that could make it more useful for poverty measurement and for other important analytical uses related to the understanding of consumption, income, and saving. It would be especially useful if improvements to the survey could be made in time for the next 10-year review of the poverty measure.

> RECOMMENDATION 5.6. **The Bureau of Labor Statistics should undertake a comprehensive review of the Consumer Expenditure Survey to assess the costs and benefits of changes to the survey design, questionnaire, sample size, and other features that could improve the quality and usefulness of the data. The review should consider ways to improve the CEX for the purpose of developing poverty thresholds, for making it possible at a future date to measure poverty on the basis of a consumption or expenditure concept of family resources, and for other analytic purposes related to the measurement of consumption, income, and savings.**

Other Issues in Poverty Measurement

Time Period

The current measure of poverty compares family income for a year with a budget that reflects a year's worth of expenditures. This annual accounting period is very familiar to policy makers and the public and is quite appropriate for evaluating the effect on poverty of provisions of the tax code (e.g., the Earned Income Tax Credit) and programs that are designed to provide long-term income support (e.g., Social Security and SSI for the elderly and disabled). We believe it makes sense for the official measure to continue to use an annual accounting period.

In addition to the official measure, however, there are needs for supplementary poverty measures with shorter and longer accounting periods than a year. Many assistance programs (e.g., AFDC and food stamps) provide benefits to people who are experiencing short spells of poverty. The use of an annual poverty measure for evaluating these programs may be misleading: an annual measure may suggest that the programs are providing benefits to people above the poverty line when, in fact, those people were poor for part of a year and hence eligible for support. An appropriate poverty measure for evaluating such programs also needs to take account of assets because of the requirement that families use up most of their accumulated assets before they can obtain program benefits.

SIPP provides data to construct subannual poverty measures that would be suitable for evaluating the effects of such programs as AFDC and food stamps. Given some of the features of the SIPP design, we suggest that a feasible measure might use a 4-month accounting period and add to income any financial assets that the family reports, such as savings accounts (after first subtracting the income from such assets). These 4-month measures might also serve as an indicator of short-term increases or decreases in economic distress, although it may be that other readily available data, such as monthly food stamp caseloads, could serve this purpose.

There are also important uses for measures that assess poverty over multi-year periods. There is strong evidence that people who experience long spells of poverty are worse off—not only economically, but also in other respects such as health status and educational attainment—than those who experience short spells. Also, long-term poverty appears concentrated in particular groups of the population, particularly minorities and the disabled. Policies and programs for ameliorating long-term poverty are likely to differ from those aimed at helping people through a temporary economic crisis.

There is no agreement on the basis of research on the best form of a long-term poverty measure. It is also not clear how often a long-term poverty measure needs to be updated. The design of SIPP makes it possible to develop estimates of the number of poor in a given year who are still poor 1, 2, and 3 years later. The Panel Study of Income Dynamics permits developing poverty measures for much longer periods, but with small sample sizes. Clearly, further research and the development of some experimental series would be useful.

> **RECOMMENDATION 6.1. The official poverty measure should continue to be derived on an annual basis. Appropriate agencies should develop poverty measures for periods that are shorter and longer than a year, with data from SIPP and the Panel Study of Income Dynamics, for such purposes as program evaluation. Such measures may require the inclusion of asset values in the family resource definition.**

Unit of Analysis

The current poverty measure defines thresholds and aggregates resources for families of various sizes and for adults who live alone or with other people not related to them.[29] In other words, the assumption is made that family members pool their resources to support consumption and thereby achieve economies of scale. Unrelated individuals, in contrast, are assumed not to share resources with others, even if they live with one or more roommates.

Although some researchers have criticized the assumption that all family members have access to their "fair share" of the family's resources, data limitations make it infeasible at this time to consider defining the unit of analysis for poverty measurement as an individual, so we recommend continuing to use the family as the unit of analysis. We also recommend that the definition of "family" be broadened to include cohabiting couples, as they maintain longer lasting relationships than other roommates and are likely to pool resources. In the case of roommates as such, there are no data on the extent of resource sharing among them. We encourage research on this topic, and more generally on resource sharing among household and family members.

> RECOMMENDATION 6.2. **The official measure of poverty should continue to use families and unrelated individuals as the units of analysis for which thresholds are defined and resources aggregated. The definition of "family" should be broadened for purposes of poverty measurement to include cohabiting couples.**

> RECOMMENDATION 6.3. **Appropriate agencies should conduct research on the extent of resource sharing among roommates and other household and family members to determine if the definition of the unit of analysis for the poverty measure should be modified in the future.**

Other Measures

Considerable thought has been given in the research literature to the development of poverty statistics that provide more information than the simple head-count ratio (the poverty rate or proportion of people who are poor). Thus, it would be useful to have a statistic that reflects the depth of poverty, by measuring, for example, the average income of the poor. It would also be useful to have a poverty statistic that increases when resources are less equally distributed among the poor.

The simple head-count ratio—although readily understandable—has some drawbacks. For example, if income were taken from some very poor people to move a few less-poor persons out of poverty, the effect would be to *reduce* the head count, even though the depth of poverty had become worse. Yet statistics that attempt to capture several dimensions of poverty in a single index

---

[29] Poverty is not defined for unrelated individuals under age 15, as no information is obtained about their income in surveys.

very quickly become impenetrable, with the result that it is hard to interpret what changes in them mean to policy makers and the public (and even to researchers).

We see the need for additional information besides the head-count ratio, but we believe it is best to provide such information in simpler, more disaggregated form, as is already done to a large extent in Census Bureau reports. These reports show the poverty gap, or the aggregate amount of income by which poor people fall below the poverty line, and it would be easy to provide the obverse, namely, the average income of the poor compared with an average weighted poverty threshold. (Because there are different thresholds for different types of families, statistics on the average income of the poor need to be calculated for each type separately or by comparing the average income for all poor people to an average weighted threshold that reflects the composition of the poor by family type.) Census Bureau reports also provide information on the proportions of people with income below varying ratios of the poverty line (e.g., below 50%, 75%, 100%, 125%), thereby indicating the distribution of poverty among the poor and, in the case of ratios of income that exceed the poverty line, the extent of near poverty.

These indicators must be interpreted carefully: for example, the poverty gap is not an actual measure of the amount of money that the government would have to spend to eliminate poverty (see below). Also, the number of people who are very far below the poverty line may be overestimated because of underreporting of income or the reporting of business losses by self-employed people. Nonetheless, such indicators can enrich understanding of the nature and scope of economic poverty in the United States and how it changes over time.

We also believe it would be useful to publish poverty statistics on the basis of measures in which family resources are defined net of government taxes and transfers. Several such measures could be useful: one in which resources are defined in before-tax terms, one in which resources are net of taxes but exclude benefits from means-tested government programs (whether cash or in-kind), and one in which resources exclude benefits from all government programs, whether means tested or not. Again, the statistics from such measures must be interpreted with care: the poverty rate in a world without government taxes or government assistance programs would likely differ from the rate under these measures. Nonetheless, when compared with the new official measure, such before-tax and transfer measures would be helpful for evaluating the effects of government policies and programs on poverty.

> **RECOMMENDATION 6.4. In addition to the basic poverty counts and ratios for the total population and groups—the number and proportion of poor people—the official poverty series should provide statistics on the average income and distribution of income for the poor. The count and other statistics should also be published for poverty**

measures in which family resources are defined net of government taxes and transfers, such as a measure that defines income in before-tax terms, a measure that excludes means-tested government benefits from income, and a measure that excludes all government benefits from income. Such measures can help assess the effects of government taxes and transfers on poverty.

Finally, we note the importance of having indicators of deprivation other than economic—physical, psychological, and social deprivation. A measure of economic poverty is undoubtedly a key social indicator. It is important in its own right as a barometer of the extent to which there is a segment of U.S. society that lacks the means to obtain basic economic necessities; it is also important because it correlates highly with other aspects of deprivation, such as poor health and low educational levels. But an economic poverty measure cannot feasibly encompass other types of deprivation. Instead, other measures need to be developed to directly assess the well-being of the population on a number of dimensions and to help focus public- and private-sector policies to ameliorate deprivation. We encourage research and development on a range of deprivation indicators.

USE OF THE POVERTY MEASURE IN GOVERNMENT PROGRAMS

The current official poverty measure plays a role in determining eligibility for a number of government assistance programs, and it is important to consider how or if the proposed measure is appropriate for program use.[30] We first examine the implications of linking the proposed measure to program eligibility. We then look at the relationship of the proposed measure to benefit standards for the AFDC program, for which we were asked to consider issues involved in establishing a national minimum benefit standard.[31]

The Poverty Measure and Program Eligibility

Need Standards for Programs That Use the Official Measure

Of 70 federal and federal-state programs that provide cash or in-kind benefits to people on the basis of an explicit test of low income, 27 programs link their need standard for eligibility to the U.S. Department of Health and Human

---

[30] The descriptions of programs and program eligibility standards are as of the time when this report was prepared; they do not reflect any changes after 1994.

[31] Another program use of the poverty measure is for allocation of federal funds to states and localities through formulas: for example, the allocation of funds for educationally deprived children to school districts on the basis of their share of children age 5 to 17 who live in poor families. This use of the poverty measure raises important issues, including that of data availability, but is beyond the scope of this report.

Services (HHS) poverty guidelines, which are derived from the official poverty thresholds. Examples include food stamps, Head Start, Legal Services, Maternal and Child Health Services, Medicaid, and the School Lunch and Breakfast Programs (Burke, 1993). Some programs (e.g., food stamps, Medicaid) have several criteria for eligibility: applicants who are already participating in another program, such as AFDC, may be automatically eligible, while other applicants can qualify on the basis of comparing their income to the poverty guidelines (or a multiple of them).

The use of the proposed poverty measure in these programs would be an improvement in several respects over the current measure for the purpose of targeting benefits to needy families. The proposed measure has an internally consistent equivalence scale by which to adjust the poverty thresholds for different types of families, it reflects geographic differences in the cost of housing in the thresholds, and its definition of family resources as disposable money and near-money income is consistent with the basic needs concept underlying the thresholds. This consistency means that two families with the same gross income would not be mistakenly treated as having the same income for consumption when one of them had nondiscretionary expenses (such as taxes or child support payments) and the other did not.

However, program agencies should carefully consider whether the proposed measure may need to be modified to better serve program objectives. For example, the proposed family resource definition is considerably more data intensive than the current definition. Full implementation would require asking about in-kind benefits and several types of expenses, as well as money income. For such programs as food stamps that require a very detailed determination of both gross and net or "countable" income in order to determine financial eligibility and benefit amounts, implementing the proposed definition of family resources would not complicate program administration—indeed, that definition, in concept, if not in precise details, is quite similar to the definition already in use.

In contrast, other programs have a simple application procedure that obtains a crude measure of gross money income for purposes of eligibility determination. Many of these programs provide an all-or-nothing service—an example is Head Start, which offers an enrichment program to preschool children in families with income below the poverty threshold. Other programs with relatively simple application procedures charge recipients for services on a sliding scale, depending on the broad income-to-poverty ratio category into which the family falls. In these cases, to fully implement the proposed family resource definition could pose a burden on applicants and program administrators. However, we believe there are ways to simplify the proposed definition for programs for which a simple application process is valued and where there is a willingness to trade off the loss of some precision in classifying an applicant's eligibility status.

With respect to the threshold or need standard component of the proposed measure, program agencies must consider whether to use 100 percent of the thresholds as the cutoff for eligibility or a multiple of them, as is now specified in many programs. Obviously, there are budgetary implications of this choice, particularly for entitlement programs that must provide benefits for all applicants who meet the eligibility criteria (in contrast to programs with a legislatively set budget that requires program administrators to put eligible applicants on a waiting list once the budget is exhausted). In this regard, it is critical to consider the implications for programs of the recommendation to update the thresholds each year for real changes in consumption of basic goods and services. The thresholds developed under this procedure will not likely increase as fast as would a purely relative set of thresholds (because the procedure considers only the categories of food, clothing, and shelter, not all goods and services). However, the thresholds developed under the proposed procedure will likely increase faster than thresholds that are simply adjusted by the CPI, like the official ones, if real growth occurs.

There are ways to address the budgetary consequences of poverty thresholds that are updated in real terms. For example, program eligibility could be limited to families with resources below a fraction of the thresholds. This type of strategy is not a contradiction in terms. Although updating the poverty thresholds for real growth in basic consumption makes a great deal of sense for a statistical measure, the design of government assistance programs must take into account many factors, only one of which is a statistical standard of need. Other considerations, such as funding constraints and competing uses for scarce tax dollars, may dictate assistance program eligibility levels that are lower than the statistical poverty thresholds.

Finally, there are some other features of the proposed poverty measure that may not be suitable for program use. For example, we propose that need be measured on an annual basis and that asset values not be included in family resources. However, many programs (e.g., food stamps) use a subannual accounting period together with an asset test because they are intended to provide immediate assistance to people who are in a crisis situation. Also, we propose that the unit of analysis be the family, as defined by the Census Bureau, but programs differ in their target populations and hence often in their definition of an eligible unit. Such differences from the proposed statistical poverty measure are quite appropriate in light of program objectives.

RECOMMENDATION 7.1. **Agencies responsible for federal assistance programs that use the poverty guidelines derived from the official poverty thresholds (or a multiple) to determine eligibility for benefits and services should consider the use of the panel's proposed measure. In their assessment, agencies should determine whether it may be necessary to modify the measure—for example, through a**

simpler definition of family resources or by linking eligibility less closely to the poverty thresholds because of possible budgetary con- straints—to better serve program objectives.

Need Standards for AFDC

In most government assistance programs, the benefit standard—that is, the maximum amount of benefits provided to people with no other income—and the eligibility or need standard are the same. People who are eligible because their countable income falls below the benefit standard are entitled to receive benefits up to the amount of the standard.[32] AFDC is unique in that federal legislation requires each state to establish a standard of need for families with no other means of support. In a separate process, each state determines the maximum benefit that it will actually pay to such families, which does not have to equal the state's need standard. As prescribed by federal statute, the need standard restricts eligibility for AFDC: currently, families must have gross income below 185 percent of the state need standard to be eligible to receive benefits. In addition, they must have net countable income (as defined by federal law) below 100 percent of either the state need standard *or* the state payment standard, whichever is lower. As of January 1994, 40 states had a maximum benefit that was below their need standard (in some states the maximum benefit was below both their need and payment standards; U.S. House of Representatives, 1994: Table 10-11; see also Solomon and Neisner, 1993:Table 1).

Historically, there has been great variation among the states in how they derive their need standard, in how often and by what method they update it, in how benefits relate to the need standard, and in the level of the need standard. The differences in state AFDC need standards are much wider than can be explained by differences in the cost of living across states, even allowing for the problems with subnational cost-of-living indicators (see, e.g., Peterson and Rom, 1990).

One could argue that the level of the need standard is irrelevant to families' welfare because states are not required to pay benefits at that level— and three-quarters do not. It is also true that welfare policy is currently in a state of flux: the AFDC program as it has operated historically may change in significant ways, possibly rendering moot the question of the soundness or adequacy of the need standard for the current program. Nonetheless, until the program is changed, there is a requirement that the states develop a need standard, which is important for several reasons: it sets limits for eligibility; it is linked to benefits, directly in those states that pay 100 percent of need and

---

[32] Strictly speaking, this statement applies to cash benefit programs (e.g., SSI, veterans' pen- sions). Near-cash programs (e.g., food stamps and assisted housing) have a benefit standard that falls below the eligibility standard because the benefit pertains to a single commodity.

indirectly in other states; and it offers a goal or target against which to assess the adequacy of benefits.

The question is whether it makes sense for states to adopt the proposed poverty measure in place of their own need standard. A related recent development in standard setting practices is that 14 states have explicitly geared their need standard to the current poverty guidelines. In many of these states, the link is more theoretical than actual in that the need standard, either by law or regulation or because of failure to adjust for inflation, is a small fraction of the poverty guidelines. In other states, the definition of the poverty guidelines has been altered to exclude some types of consumption. Still, a growing number of states have found it convenient to link their AFDC need standard in some fashion to the poverty guidelines. We believe the proposed measure represents an improvement over the current measure for this purpose, and we encourage states to consider its use.

The proposed budget concept correlates well with the objectives of the AFDC program to provide the means for low-income families to obtain basic necessities. The exclusion of medical care needs from the proposed budget concept is consistent with the separate provision of medical care to AFDC families through the Medicaid program. In many respects, the proposed definition of family resources is similar to the AFDC definition of countable income, such as the treatment of work-related expenses, including child care, as deductions from family resources rather than as part of the poverty budget. In addition, the proposed measure includes an improved equivalence scale and reflects area differences in housing costs.

The 1988 Family Support Act requires states to review their need standard every 3 years and report to HHS. In the next review, states could consider the possible use of the proposed poverty measure as a need standard for AFDC. In their review, the states would need to look at the implications of the proposed measure—both the thresholds and the definition of family resources—in relation to their current need standards (whether the current poverty guidelines or the states' own standards). They would also need to consider whether the proposed measure may need to be modified in one or more respects to be more suitable for program purposes. It may be that, for budgetary or other reasons, states will decide to set the need standard at different fractions of the poverty threshold. Nonetheless, having a link between state need standards and the proposed poverty measure would be a major step toward providing a common framework for determining AFDC eligibility and evaluating eligibility levels across states.

RECOMMENDATION 8.1. **The states should consider linking their need standard for the Aid to Families with Dependent Children program to the panel's proposed poverty measure and whether it may be necessary to modify this measure to better serve program objectives.**

The Poverty Measure and AFDC Benefit Standards

State AFDC benefit standards vary even more widely than do state AFDC need standards, and no state provides benefits as generous as the official poverty thresholds. From time to time, there have been efforts to enact a federal minimum benefit standard for AFDC. These efforts have invariably come to naught, largely because of the cost implications of raising the benefit standard in states with low benefits. Changes in the percentage of benefits that the federal government will reimburse the states have been enacted with the intent of providing incentives for low-benefit states to increase their benefits; however, these changes in the matching formula have had little effect on the variation in benefit levels among the states (Peterson and Rom, 1990).

AFDC recipients are eligible for food stamps, and the nationalization of the Food Stamp Program has served to reduce the disparities in combined AFDC and food stamp benefits across the states.[33] However, significant differences still remain that exceed what can be reasonably attributed to cost-of-living differences among the states. Thus, the maximum combined AFDC and food stamp benefit for a three-person family in January 1994 varied from $1,208 in Alaska to $415 in Mississippi; the median benefit was $658, which is 69 percent of the corresponding official 1993 poverty threshold (U.S. House of Representatives, 1994:Table 10-11).

Currently, a de facto national minimum level of available benefits exists for AFDC recipients, namely, the maximum food stamp allowance combined with the maximum AFDC benefit in the lowest benefit state. (In January 1994, this amount for a three-person family was 43% of the corresponding official 1993 poverty threshold.) Hence, the issue of a national minimum benefit standard for AFDC really comes down to an issue of raising this de facto standard. Arguments for adopting such a nationwide minimum benefit standard for AFDC have been made on the basis of equity—namely, that low-income families with children should not be disadvantaged simply by reason of their state of residence. Arguments have also been offered that differences in benefits encourage low-income families to migrate from low-benefit to high-benefit states. The studies that have been done on the migration effects of AFDC suffer from serious data and methodological problems, but they suggest that the effect on migration of low-income families is quite small.

The question of how or if the proposed poverty measure, for which the thresholds vary much less across states than do AFDC need and benefit standards, should be linked with program benefits (for AFDC or a combination of assistance programs) is a difficult one. There are several reasons that a benefit

---

[33] This evening-out occurs because the food stamp benefit formula decreases food stamp benefits by 30 cents for every dollar increase in AFDC benefits and, conversely, increases food stamp benefits by 30 cents for every dollar reduction in AFDC benefits.

standard could differ from a poverty standard and, more generally, why the design of an assistance program could deviate from the goal of helping everyone who is classified as poor. First, scarce budget resources (and competition for them from other programs) may well limit the extent to which payments can approach the poverty threshold; in state-federal programs (such as AFDC), the nature of the state-federal cost sharing provisions has an important effect on funding constraints.

Second, there may be reasons to target payments on particular groups in order to maximize the effectiveness of limited funds and achieve other policy goals. For example, because of the social cost of children growing up in economic deprivation, it may be sensible to concentrate assistance dollars on poor families with children, even though other groups have measured need that is just as great. Or it may make sense to concentrate scarce assistance dollars on the poorest families, even though helping the families closest to the poverty line would achieve the fastest reduction in measured need.

Third, the existence of multiple assistance programs can affect the level of the benefit standard that makes sense for any one of them. For example, AFDC interacts with food stamps and public housing, among other programs, and it makes little sense to think of an AFDC benefit standard in isolation from other programs. Finally, incentive effects drive a wedge between measured need and the amount of program dollars needed to alleviate need. For example, families who are provided benefits designed to raise them above the poverty line may reduce their work effort so that the net effect is to leave them in poverty. Behavioral effects of program benefits are, indeed, the reason that it is misleading to describe the aggregate "poverty gap"—the difference between the poverty line and a family's resources, aggregated over all families—as the dollar amount that the government would have to spend to eliminate poverty.

The question of incentives is one of the most difficult issues that policy makers face in designing assistance programs to serve multiple goals, such as alleviating need while containing costs and discouraging dependency. The task is made more difficult by the fact that research findings on incentive effects are sometimes incomplete or inconclusive. Issues of program incentives have been at the center of the policy debate about AFDC, which is directed to families that the public would like to see increasingly responsible for their own support. Consequently, there has been considerable experimentation with changes in benefit levels and formulas for calculating disposable income to try to induce AFDC families to become more stable and self-supporting. To date, results show limited effects of changes in benefit levels and the tax rate on earnings on such behaviors as work effort. The findings are not yet available on more recent state initiatives, such as not increasing benefits when another child is born or reducing benefits if parents do not stay in school or fail to have their children vaccinated. It is important also to note that other programs besides AFDC raise concerns about incentives; for example, Social Security and SSI have negative effects on work effort (see Chapter 8).

For all of these reasons, it is not possible, on any theoretical or strictly scientific grounds, to link poverty thresholds directly to benefits. To the many people involved in evaluating and designing public assistance programs, this conclusion may seem obvious. However, we believe it is worth restating the obvious to underscore the point that measuring need, by determining how many people have resources below a reasonable poverty standard, is different from determining the proper societal response to that need.

In sum, many factors properly enter into a determination of program benefit standards, including judgments about the extent to which society is prepared to allocate scarce resources to support low-income people and the mix of goals that society wants government assistance programs to serve. The critical role of such judgments is the reason that a panel such as ours, chosen for expertise in measurement issues, cannot make recommendations about appropriate benefit levels for specific assistance programs. However, the fact that we do not make a recommendation about national minimum benefit standards for AFDC (or other programs) should not be taken to mean that there is no case for reducing the wide variation in AFDC benefits across the states. Rather, as a panel on poverty measurement, our position on the issue of benefit levels for assistance programs is necessarily neutral.

In conclusion, we urge policy makers at the federal and state levels to carefully consider all of the issues involved in the current debate about the nation's welfare policy. Ultimately, the determination of appropriate programs and policies to alleviate poverty involves "politics" in its best sense—namely, the consideration of competing public objectives against the constraints of scarce public resources within the framework of a nation's social and political system.

Poverty Thresholds

2

$\mathbf{A}$s we describe in Chapter 1, we conclude that the current measure of poverty should be revised for several reasons. First, the measure is flawed in the definition of family resources. The resource definition counts taxes as income, although taxes are not available for consumption. A before-tax income definition is also inconsistent with the original threshold concept, which was derived on an after-tax basis. In addition, the resource definition does not count in-kind benefits as income, although such programs as food stamps are designed to provide for consumption.

Second, the measure is flawed in the adjustments to the thresholds for different family circumstances. There are anomalies in the adjustments for family type and size (i.e., in the implicit equivalence scale), and there are no adjustments of any kind for geographic cost-of-living differences. Third, the measure does not distinguish between parents who work outside their homes and workers generally versus nonworkers, or between people with higher versus lower health care needs and costs—either by adjusting the thresholds or (as we propose) by deducting nondiscretionary expenses from income. Changes over the past three decades, including socioeconomic changes (such as the increase in the proportion of working mothers), demographic changes (such as the growth in elderly households), and government policy changes (such as changes in tax laws and the growth of in-kind benefit programs), have made all of these aspects of the current measure increasingly problematic for its primary purpose of informing policy makers and the public of differences in poverty rates across time and among population groups and areas.

Fourth, the concept for the official poverty thresholds is problematic. That concept originally was the cost of a minimum diet times a multiplier to allow for all other expenses; however, as implemented, the concept is simply the threshold value that was set for 1963 updated for price changes. Hence, whether the concept is still relevant today, given the increase in the U.S. standard of living over the past 30 years, is very much a question.

THRESHOLD CONCEPTS

The measurement of economic poverty involves two primary components: a budget or threshold below which people are considered poor and an estimate of resources available to people to compare with that threshold. Although the two components work in conjunction with one another—indeed, they need to be defined in a consistent manner in order to have a defensible measure of poverty—for reasons of analysis and presentation we discuss each component in turn.

In this chapter we consider concepts for a poverty threshold for a reference family type, including the implications for how that threshold is updated over time. (Chapter 3 discusses adjustments to the reference family threshold for other family types.) We also consider levels for the reference family threshold with which to initiate a new series of poverty statistics under the proposed measure.

Analysts often use the terms "absolute" and "relative" poverty thresholds. Absolute thresholds are fixed at a point in time and updated solely for price changes, as is the case for the current U.S. poverty measure. Relative thresholds, in contrast, are updated regularly (usually, annually) for changes in real consumption.

Absolute thresholds also generally carry the connotation that they are developed by "experts" with reference to basic physiological needs (e.g., nutritional needs) for one or more budget elements. Relative thresholds, as commonly defined, are developed by reference to the actual expenditures (or income) of the population. For example, a relative measure might set the poverty threshold for a four-person family at one-half the median income or expenditure of families, adjusted for the composition of the population by family type.

Relative thresholds are often criticized on the grounds that the choice of the expenditure or income cutoff is arbitrary or subjective rather than reflecting an objective standard of economic deprivation. It is also argued that relative poverty thresholds do not provide a stable target against which to measure the effects of government programs because they change each year in response to real increases or decreases in consumption levels. In practice, however, relative poverty thresholds are not so different from thresholds developed according to expert standards of need: the latter also embody a great deal of relativity and subjectivity. Moreover, it is rare for expert (or other) standards to be maintained in absolute terms (i.e., to be updated solely for price changes) over long periods of time. The more common experience is that an old standard is replaced after some period of time by a new standard that is higher in real terms.

Our review below of poverty threshold concepts begins with an overview of our recommended concept, which leads us also to propose that the current level of the reference family threshold be reassessed (although we do not make a recommendation on the level). We then discuss in detail both expert-based poverty budgets and relative concepts developed both here and abroad. Because expert budgets are typically updated on a sporadic rather than a regular basis, with price adjustments made between realignments, we discuss types of price updating. We also review "subjective" poverty concepts, which derive poverty thresholds from survey questions. Finally, we return to the proposed concept, which is a hybrid of the budget and relative approaches and for which there is support provided by a time series of subjective thresholds developed for the United States.

Our conclusions about the threshold concept and the need to reevaluate the level of the current reference family threshold involve considerable elements of judgment. Although judgment enters into nearly all aspects of the poverty measure—from how to value in-kind benefits to how to specify the particular form of an equivalence scale—questions of the threshold concept and level are more inherently matters of judgment than other aspects of a poverty measure. In our deliberations on the threshold concept, we used the criteria we developed in Chapter 1 for a poverty measure—namely, that it be understandable, statistically defensible, and operationally feasible. Also, to the greatest extent possible, we used historical and statistical evidence about the implications of alternative concepts for official poverty statistics in the United States.

In this regard, we note that our review was largely limited to poverty measures that, like the current measure, relate to economic or material needs and resources and to threshold concepts that, correspondingly, express the poverty threshold in monetary terms. In other words, we reviewed measures of economic deprivation, in which poverty is defined as insufficient economic resources (e.g., money or near-money income) for minimally adequate levels of consumption of economic goods and services (e.g., food, housing, clothing, transportation).

Such measures have been criticized as too narrow in focus, even considered as measures of economic poverty. Townsend (1992:5, 10), for example, comments that people are "social beings expected to perform socially demanding roles as workers, citizens, parents, partners, neighbors, and friends." He argues that economic poverty should be defined as the lack of sufficient income for people to "play the roles, participate in the relationships, and follow the customary behavior which is expected of them by virtue of their membership of society." Toward this end, Townsend (1979, 1992) has worked to derive a monetary poverty standard that corresponds to low scores on a "deprivation index." Other researchers (e.g., Mack and Lansley, 1985; see also Callan, Nolan, and Whelan, 1992) have developed deprivation indexes to measure socioeconomic deprivation directly—that is, they define socioeconomic poverty as low scores on the index itself. Deprivation indexes commonly include a dozen or more behaviors and types of ownership that are viewed as indicative of full participation in one's society: for example, whether people have certain appliances for household maintenance, new (not second-hand) clothing, access to items necessary for getting and keeping a job (e.g., a telephone or a car or other transportation), or the ability to take a vacation.[1]

We agree with Townsend and others about the limitations of economic poverty measures as commonly defined. We argue in Chapter 1 for the need for measures of other forms of deprivation. It is important to have direct indicators of such types of deprivation as physical and mental illness, family abuse, unemployment, hunger, homelessness, risk of criminal victimization, and others. It is also important to have measures that characterize the standard of living, such as the extent to which certain types of consumption (e.g., automobiles, televisions) have diffused throughout society (see, e.g., the work of Mayer and Jencks, 1993) or the extent to which people engage in leisure activities.

Our charge, however, was to consider the official U.S. poverty measure, which compares economic resources with a monetary threshold for economic consumption. We saw our primary task as twofold—to evaluate the usefulness of the current measure for informing policy makers and the public and to review alternative measures of economic or monetary poverty that could represent an improvement over the current measure. Although we did not do so, we certainly encourage work on measures of other kinds of deprivation, as well as work on measures (such as the Townsend deprivation index) that relate to, but are not the same as, an economic measure of poverty.

RECOMMENDATIONS

We recommend a revised threshold concept for the official U.S. measure of poverty. Two aspects of the proposed threshold concept need to be kept in mind when comparing it with other concepts: the definition of a reference family and the treatment of nondiscretionary expenses.

---

[1] Sen (1983, 1987) and Atkinson (1985, 1989) discuss the philosophical basis for deprivation indexes that reflect specific, socially influenced types of activities and consumption that are needed to achieve basic capabilities (e.g., literacy, the ability to obtain a job). In the version developed by Mack and Lansley (1985), the index is limited to items that at least one-half of the respondents to a national survey claim to be "necessary" for minimal participation in society, and people who lack a given item because they do not want it are distinguished from people who lack it because they cannot afford it.

The Two-Adult/Two-Child Reference Family

We recommend that the poverty threshold concept apply to a reference family of two adults and two children, with the thresholds for other types of families developed by means of a formal equivalence scale that recognizes the different needs of adults and children and the economies of scale for larger families. An alternative approach would be to develop thresholds for each family type on a separate basis, by building up a budget with specific assumptions about scale economies and the needs of different types of family members for each item (e.g., food, housing). The current thresholds were originally developed by Orshansky in this manner, although food was the only budget item specifically determined for each family type. Renwick (1993a, 1993b) also proposes such an approach for constructing budgets for a number of major commodities. This approach, however, involves making many specific judgments about each item and each type of family. Such judgments are inevitably arbitrary (as is evidenced by the anomalies in the current thresholds across family types), and, in our judgment, it is better to have the arbitrariness expressed in a formal equivalence scale. (See Chapter 3 for a detailed discussion of alternative equivalence scales with which to adjust the reference family threshold and methods to adjust the thresholds for geographic area differences in the cost of living.)

Any proposed equivalence scale will, of course, produce different thresholds for various types of families than the scale implicit in the current thresholds. Hence, it is desirable for the reference family to fall near the center of the family size distribution rather than at one of the extremes: this tends to reduce the sensitivity to the equivalence scale. Also, it is preferable for the reference family to be one that accounts for a relatively large proportion of the population because its spending patterns observed in a sample survey will be the basis for the poverty thresholds under the proposed concept.

The two-adult/two-child family meets these criteria. Although it is no longer the predominant living arrangement in U.S. society, it represents the largest number of people. Of all households (including family households and those headed by unrelated individuals), the single largest type today consists of one-adult households (25% of total households in 1992), followed by married couples with no other family member (22%). The four-person family, comprising a married couple and two other family members, is the third largest household type (13%). However, these four-person families are the modal type in terms of the number of people they represent: in 1992, they accounted for 20 percent of all people, compared with 17 percent for married couples with no other family members, and 10 percent for one-adult households (Rawlings, 1993:Table 16).

Nondiscretionary Expenses

In addition to accounting for different needs of families by number of adults and children and geographic area of residence, we recommend that the poverty measure take account of different needs due to the fact that some families incur nondiscretionary expenses that are not available for consumption. For example, some families pay for child care in order to earn income, while other families (and individuals) make no such payments, yet the current thresholds are the same for both situations. One way to recognize these different circumstances is to develop additional thresholds, such as thresholds for nonworking families, working families with children who pay for child care, and other working families (see Renwick 1993a, 1993b, for an example of such an approach). We recommend instead that nondiscretionary expenses—which we define as taxes, child care and other work-related expenses, child support payments to other households, and out-of-pocket medical care expenditures (including health insurance premiums)—be deducted from the incomes of families with such expenses.

This approach will more accurately capture the poverty status of families in different circumstances than would the approach of trying to develop a range of different thresholds (see Chapter 4). However, the proposed approach has implications for comparing poverty thresholds across concepts: a reference family threshold developed as we propose will necessarily exclude some expenses that are typically averaged in for all such families.

Updating the Thresholds

The major reason, in our view, to revise the threshold concept for the U.S. poverty measure is its implications for updating the thresholds over time. In this regard, it is important to understand the nature of the current poverty measure. As described below ("Expert Budgets"), the method originally used to develop the official thresholds involved taking the cost of a minimum food diet and applying a multiplier that reflected the share of food in the total expenditures of the average family, but that method has never been used to update the thresholds (although its original author, Mollie Orshansky, urged several times that this be done). The thresholds have been updated only for price changes. In other words, the poverty line of about $3,100 for a two-adult/two-child family that was originally set for 1963 has been treated as an absolute standard of need and kept fixed in real terms ever since. Thus, it no longer represents a current estimate of the cost of the food budget times a food-share multiplier. In fact, neither the cost of that original food basket nor the food share underlying the multiplier of three has remained constant over time. The share of food in the typical consumer bundle has declined with economic growth, and the cost updating using the overall Consumer Price

Index (CPI) does not necessarily reflect changes in the price of food. Moreover, the composition of the minimum food diet has not been reevaluated on the basis of new information about the food-buying preferences of low-income families.

If one believes that it is appropriate to have an absolute poverty line that is updated solely for price changes, there is little need to revisit the threshold concept. However, we believe that to maintain a standard in absolute terms becomes increasingly problematic as living standards change over time. The historical evidence supports the conclusion that poverty standards reflect their time and place. This is true not only when poverty standards are set in an explicitly relative fashion (e.g., as a percentage of median income or expenditures), but also when they are developed according to expert criteria for various needs. Similarly, when surveys ask people questions about minimum income levels, their answers generally reflect prevailing levels of consumption.

Hence, we conclude that the relevant question is not whether poverty thresholds should be updated for changes in real consumption, but whether they should be updated on a sporadic or on a regular basis. The former choice would suggest revisiting the standards periodically, perhaps every 10-20 years, and making price adjustments in between major realignments. The latter choice would suggest an automatic mechanism for recalculating the thresholds annually to reflect real consumption changes. We believe that an automatic, regular adjustment is preferable to sporadic adjustments. An automatic adjustment will avoid major breaks in the time series of poverty statistics and also will obviate the controversy that is likely to occur with periodic readjustments.[2]

A decision to recommend a regular adjustment of the thresholds entails careful consideration of the updating properties of alternative concepts, particularly the implications for the magnitude of the adjustment that is made. We believe that a conservative adjustment is preferable—that is, one that updates them for real growth in consumption of basic goods and services that pertain to a concept of poverty, rather than to update them for real growth in total consumption or income. There is support for a conservative approach from ideas of poverty levels derived from surveys, specifically, those developed on the basis of responses to questions about minimum income amounts needed to "get along." Over time, such levels have reflected growth in real income but less than proportionately with overall growth (see below). Also, a conservative updating approach will make less of a break with the historical time series.

---

[2] Of course, even an "automatic" updating procedure should be reviewed periodically to determine if it is performing as intended or whether it needs to be modified. Such a review, which would include the data source and methodology, should be part of the regular reviews of the poverty measure that we recommend be carried out every 10 years by the U.S. Office of Management and Budget (see Chapter 1).

A way to implement a regular adjustment of the thresholds would be to return to the original concept for developing the poverty line and apply it afresh each year, namely, determine a minimum food budget and apply a multiplier that is equal to the inverse of the share of food in the total expenditures of the average family. If that procedure was correct for 1963, then it should be correct for every other year. The advantages of this method of updating mirror its initial attractiveness: it rests on a commodity, namely food, that all would agree is a necessary item of consumption; it is understandable ("food times a multiplier"); and it is easy to implement with available consumer expenditure data. However, we believe that its problems outweigh its advantages.

One problem is the reliance on experts to determine the minimum food budget. As we show below, judgment inevitably enters into the determination of a poverty level for any basic need, whether food, housing, or anything else. We believe it best if these judgments are introduced explicitly and not with an apparent reliance on experts. A more important problem is the use of only one commodity with a large multiplier and, moreover, a multiplier that reflects total expenditures of the *average* family. This approach is not conservative with respect to adjusting the thresholds over time because the multiplier, which drives the thresholds, will reflect increased spending on luxuries as well as on basic commodities. In other words, continued application of the original threshold concept is more akin to a completely relative concept, like one-half median family income or expenditures.

We sought a concept that would retain the attractive features of the original concept, namely, its understandability and grounding in familiar, basic commodities, but improve on it. Our recommendation is that the reference family poverty threshold be developed by specifying a percentage of median expenditures on the sum of food, clothing, and shelter (including utilities) by two-adult/two-child families in the Consumer Expenditure Survey (CEX), and applying a multiplier to that dollar value so as to add a small amount for other needed expenditures (e.g., personal care, household supplies, non-work-related transportation). This approach builds the budget on three categories of basic goods and services plus a little more, and it uses actual expenditure data directly in the derivation.

Having specified a percentage of median expenditures and a multiplier, these values would then be used to update the poverty threshold for the reference family each year on the basis of more recent CEX data. To smooth out year-to-year fluctuations and to lag the adjustment to some extent, we propose to perform the calculations for each year by averaging the most recent 3 years' worth of CEX data, with the data for each of those years brought forward to the current period by using the change in the CPI. Once the threshold is updated for the reference family, the thresholds for other family types can be calculated (see Chapter 3).

The proposed concept has an important advantage for updating the poverty thresholds over time. Historically, spending on food, clothing, and shelter has increased at a slower rate in real terms than has total spending; hence, the proposed updating procedure will tend to update the thresholds in a conservative or a quasi-relative rather than a completely relative manner. However, because the proposed procedure is new, it will be important to evaluate the behavior of the resulting thresholds in relation to the thresholds that would result from a simple adjustment for the change in the Consumer Price Index.

RECOMMENDATION 2.1. **A poverty threshold with which to initiate a new series of official U.S. poverty statistics should be derived from Consumer Expenditure Survey data for a reference family of four persons (two adults and two children). The procedure should be to specify a percentage of median annual expenditures for such families on the sum of three basic goods and services—food, clothing, and shelter (including utilities)—and apply a specified multiplier to the corresponding dollar level so as to add a small amount for other needs.**

RECOMMENDATION 2.2. **The new poverty threshold should be updated each year to reflect changes in consumption of the basic goods and services contained in the poverty budget: determine the dollar value that represents the designated percentage of the median level of expenditures on the sum of food, clothing, and shelter for two-adult/two-child families and apply the designated multiplier. To smooth out year-to-year fluctuations and to lag the adjustment to some extent, perform the calculations for each year by averaging the most recent 3 years' worth of data from the Consumer Expenditure Survey, with the data for each of those years brought forward to the current period by using the change in the Consumer Price Index.**

RECOMMENDATION 2.3. **When the new poverty threshold concept is first implemented and for several years thereafter, the Census Bureau should produce a second set of poverty rates for evaluation purposes by using the new thresholds updated only for price changes (rather than for changes in consumption of the basic goods and services in the poverty budget).**

Setting the Initial Threshold

Although we recommend a threshold concept and a procedure for updating the poverty thresholds, we do not recommend an initial level with which to initiate a new series of official poverty statistics under the proposed measure.

Specifying a poverty line is the most judgmental of all the aspects of a poverty measure, and we did not think it appropriate for us to make that final, ultimately political, judgment.

We do, however, recommend that the level of the current threshold for a two-adult/two-child family be reevaluated in light of both the proposed poverty concept (which treats nondiscretionary expenses as deductions from income rather as elements of the poverty budget) and the increase in the standard of living since 1963, when the current threshold was first fixed in real terms. We also offer a conclusion about what we believe is a reasonable range for the initial reference family threshold. This conclusion is informed by our analysis of thresholds that result from a variety of concepts in the published literature and is consistent with our recommendation to update the thresholds in a conservative manner.

We conclude that reasonable values for the starting threshold for a two-adult/two-child family lie in the range of $13,700 to $15,900 (in 1992 dollars). In terms of the proposed budget concept, the lower end of the range can be expressed as 1.15 times the spending on food, clothing, and shelter of two-adult/two-child families at the 30th percentile of the distribution of such spending. The upper end of the range can be expressed as 1.25 times the spending on food, clothing, and shelter of two-adult/two-child families at the 35th percentile of the distribution. In overall terms, the range of $13,700 to $15,900 is 14 to 33 percent higher than the current 1992 reference family threshold, when it is converted (as best as can be done) to the proposed budget concept (i.e., when an amount for nondiscretionary expenditures is removed). The updating that these figures represent is conservative when compared with thresholds developed for 1992 with other approaches and converted to the proposed concept (see below, "Implementing the Proposed Approach").

RECOMMENDATION 2.4. **As part of implementing a new official U.S. poverty measure, the current threshold level for the reference family of two adults and two children ($14,228 in 1992 dollars) should be reevaluated and a new threshold level established with which to initiate a new series of poverty statistics. That reevaluation should take account of both the new threshold concept and the real growth in consumption that has occurred since the official threshold was first set 30 years ago.**

In the remainder of this chapter we describe in greater detail the nature of and reasoning behind our choice of a poverty threshold concept and procedure for updating the thresholds. We describe the major alternatives, including expert budget concepts, relative concepts, and subjective (survey-based) concepts of poverty. We give our reasons for preferring our recommended approach to the others. We note that other approaches support the appropriateness of regularly adjusting the poverty thresholds for real changes in consumption of basic goods and services.

EXPERT BUDGETS

Expert-based poverty thresholds, as they have been developed in recent decades, generally derive from one of several approaches that fall along a continuum: expert-defined budget allotments for one or a few categories of expenditures with a large multiplier to allow for other needed expenditures (i.e., the Orshansky multiplier method); expert allotments for a larger number of categories with perhaps a small "other" or miscellaneous category; and expert allotments for a comprehensive, detailed list of budget items (e.g., specific types of clothing instead of clothing as a broad category).[3] Thresholds developed in this manner have the appeal of being based on the notion of minimum standards of physical needs. Food is almost always specified in expert budgets since it is biologically required for survival. Emphasis is also typically placed on other goods necessary for survival, such as shelter and clothing.

Although expert budgets are generally intended to be derived in an objective manner, with a strong grounding in human physiological requirements, large elements of relativity and subjective judgment invariably enter the process. Thus, for every category for which an explicit budget figure is developed, judgments must be made about the composition of the category and the dollar value that is appropriate for a poverty standard. In a developed country such as the United States, there is usually a wide variety of specific items at varying quality and price levels for any category, almost any of which are adequate for sheer survival. To decide, for example, that a minimally adequate diet must include meat as well as rice and beans and how much of each foodstuff, or that a minimally adequate house or apartment must include at least one bedroom for every two children, is to make a set of judgments that are inevitably influenced by the mores and experiences of the expert's own society. Similarly, to decide what quality of meat (hamburger or ground sirloin) or clothing (polyester or cotton) to price as the poverty standard is to make another set of judgments. Moreover, the people who are defined to be in poverty according to the standards developed by the experts may or may not agree with the experts' choices.

Experts can decide to eschew the valuation of a specific item, such as a haircut, in favor of a broader category, "personal care." This approach will reduce the number of specific judgments required, but it will also inevitably

---

[3] The term for expert budgets in earlier literature is "standard budget" (see, e.g., de Neufville, 1975; Orshansky, 1959). The approach of applying a large multiplier to a budget for one or a few categories was originated by Orshansky in her work on the U.S. poverty measure.

lead to consideration of the distribution of actual expenditures on those categories. The process will again introduce elements of relativity to time and place and judgment in that a choice must ultimately be made of a specific dollar level to serve as the poverty standard.

The use of a multiplier introduces other elements of judgment and relativity. The advantage of a multiplier is that it is another way to reduce the number of budget categories for which explicit decisions must be made. But there is no method for scientifically or objectively determining a multiplier. Hence, experts are again inevitably driven to look at actual expenditures.

It is not a criticism of the poverty thresholds that result from expert-based approaches to say that they embody judgments that almost always reflect the conditions of the society for which those judgments are made. This statement is true of other poverty thresholds as well. Indeed, Adam Smith's definition of "necessaries" captured the essence of the matter: they include "not only the commodities which are indispensably necessary for the support of life, but whatever the custom of the country renders it indecent for creditable people, even of the lowest order, to be without" (1776:Book V, Chap. II, Pt. II, Article 4th). The definitions of "custom of the country," "indecent," "the lowest order," and even "indispensably necessary" all clearly involve judgment. The problem with expert approaches is that people may not recognize the elements of judgment involved and may prefer the experts' budgets because they appear more objective.

Multiplier Approaches

The official U.S. poverty thresholds were originally developed by setting expert standards for one commodity, food, and applying a large multiplier to allow for other needed expenditures. In this section, we review the methods underlying those original thresholds (see Fisher, 1992a, 1992b, for more detail on their history and derivation), along with a few other examples of the multiplier approach.

The Original U.S. Poverty Thresholds

The original U.S. poverty thresholds were those developed by Mollie Orshansky in the 1960s on the basis of the Economy Food Plan, the least expensive of four food plans designed by the U.S. Department of Agriculture (USDA).[4] This plan was developed in 1961 with data from the USDA 1955

---

[4] Orshansky actually developed two sets of thresholds—one derived from the Economy Food Plan and another derived from the somewhat more generous Low-Cost Food Plan. The lower set of thresholds was designated for official government use.

Household Food Consumption Survey (as a plan for temporary or emergency use) by examining the food-buying patterns of lower income households, modifying these preferences to develop a nutritionally balanced food plan, and costing out the items in the plan. Orshansky calculated the cost of the Economy Food Plan for families of various sizes and compositions. Specifically, her budgets varied by total family size, number of family members who were children, sex of the family head, and whether the head of a one-person or two-person family was over or under age 65. She developed thresholds for families residing on farms as a percentage of the corresponding nonfarm thresholds. Later, the distinctions by sex of head and farm or nonfarm residence were dropped.

To get from minimum food costs to estimates of minimum total living costs for families of three or more persons, she multiplied the food budgets by three. This multiplier was based on evidence from the 1955 Household Food Consumption Survey that the average family of three or more persons spent one-third of its total after-tax income on food. (Orshansky used somewhat different procedures to develop thresholds for families of one and two persons; see Chapter 3.)

In focusing on the two-adult/two-child threshold developed by Orshansky, which was about $3,100 for 1963, one can see the elements of relativity and judgment in its derivation. First, although nutritional experts at the USDA made use of their knowledge in developing the Economy Food Plan, the basis of the plan was the food-buying patterns of households deemed to be "lower income" from the 1955 survey. The USDA experts could readily have developed an "economy" plan at a lower cost that was still nutritionally adequate if they had been willing to ignore the preferences of Americans, even at lower income levels, for some variety and taste in their diet. Alternatively, they could have readily developed an "economy" plan at a somewhat higher cost with more variety than that provided in the plan they actually developed. The USDA experts also made other judgments in developing the Economy Food Plan: that low-income households had adequate time and knowledge to minimize waste by very careful management of their food storage and preparation and that all meals would be prepared at home.

Second, the multiplier was based on the share of total after-tax money income spent on food by the average family of three or more persons. This approach assumed that all kinds of expenditures should be included in the multiplier. It has also been criticized for using the expenditure patterns of the average family as the basis for deriving a budget for poor families. Thus, Friedman (1965) argued that poor families spend a higher proportion of their income on food than do average families.

Again, our point is not that the judgments that underlay the original poverty thresholds were necessarily more or less preferable than other judgments that could have been made, but rather, that Orshansky's approach involved judgments that are ultimately subjective in nature.[5] As we have seen, the particular judgments were strongly influenced by the spending patterns at that time—of lower income families for the food budgets developed by the USDA and of average-income families for the multiplier. As a consequence, the thresholds were higher in real terms than minimum budgets that were developed earlier in the twentieth century. For example, the Economy Food Plan was more generous in terms of allowed quantities than the food components of minimum budgets that were derived for major American cities between 1906 and 1929; also, the implicit allowance for nonfood items in the Orshansky multiplier was considerably more generous than the allowance in pre-1929 budgets, when incomes were lower and the percentage spent on food was, consequently, higher (Appelbaum, 1977; see also Fisher, 1993).

The Orshansky Multiplier over Time

The multiplier method developed by Orshansky has been used only once in the history of the official U.S. poverty thresholds—when the thresholds were first derived. The method was never used again to revise the thresholds, although Orshansky and others recommended its use several times (see, e.g., Fendler and Orshansky, 1979; see also Fisher, 1992b). Instead, the thresholds have been kept constant in real terms over the years through a price adjustment.

One can argue, in fact, that Orshansky's thresholds were adopted as the official thresholds not because her basic method had such widespread support, but for two other reasons. First, her central threshold for 1963 of $3,100 for a two-adult/two-child family accorded well with other views about the level for a poverty line at the time (see Vaughan, 1993; see also Fisher, 1992b, 1993). Also, unlike a number of other contemporary attempts at developing a poverty measure, she provided a matrix of thresholds that reflected different family circumstances, instead of one threshold for all families and another for unrelated individuals. Thus, the more lasting influence of her work on the official thresholds has been her implicit equivalence scale rather than her basic concept of a minimum food budget times a multiplier.

The application of Orshansky's method to update the thresholds would involve two steps: first, revising the food budget to reflect more recent data on the buying patterns of lower income families and, second, recalculating the multiplier. Each of these steps presents some problems.

In terms of the food budget, the USDA has revised its food plans several times since it developed the Economy Food Plan in 1961. (In between revisions, it uses changes in the Consumer Price Index for specific food

---

[5] Indeed, we want to acknowledge Orshansky's pioneering efforts in developing a poverty measure that proved broadly acceptable and widely useful. Having struggled with the issues and with the problems of available data, we realize full well the task that she faced.

categories to update the plan costs.) In 1975 USDA published revised food plans based on data from a 1965-1966 Household Food Consumption Survey and revised recommended dietary allowances (RDAs) from the National Research Council.[6] The lowest cost plan was renamed the Thrifty Food Plan. In 1983, USDA published a revision of the Thrifty Food Plan based on data from the 1977-1978 Nationwide Food Consumption Survey, further revisions to the RDAs, and new information about the nutrient content of various foods.

For the 1975 and 1983 Thrifty Food Plans, however, USDA relied much less heavily than in the original Economy Food Plan on the food-buying patterns of lower income households. Instead, it gave greater weight to cost constraints, namely, a decision to keep the costs of each revision about the same in real terms as the costs of the previous plan. This decision was made because a revised plan reflecting newer data on food-buying patterns would have resulted in a considerable cost increase (24% for the 1983 plan), and the Economy and then Thrifty Food Plan had been mandated as the basis for benefit allotments under the Food Stamp Program, so cost increases would have affected program costs to an extent that was viewed as unacceptable (Peterkin et al., 1983; Greger, 1985:3-4; Orshansky, 1986; see also Ruggles, 1990:179-180). Thus, changes in the mix of foodstuffs in the plan for reasons of nutrition or variety were made to stay within these cost limits. In terms of real dollar costs, the Thrifty Food Plan has been held about constant over time.

We estimated the effects on the reference family poverty threshold of implementing the Orshansky approach for selected years from 1950 to 1992, expressing the results in constant 1992 dollars; see Table 2-1.[7] We first determined the share spent on food (consumed at home and away from home) in each year by four-person families as a percentage of their total after-tax expenditures and the corresponding multiplier (the inverse of the share). We then determined the ratio of the multiplier in each year to the multiplier in 1960 and applied that ratio to the official poverty threshold in 1992 dollars for a two-adult/two-child family.[8] By definition, the official threshold and the

---

[6] The RDAs are based on the scientific findings of nutritional research, but they also involve judgment.

[7] We used 1992 as the reference year because our analysis of the effects on poverty rates of implementing the proposed measure used 1992 income data from the March 1993 Current Population Survey (see Chapter 5).

[8] We did not take the more straightforward approach of simply applying the multiplier we derived for each year to the food budget (i.e., one-third of the official threshold) because the multiplier in 1960 from CEX data was higher than that used by Orshansky from the 1955 USDA survey (4.56 for four-person families or 4.12 for all families, compared with her multiplier of 3.00 for families of three or more persons). Hence, to apply each year's multiplier as is would overadjust the thresholds relative to the change in the multiplier that occurred over the 1960-1992 period (the multiplier for four-person families increased from 4.56 in 1960 to 6.62 in 1991); see Table 2-1 for sources.

TABLE 2-1   Comparison of Updated Poverty Thresholds for a Two-Adult/Two-Child Family Using the Orshansky Multiplier, the Official Threshold, and Two Relative Thresholds, 1950-1992, in Constant 1992 Dollars

Year	Official Threshold	Orshansky Multiplier Threshold[a]	One-Half Median Four-Person Family Income	
			Before-Tax[b]	After-Tax[c]
Dollar Amount				
1950	14,228	11,681	10,697	10,106
1960	14,228	14,228	14,919	13,030
1963	14,228	14,228	16,364	14,120
1972–1973	14,228	16,874	21,661	18,236
1980	14,228	16,163	20,715	16,629
1989	14,228	20,659	23,062	18,990
1991	14,228	20,659	22,174	N.A.
1992	14,228	N.A.	22,308	18,018
Percent of Official Threshold				
1950	100.0	82.1	75.2	71.0
1960	100.0	100.0	104.9	91.6
1963	100.0	100.0	115.0	99.2
1972–1973	100.0	118.6	152.2	128.2
1980	100.0	113.6	145.6	116.9
1989	100.0	145.2	162.1	133.5
1991	100.0	145.2	155.8	N.A.
1992	100.0	N.A.	156.8	126.6

NOTES: The official 1992 threshold for a two-adult/two-child family (which, in constant 1992 dollars, applies to all earlier years) from Bureau of the Census (1993c:Table A).

[a]Based on calculating the share of food in the total after-tax expenditures of four-person consumer units, determining the multiplier (the inverse of the share), calculating the ratio of the multiplier in each year to that in 1960, and applying the ratio for each year to the official 1992 poverty threshold. The procedure assumes that the cost of the food component of the threshold remained constant in real terms and that Orshansky would have used the same food share and multiplier for a base year of 1960 as she did for her base year of 1963. Food shares and multipliers were obtained for 1960, 1972, 1980, and 1991 from tabulations provided to the panel from the 1960-1961, 1972-1973, 1980, and 1991 Consumer Expenditure Survey by the Bureau of Labor Statistics. The food share and multiplier for 1989 are assumed to be unchanged from 1988 (from Bureau of the Census, 1991:Table 718 for four-person consumer units). The food share and multiplier for 1950 were derived relative to 1960 by comparing food shares for these years for all urban families from Bureau of the Census (1975:323).

[b]For 1950, 1960, 1963, 1973, and 1989, calculated from Vaughan (1993:Table 1); for 1991 and 1992, calculated from Bureau of the Census (1993b:Table 13). All amounts were converted to 1992 dollars using the CPI-U (the CPI for urban families; from Bureau of the Census, 1993c:Table A-2).

[c]For 1950, 1960, 1963, 1973, and 1989, calculated from Vaughan (1993:Table 1), who estimated taxes for a two-adult/two-child family; for 1992, calculated from the March 1993 Current Population Survey; all amounts were converted to 1992 dollars using the CPI-U.

threshold as we calculated it are the same for the base year for Orshansky's original work.[9]

There are at least two ways of expressing the comparison between columns 1 and 2 of Table 2-1. First, since the method of setting the threshold was applied only once, the base year for which it was applied is critically important. If the official poverty level had been defined for 1950 instead of for 1963, the threshold would have been considerably lower than it is—about 18 percent lower—throughout the past 40 years. Yet if the official level had been defined for 1972-1973 instead of for 1963, using the identical logic and relevant data, the threshold would have been consistently higher than it is— about 19 percent higher—throughout the past 20 years.[10] Thus, pegging the threshold at one point in time—whether 1950, 1963, or 1972-1973—and then only updating for price changes means that the level of the threshold will be affected by the historical accident of the base year for which it is set.

Second, if the method of setting the threshold had been applied annually or periodically, the threshold would have risen dramatically as real income rose over the past 40 years. That is, the application of the same method for 1950 and for 1991 would have yielded a reference family poverty threshold of $11,681 for 1950 and $20,659 for 1991.

Even if the method for determining the poverty threshold for 1963 is considered flawless, there is no logical argument why 1963 was the historically correct time at which to apply that method to set a level for all years thereafter. Yet to apply that same method in subsequent years would have had a very large impact on the threshold. So one is faced with the uncomfortable conclusion that the current U.S. poverty threshold today cannot be right: if it was right for 1963, a year selected by historical accident, then it cannot also be right today.

For comparison purposes, we also developed two sets of relative thresholds (drawing on Vaughan, 1993): one set represents one-half the median before-tax four-person family income and the other set represents one-half the median after-tax four-person family income (see Table 2-1). Both thresholds are considerably below the 1950 equivalent of the official threshold (by 25-29%), while they are reasonably close to the official threshold for 1963 (the before-tax threshold is 15% above and the after-tax threshold is 1% below the official threshold for that year). Subsequently, both relative thresholds exceed

---

[9] That year was 1963; for our calculations, we assumed that the multiplier she used would have been the same for 1960 as for 1963.

[10] These percentage increases are somewhat higher than would result from applying an estimate of the change in the food multiplier to poverty thresholds that were updated by the change in the cost of the Economy/Thrifty Food Plan instead of the CPI (see below). However, they are lower than would result from applying an estimate of the change in the food multiplier to poverty thresholds based on an update of the Economy/Thrifty Food Plan to reflect new data on food-buying patterns of lower income families.

the official threshold—by amounts that now bracket the Orshansky multiplier threshold.

Because of problems of data comparability over time and measurement error, one should not make too much of the specific threshold values shown in Table 2-1 (or below). They are illustrative and broadly accurate, and we present them only to emphasize the overall patterns. In this set of comparisons, what is clear is that the relativity in the application of the Orshansky approach, which stems from the large multiplier that includes all other non-food spending, produces thresholds that mirror changes in real consumption above and beyond price changes.

Other Multiplier Approaches

Ruggles (1990:Table A.5) derived poverty thresholds by using a multiplier approach but applying the multiplier to a poverty standard for housing rather than food. Her foundation for this measure was the fair market rents developed by the U.S. Department of Housing and Urban Development (HUD) for use in determining rent subsidies to eligible families under the Section 8 Housing Assistance Payments Program, established in 1975.

HUD develops fair market rents by analyzing rent distributions in metropolitan areas and nonmetropolitan counties for two-bedroom apartments occupied by recent movers that meet specified quality standards. (The data sources for the rent distributions include the decennial census, the American Housing Survey [AHS], and local-area random digit dialing telephone surveys; see Chapter 3.) The Section 8 program subsidizes tenants by making up the difference between a rental amount, which generally cannot exceed the applicable fair market rent, and a percentage of the family's income. Currently, fair market rents are set at the 45th percentile of the rent distribution in each area, and eligible families are expected to contribute 30 percent of their net countable income toward the rent. (Prior to 1983, fair market rents were set at the median or 50th percentile of the distribution, and prior to 1981, families were expected to contribute only 25% of their net countable income toward the rent.)

To calculate poverty thresholds, Ruggles divided the annualized value of the fair market rent for the nation as a whole by the applicable percentage of income: 25 percent, corresponding to a multiplier of 4.00, or 30 percent, corresponding to a multiplier of 3.33; see Table 2-2. Thresholds developed in this manner are not available prior to the initiation of the Section 8 program; for the period 1977-1992, such thresholds have exceeded the official threshold by 45-55 percent.

Weinberg and Lamas (1993) developed a set of poverty thresholds for 1989 by budgeting amounts for both food and housing and applying a multiplier. They took the annual cost of the Thrifty Food Plan, added the 25th percentile value of the distribution of all nonsubsidized rented units from the

TABLE 2-2 Comparison of Poverty Thresholds for a Two–Adult/ Two–Child Family Using Two Multiplier Approaches, Selected Years, in Constant 1992 Dollars

Year	Official Threshold[a]	Housing Multiplier Threshold (45th or 50th percentile)[b]	Housing and Food Multiplier Threshold[c]	
			25th percentile	35th percentile
Dollar Amount				
1977	14,228	20,781	N.A.	N.A.
1980	14,228	21,331	N.A.	N.A.
1982	14,228	21,205	N.A.	N.A.
1985	14,228	20,758	N.A.	N.A.
1988	14,228	22,154	N.A.	N.A.
1989	14,228	21,815	20,267	21,790
1992	14,228	21,640	N.A.	N.A.
Percent of Official Threshold				
1977	100.0	146.1	N.A.	N.A.
1980	100.0	149.9	N.A.	N.A.
1982	100.0	149.0	N.A.	N.A.
1985	100.0	145.9	N.A.	N.A.
1988	100.0	155.7	N.A.	N.A.
1989	100.0	153.3	142.4	153.1
1992	100.0	152.1	N.A.	N.A.

[a]The official 1992 threshold for a two–adult/two–child family (which, in constant 1992 dollars, applies to all earlier years) from Bureau of the Census (1993c:Table A).

[b]The housing multiplier is based on obtaining the nationwide HUD fair market rent value for two-bedroom rental units (calculated for such units occupied by recent movers and having other specified characteristics) and applying a multiplier (the inverse of the percent of net countable income that subsidized tenants are expected to contribute toward rent). For 1977-1982, fair market rents were set at the 50th percentile of the distribution of all two-bedroom units including subsidized units and new construction; for subsequent years, fair market rents were set at the 45th percentile of the distribution of two-bedroom units excluding subsidized units and new construction. For 1977-1980, the multiplier was 4.0 (inverse of 25%); for 1982, the multiplier was 3.85 (inverse of 26%, reflecting a phase-in to 30%); for 1985 and later, the multiplier was 3.33 (inverse of 30%). The estimated thresholds for years 1977-1988 are from Ruggles (1990:Tables A.3, A.5); for 1989 and 1992 derived by using Ruggles' method with fair market rent(s) provided by HUD; all values were converted to 1992 dollars using the CPI-U (from Bureau of the Census, 1993c:Table A-2).

[c]The housing and food multiplier was originally developed by Weinberg and Lamas (1993:32-35) by calculating the value for the 25th or 35th percentile of the distribution of all nonsubsidized rental units by region and type of place (central city, suburb, nonmetropolitan) from the American Housing Survey, adding the value of the Thrifty Food Plan for a three-person family, and applying a multiplier of 2.0. The estimated thresholds for 1989 were calculated by taking the simple average of the Weinberg and Lamas region-place-specific thresholds times 1.282 (the ratio of the weighted average four-person official threshold to the weighted average three-person official threshold) to convert to four-person thresholds; all values were converted to 1992 dollars using the CPI-U.

AHS, and multiplied the result by two. The basis for their multiplier was the HUD limit of 30 percent on the amount of income families who receive rent subsidies are expected to contribute to the rent plus an estimate from CEX data that food accounts for about 20 percent of total expenditures. (This method follows Orshansky's approach of using the spending of average families to determine the food component of the multiplier but then determines the housing component of the multiplier on the basis of program standards for lower income families.) They computed another set of thresholds in the same manner but using the 35th percentile value of the rental distribution (see Table 2-2). Their thresholds are, respectively, 42 and 53 percent higher than the official threshold for 1989.

Several points emerge from the work by Ruggles (1990) and Weinberg and Lamas (1993). First, the level of the poverty threshold is obviously affected by the choice of the standard.[11] In the case of the food component, several analysts have argued that the Thrifty Food Plan is unrealistically restrictive and that the Low-Cost Food Plan should be used instead.[12] Second, over time, if the developers of poverty thresholds rely on program standards that are set by legislation, the standards may change for many reasons other than an evaluation of need (such as the desire to cut program costs). This problem is evident in Ruggles' HUD-based thresholds, for which changes were legislated in the early 1980s for both the housing standard (from the 50th to the 45th percentile) and the basis for the multiplier (from a 25% to a 30% share of income).[13] Had these changes not been made, it is likely that the HUD-based thresholds in Table 2-2 would have increased as a percent of the official threshold in the late 1980s rather than remaining flat.

Categorical Approaches

Renwick and Bergmann (1993) took a categorical approach to defining a poverty budget, which they refer to as a basic needs budget (BNB). Their approach is based on adequacy standards, not only for food, but also for housing and household operations, transportation, health care, clothing, child

---

[11] Why there is not more of a difference between the Weinberg and Lamas (1993) thresholds and the Ruggles (1990) thresholds, which are based on different percentiles of the rent distribution (see Table 2-2), is not clear. Weinberg and Lamas calculated the 25th and 35th percentiles of the rent distribution of all nonsubsidized rental units, while the HUD fair market rents used by Ruggles represent the 45th or 50th percentile of two-bedroom units occupied by recent movers and having other specified characteristics. In addition, the data sources were somewhat different.

[12] Indeed, Orshansky herself developed two sets of poverty thresholds, one based on the Economy Food Plan and the other on the Low-Cost Food Plan.

[13] Indeed, CEX data for 1991 indicate that the housing share of total after-tax expenditures was about 24 percent (for all consumer units and four-person units), not 30 percent (Bureau of the Census, 1993d:Table 708).

care, and personal care. To date, they have developed BNBs for single-parent and two-parent families with varying numbers of children (see Renwick and Bergmann, 1993; Renwick, 1993a, 1993b). Their budgets vary by whether the parent(s) work and by whether they receive such in-kind benefits as food stamps, school meals, free or subsidized child care, and medical care benefits. Their budgets also vary by region and type of place (central city, suburb, rural). The final step in their procedure is to determine the before-tax income required to be out of poverty on the basis of the BNB dollar level together with an estimate of payroll and income tax liabilities.

In constructing the basic needs budget, Renwick and Bergmann used previously defined standards whenever they considered them appropriate. Their food standard is based on the USDA Low-Cost Food Plan, the second least expensive of the four food plans, which incorporates some economies of scale for families of larger sizes. For housing, they assumed that parents have a separate bedroom from children and that no more than two children share a bedroom. For two-bedroom units they analyzed AHS data to determine the 25th percentile of the distribution of all such units, separately by the four regions and by central city, suburban, and rural locations. They allowed for a telephone and household supplies in the budget (updating the latter from the Bureau of Labor Statistics (BLS) lower level family budget—see below), but they did not allow for household furnishings or equipment, assuming that families would make do with what they had during a poverty spell. They assumed the use of public transportation by central city and suburban families and developed a weekly allowance for work trips for each adult earner plus an allowance for shopping and errands. In the budget for rural families, they allocated the cost of operating a second-hand car, using data from a 1977 survey on distance to work and the mileage allowances of the Internal Revenue Service (IRS) to estimate the cost of work trips for these families. They based their allowance for health insurance on the average total premium cost of group health insurance covering lower income families as reported in the National Health Care Expenditure Survey, and their allowance for out-of-pocket medical care expenditures was based on typical expenditures of moderate-income families with health insurance from the same source.[14] They developed a child care budget (for the case of no parent at home) by using the IRS dependent care tax credit limits on eligible expenses in full or in part, depending on the assumed age of the children and an assumption about use of free or subsidized care. For the clothing portion of the budget, they updated the lower level family budget allowance from the BLS. Finally, for personal care, they updated the BLS lower level family budget allowance, omitting the services component (principally, haircuts) and adding an allowance for dispos-

---

[14] It is not clear, but presumably the survey they used is the 1987 National Medical Expenditure Survey.

able diapers for children under age 2. They made no provision for other or miscellaneous expenses, thus excluding such BLS categories as reading materials, recreation, educational expenses, alcohol, and miscellaneous.

In the case of two-parent families with at least one wage earner, Renwick (1993a:Table 2, Appendix) made a further adjustment to the basic needs budget by deducting an estimated employer contribution to the health insurance premium. For a two-adult/two-child family in 1992, the resulting BNB (assuming the use of public transportation and weighted average housing costs) was $16,044, which was 113 percent of the official poverty threshold. For the same family with two adult earners (and hence higher work expenses and a need for child care), the resulting BNB was $21,132, or 149 percent of the official threshold.

Watts (1993) also proposed a categorical approach to the definition of poverty thresholds based largely on the work of Renwick and Bergmann. He concluded that the categorical approach is more feasible, understandable, and acceptable than either budgets with a large multiplier applied to only one or two categories or very detailed budgets.[15] Watts' proposal differs from the Renwick and Bergmann approach in a number of ways. First, he recommended that actual work-related transportation expenses be deducted from family resources rather than accounted for in the budget. Second, he argued that adequate medical insurance should be assumed for people with coverage. For households that lack such coverage, the cost of a standard insurance package should be deducted from resources. Employee contributions to medical insurance should also be deducted from resources. That is, the budget itself should only allow for estimated out-of-pocket medical costs (other than premiums). Third, since child care is an expense of work, he recommended that it too be deducted from resources. Fourth, he proposed that a new look be taken at the BLS family budget standards for clothing and personal care.

To develop what he termed a "modest proposal budget," Watts simply deducted the work and child care expense and medical insurance components from budget thresholds presented by Renwick (1993a). Implementing these calculations for 1992 produces a two-adult/two-child poverty threshold of $14,580, or 102 percent of the official threshold.

Watts' adaptation of the Renwick and Bergmann categorical budget approach has the advantage, in our judgment, of treating such expenses as child care that pertain to specific situations (namely, working) as deductions from family resources rather than as components of the budget. At the time Orshansky originally developed her thresholds, the treatment of such a category as child care expenses was largely not an issue because most families with

---

[15] Watts also found attractive the feature of the BNB approach that a budget is developed explicitly for each family type (in terms of the number of adults and children) rather than by applying a formal equivalence scale. We believe, however, that this feature is problematic, just as it is problematic for the official thresholds (see Chapter 3).

children had a parent at home to provide care. Today, many working families need to pay sometimes sizable amounts for child care in order to earn income. It seems preferable to deduct actual expenses from the income of those who pay for child care rather than to develop separate budgets for working families who pay for day care, working families who do not, and nonworking families. It also seems preferable to deduct from families' resources their actual out-of-pocket medical care expenses, which vary widely across the population (see Chapter 4 on these points).

In comparing the categorical approach with the multiplier approach, the categorical method does not require setting a multiplier; also, it does not allow changes in the multiplier to drive the behavior of the thresholds over time. On the negative side, the categorical approach requires making a larger number of individual judgments about standards (e.g., how many family members should be expected to share a bedroom or whether to provide for disposable diapers or assume that the family has a washing machine). One can anticipate disagreements about the assumptions for each category and also the particular dollar levels that are chosen.

Detailed Budget Approaches

Extensive work on detailed budgets has been done abroad; one example is the work of the York Family Budget Unit in the United Kingdom. The United States also has experience with detailed budgets, most recently through the BLS Family Budgets Program.[16]

York Family Budget Unit

The Family Budget Unit of York was established in 1985 to conduct research on the cost of living throughout the United Kingdom and on the economic requirements and consumer preferences of families of different compositions. The research on budget standards has sought to construct a series of "modest-but-adequate" and "low-cost" budgets for families in the United Kingdom, develop a means of updating the budgets, explore the relationship between living levels, develop equivalence scales from the budgets, and assess the practical and political applications of the budgets approach (Bradshaw, 1991).

In developing the modest-but-adequate budget, the York analysts included such items as durable goods that were owned by more than half of the population. For the low-cost budget, they included items that more than two-thirds of the population viewed as "necessary" or that were owned by at least 75 percent of the population (Yu, 1992). The budgets comprise amounts

---

[16] Extensive work on expert (or "standard") budgets was done in the United States from 1900 to 1940, although mostly outside the federal government (see Fisher, 1993).

for housing, which include shelter costs, fuel (with slightly higher allowances in the modest budget), interior decoration, and maintenance (the latter only in the modest budget); food at home, food away from home, and alcohol (the latter two categories in the modest budget only); clothing; household goods and services (including such things as furniture, kitchenware, stationery, postage, telephone services, and dry cleaning); personal care; medical care; transportation; leisure goods and services (including such goods as a television, sporting equipment, toys, Christmas decorations, and such services as home-based activities, sport and physical exercise, and social and cultural activities). Standards were drawn from a combination of government standards (e.g., for housing) and expenditure patterns.

BLS Family Budgets Program

The modern BLS Family Budgets Program had its origins in a 1945 directive from the Committee on Appropriations of the U.S. House of Representatives for BLS to determine how much it cost workers' families in large U.S. cities to live. Since the turn of the century, private groups and some local and state agencies had developed detailed budgets for various types of families and geographic locations (generally individual cities), for such purposes as determining relief payments and government pay scales. A few such budgets were also developed by BLS and later the Works Progress Administration (WPA) (see Expert Committee on Family Budget Revisions, 1980; Fisher, 1993). After World War II, Congress wanted BLS to revamp the old WPA budgets, and this resulted in a series of budgets. In 1948 BLS published a "modest but adequate" budget for 1946 for urban working families, priced separately for 34 cities. In 1960 BLS published a revision of this budget for 1959, which was derived using data from the 1950 CEX. In 1967 BLS published a further revision of the budget for 1966, which it termed a "moderate living standard" and derived using data from the 1960-1961 CEX. Finally, in 1969, BLS published a revision of the moderate budget for 1967 (also derived using 1960-1961 CEX data), together with higher and lower budgets developed by scaling the moderate budget up and down.[17] Between revisions, the budgets were repriced by using augmented price data collected for the CPI, or, after 1966, by using changes in the appropriate components of the CPI (see Bureau of Labor Statistics, 1969; Sherwood, 1977). In 1981 BLS discontinued the Family Budgets Program for lack of funds to improve it.

BLS initially developed the higher, moderate (or intermediate), and lower budget levels for two family types: a four-person family with a husband aged 38 and employed full-time, a homemaker wife (with no age specified), a girl of 8, and a boy of 13; and a retired couple aged 65 or over in reasonably good

---

[17] The moderate budget was later termed the intermediate budget level.

health. Budget levels for other family types were set by the use of an equivalence scale (see Chapter 3). BLS also varied the budgets by region of the country and size of area, publishing budgets over the years for 25-40 specific urban areas, together with regional averages. Examples of geographic differences included an assumption of use of public transportation in larger cities, different foodstuffs reflecting regional variations in food-buying patterns, and adjustments in utility costs for climate differences.

The detailed family budgets included food, transportation, clothing, personal care, medical care, and specific other consumption items, gifts and contributions, and occupational expenses. The budgets also allowed for income and payroll taxes. The food-at-home allowance for the intermediate budget was based on USDA's Moderate-Cost Food Plan. The housing component was based on recommendations on number of rooms, essential household equipment, adequate utilities, and neighborhood location, originally made by the American Public Health Association and the U.S. Public Housing Administration. The intermediate budget used the average for the middle third of the distribution of housing prices for houses and apartments meeting the designated requirements.

For additional components of the budget for which no expert standards had been developed—such as food away from home, furniture, transportation, clothing, personal care items, medical care, reading and recreational materials, education, tobacco, alcohol, gifts and contributions, life insurance, and miscellaneous consumption items—BLS used a statistical procedure known as the quantity-income-elasticity (q-i-e) technique. This method attempted to determine at what point an increase in income resulted in a decrease in the rate at which expenditures rose for each category of goods. This technique "sought to determine the income level at which elasticity, defined as the percentage change in the quantity purchased divided by the percentage change in income, reached a maximum. The associated quantities were then used to form the budget list" (Expert Committee on Family Budget Revisions, 1980:21). The results of applying the q-i-e method, however, were often uninterpretable, and the BLS analysts ultimately had to use their judgment to set budget levels. Generally, each time that the moderate or intermediate budget was revised, the budget level equated closely to median family income.

To develop the lower budget, BLS adapted the intermediate budget in several ways. For food at home, BLS used the USDA Low-Cost Food Plan (the second lowest cost of the four USDA plans). For housing, it used the mean contract rent for the bottom third of rental units that met specified requirements (excluding all owned units). For the items for which no standard existed and the q-i-e approach was used, BLS generally derived the lower budget from the income interval below the interval in which maximum elasticity was estimated to have occurred. As a whole, the lower budget amounted to about two-thirds of the intermediate budget.

In 1981, the last year for which BLS published family budget estimates (Bureau of Labor Statistics, 1982:Table A), the lower level budget for urban four-person families excluding taxes was $19,587 (in 1992 dollars), or 138 percent of the official poverty threshold for a two-adult/two-child family. Excluding gifts, contributions, insurance, and work expenses, the lower budget was $18,629, or 131 percent of the official poverty threshold.

Schwarz and Volgy Budget

Schwarz and Volgy (1992:Table 4) took an approach similar to, although less detailed than, the original BLS Family Budgets Program to develop an "economy budget" for a family of two adults and two children for 1990. Their market basket of goods contains those things that they consider to be "basic necessities," defined as goods and services directly and indirectly necessary to sustain life and health. Direct necessities include food, medical care, housing, clothing, and personal care and cleaning products. Indirect necessities include transportation, clothing adequate for employment of the adults and for school for the children, and such smaller items as school supplies and postage stamps. They also included items needed to participate in the wider community and express one's feelings, such as a telephone, a television, newspapers, stationery, and a gift fund. Their budget allows for the payment of federal and state income taxes and Social Security contributions.

The food component of the budget was based on the USDA Thrifty Food Plan. The housing component used the Department of Housing and Urban Development's fair market rent standard, based on the 45th percentile of two-bedroom rental units in an area that met specified characteristics. Transportation and medical care were based on national averages. Allowances for additional items, such as clothes, toys and presents, dishes, utensils, bedding, and used furniture, as well as other personal items and incidentals, appear to be based solely on the authors' judgments.

The resulting budget constructed by Schwarz and Volgy for a four-person family for 1990, including payroll and state and federal income taxes, was $22,176 in 1992 dollars; excluding taxes, the budget was $18,983. These figures are, respectively, 156 percent and 133 percent of the official four-person poverty line.

Conclusions

Detailed budgets avoid the problem of specifying a multiplier, which is inevitably done by reference to actual expenditure patterns. Such budgets, however, entail a myriad of judgments about many different goods and services. Moreover, inevitably such judgments also make reference to actual spending patterns as opposed to strictly physiologically based standards of need. This is true even when the budget makers adopt expert standards from another source, such as the USDA food plans or HUD fair market rents: we have seen the elements of relativity (and, indeed, political considerations) that enter into those standards.

BLS attempted to introduce some objectivity into standards for such commodities as clothing by the q-i-e approach, which assumed that the point at which the rate of increase in expenditures on the commodity relative to income slowed down was the point at which families no longer "needed" so much of the item. For most categories for which this approach was initially applied, however, there was no such inflection point or it came at a level that was not believable. Moreover, it is unclear whether the theory underlying this approach can be rigorously defended (see Expert Committee on Family Budget Revisions, 1980:30-34, for a detailed critique). Again, the BLS analysts had to make their own judgments, which, again, inevitably referred to actual spending patterns.

Updating for Price Changes

Until a new budget standard is adopted, expert budgets are usually updated for price changes to keep the dollar levels constant in real terms. An important issue in deciding to maintain a poverty line as an absolute standard—whether the line is originally developed from an expert budget or from another concept—is what type of price index to use. We have used values of the CPI-U (the Consumer Price Index for urban consumers) to express poverty thresholds developed under various methods for earlier years in constant 1992 dollars, because the original official poverty thresholds have historically been updated by the CPI-U, and we wanted to maintain the real dollar relationship between the 1963 two-adult/two-child family threshold of about $3,100 and the 1992 threshold of $14,228. But our purpose is purely illustrative.

For use in maintaining an absolute poverty standard, one can argue for other price indexes. Historically, the CPI-U overestimated inflation due to its treatment of housing costs, although this problem was corrected in the last revision, introduced beginning in 1983.[18] For years prior to 1983, BLS developed an experimental index, CPI-U-X1, which closely approximates the methodology of the current, improved CPI-U.[19] If a combination of the

---

[18] Prior to 1983, the measurement included changes in the asset value of homes; subsequently, it was modified to consider just the consumption aspects of home ownership by measuring changes in the equivalent rental costs for owned homes (see Bureau of the Census, 1993a:Appendix H). It is likely that, for other reasons, the CPI-U still overestimates inflation, but the extent is not known.

[19] The CPI-U-X1 shows less inflation prior to 1983 than the CPI-U (particularly in the period 1978-1981, when sale prices of housing were rising significantly faster than equivalent rental costs). Values of the CPI-U-X1 have been created back to 1947, although for years prior to 1967 they are not an actual calculation using the BLS procedures, but a ratio adjustment to the CPI-U; see Bureau of the Census (1993b: Table B-1).

CPI-U-X1 and CPI-U for the years before and after 1983 had been used to update the official poverty thresholds, then the threshold for a two-adult/two-child family in 1992 would have been $13,082, or 92 percent of the official threshold for that year.

If the poverty thresholds had continued to be updated by the cost of the Economy Food Plan (as occurred prior to 1969), the thresholds would also have increased less than has been the case with the CPI-U: the two-adult/two-child threshold in 1992 would have been $13,072, or 92 percent of the official 1992 threshold.[20]

The use of a Consumer Price Index specific to the low-income population has sometimes been discussed (see, e.g., King, 1976). Low-income people have different consumption patterns from high-income people: they spend a larger fraction of their budgets on necessities and a smaller fraction on luxury goods. Hence, if the relative prices of necessities and luxuries change over time, as has happened in some periods in the past, the use of the CPI will not give an accurate picture of real adjustments for poor people. In practice, however, the use of a low-income price index would probably not have made much of a difference over the period from 1963 to 1992 taken as a whole. (As we have noted, the cost of the Economy/Thrifty Food Plan increased about as much over this period as the overall CPI-U-X1.) Hence, we believe that work on a low-income price index is not a priority, although circumstances might arise in the future that could make it advisable to investigate the issue further. (To develop a reliable low-income price index could require improvements to both the CEX and the BLS price database.) We note that our proposed updating method has the advantage of relying very little on a price index: the only use of an index is to express the expenditure data for the prior 3 years that will be used to develop each year's reference family threshold in current dollars.

RELATIVE THRESHOLDS

Relative poverty thresholds—thresholds that are derived from the outset in a relative fashion—are based on comparing the income or consumption of a family to that of other typical families. The relative approach, as commonly implemented, designates a point in the distribution of income or expenditures to serve as the poverty line for a reference family. (Thresholds for other family types are developed by use of an equivalence scale.) Although a relative threshold, once chosen, could be kept constant in real dollars over a period of

---

[20] This is derived from changes in the cost of the Economy and Thrifty Food Plans, 1963-1992: the 1963 cost figure is from Ruggles (1990:Table A.4); the 1992 cost figure is from unpublished tables provided by the Food and Nutrition Service, U.S. Department of Agriculture.

years (i.e., be turned into an absolute threshold), relative thresholds are usually updated automatically on the basis of new information about the distribution of income or expenditures.

The conceptual argument that is often made for relative thresholds is that people are social beings and operate within relationships. Full participation within those relationships and within society requires that they "fit in" with others. Those whose resources are significantly below the resources of other members of society, even if they are able to eat and physically survive, are not able to participate adequately in their relationships, and therefore are not able to participate fully in society.[21] A relative approach to deriving poverty thresholds recognizes the social nature of economic deprivation and provides a way to keep the poverty line up to date with overall economic changes in a society.

There are several advantages to relative thresholds. First, they are easy to understand and fairly easy to calculate. Indeed, convenience is often as important a reason for choosing a relative approach as is any theoretical argument. The convenience factor is particularly compelling in the case of international comparisons of poverty, for which it can be difficult to develop comparable expert budgets or other types of poverty thresholds for different countries. Second, relative thresholds are explicitly arbitrary. They do not represent any type of budget, but simply a point in the distribution of income or expenditures. That point is usually one-half the median. As we have seen, expert budgets have large elements of relativity and judgment in them, but are typically couched as representing something more objective. Third, relative thresholds are self-updating, so their use avoids the need for periodic—and often controversial—reassessments of budgets or other types of thresholds to determine if they need to be revised for other than price changes.

Yet the very advantages that some find in the relative, arbitrary, and self-updating features of relative thresholds are drawbacks to others. For example, some argue that relative thresholds offer too much of a moving target for policy makers attempting to ameliorate poverty. Such arguments can be overstated—it is not, as is sometimes said, impossible to reduce poverty with a relative threshold. If the reference family threshold is defined as a percentile of the distribution of income or expenditures (e.g., the 25th or 35th percentile), that would be true. By definition, 25 or 35 percent of the population is always below the 25th or 35th percentile. However, if relative thresholds are defined as a percentage of the median value (as is commonly done), then it is possible to reduce poverty, and this seems the appropriate approach. Defined in such terms, relative thresholds will move with the median (as, indeed, expert budgets tend to move, although sporadically rather than on a continuous basis).

---

[21] See Townsend (1992) for an argument that poverty has a social as well as a physical dimension and, furthermore, that people evaluate their own situation in relation to others, not by reference to an absolute standard of need.

But changes in the distribution of income or expenditures below the median can lower the poverty rate even when the median value (and hence the value of the poverty line as a fixed percent of the median) increases.

However, there are serious concerns about the behavior of relative thresholds over time, not only in periods of economic growth but also in periods of recession or depression, when relative thresholds may decline in real terms. Many people are uncomfortable with a poverty measure that could possibly show a lower poverty rate in a recession that makes everyone worse off or that could fail to show a decrease in the rate in response to a policy change that makes everyone better off, including the poor. While decreases in relative thresholds in real terms will not necessarily lead to decreases in the poverty *rate* (just as increases in the thresholds in real terms will not necessarily lead to increases in the rate), it may be difficult to explain and justify frequent changes in the thresholds that are not simply a reflection of price changes.

International Examples

The United States is one of the few developed countries with an official poverty measure (see Will, 1986), but many countries and international organizations have undertaken poverty measurement. Often, individual countries use their benefit standards for public assistance programs as unofficial poverty lines. For comparative work across countries, however, poverty thresholds are often defined in relative terms. Thus, the Social Indicator Development Program of the Organization for Economic Cooperation and Development (OECD) includes an indicator of "material deprivation" in its list of 33 indicators. That indicator defines households facing material deprivation as those with incomes or expenditures below a proportion of median disposable (i.e., after-tax, after-transfer) household income, adjusted for differences in household composition (Organization for Economic Cooperation and Development, 1982). No suggestion is made for the specific proportion of median income below which a household would be considered materially deprived.

Work by the European Community to compare poverty rates among member nations has often used relative poverty thresholds. As an example, O'Higgins and Jenkins (1990) at the request of the European Commission worked with consultants from each member country to develop comparable poverty estimates for 1980 and 1985. O'Higgins and Jenkins specified poverty thresholds at 40, 50, and 60 percent of average equivalent disposable income of households. This represents household income adjusted by means of an equivalence scale to produce a threshold for one-person households, with thresholds for households of other sizes developed by means of the same scale.[22]

---

[22] The adjusting procedure works as follows: if the equivalence scale says that families of four need two (or three) times as much income or consumption to sustain the same living standard as

The United Kingdom recently began to publish estimates of the proportion of households with incomes below various proportions of average income. Analysts most commonly cite the estimates based on 50 percent of average income, using them in place of the earlier practice of using the welfare benefit ("supplementary benefit") standard as an unofficial poverty line (Johnson and Webb, 1992).

In Canada, Statistics Canada has for a number of years published a time series of statistics on the low-income population that is similar to a poverty rate series. The determination of low-income status has been based on a set of "low income cut-offs" (LICOs), which were developed by means of a hybrid approach that involved a set of quite complex procedures (Wolfson and Evans, 1989). The LICOs were developed by first determining the average expenditure of all families on food, shelter, and clothing as a percent of gross income. To this percentage was added an arbitrary 20 percentage points. Then, log-linear curves were fit between food, shelter, and clothing on one side and before-tax income on the other, taking account of variations in family size and urbanization (size of community).[23] Finally, on the basis of these curves, the LICO for each family type that corresponded to the designated proportion of spending on food, shelter, and clothing was determined.

The idea behind the LICOs, originally developed by Jennie Podoluk on the basis of a 1959 Survey of Family Expenditures, was that families spending more than the specified proportion on "necessities" (i.e., the average proportion plus 20 percentage points) were constrained in their spending on other items and hence could be considered "low income." The LICOs were revised subsequently on the basis of new expenditure data for 1969 and 1978.[24] The "straitened circumstances" proportion (i.e., the average plus 20 percentage points spent on food, shelter, and clothing) was estimated at 70 percent of income in 1959, 62 percent in 1969, and 58.5 percent in 1978, thus adjusting the LICOs for changes in real consumption. Between revisions, the LICOs were adjusted for price changes. The approach is a hybrid in that it refers to specific types of goods as necessities but determines the key parameter for the

---

a single person, then the income (or expenditures) of four-person families would be divided by two (or three) to produce a per capita equivalent amount, and so on for other family sizes. Median or average adjusted income for one-person households would then be produced from the distribution of equivalent per capita amounts. This procedure can be adapted to set a reference threshold for any size family. Thus, for a four-person reference family, income amounts for other families would be converted to four-person equivalent amounts (e.g., the income for a single person would be multiplied by two or three, depending on the ratio of the equivalence scale value for a four-person family to that for a single person).

[23] This curve-fitting approach is similar to the Engel or iso-prop method of developing equivalence scales; see Chapter 3 for a critique.

[24] Most recently, the LICOs were revised on the basis of 1986 expenditure data (see Statistics Canada, 1991:App.).

procedure (the maximum proportion spent on necessities) by reference to actual spending patterns, so that both that proportion and the implicit allowance in the LICOs for other spending are determined in a relative manner.[25]

Recently, Statistics Canada decided to publish another series, on an experimental basis, in which the determination of low-income status is based on a set of "low-income measures" or LIMs, which are derived in an explicitly relative manner (Statistics Canada, 1991:App.; see also Wolfson and Evans, 1989, who reviewed a range of alternative measures, including LIMs). The decision to add this series (and possibly in the future to publish it as the main or preferred series) stemmed mainly from Statistics Canada's conclusion that no type of low-income measure is clearly superior to others and that all measures have arbitrary components. In that agency's view, it seems best to minimize the number of arbitrary judgments and to make them as clear and explicit as possible.

Wolfson and Evans (1989) note that a relative measure can be tied to a number of national measures, such as an average wage index, per capita gross domestic product (GDP), median consumption or expenditures, or median family income. Statistics Canada chose to tie the Canadian measure to median family income adjusted for family size by means of an equivalence scale, setting one-half the median as the low-income line. Although an average wage index is a reasonable indicator of changes in the average income per person, it fails to account for the trend toward an increasing number of wage earners per family and decreasing family size. Average per capita GDP (or personal income or consumption from the national accounts) has a similar failing. Additionally, GDP is subject to historical revisions and includes non-household income. Median adjusted family income, in contrast, directly measures family income and adjusts for the needs of families of different sizes through an equivalence scale. (Median adjusted family consumption or expenditures could also be used, but expenditure surveys are conducted only periodically in Canada, while income surveys are conducted annually.)

U.S. Expert Committee on Family Budget Revisions

The Expert Committee on Family Budget Revisions (1980), when assigned the job of assessing the BLS Family Budgets Program (described above), recommended abandoning the budgets that had been built commodity by commodity and substituting a relative set of standards. The committee asserted that a scientific basis does not exist by which to develop commodity-

---

[25] A variant of the approach used to develop the LICOs is based on the idea that the smaller the proportion of total income that is spent on necessities, the better off the household is. Hence, a maximum on the proportion of total income that is devoted to fixed costs (such as food and shelter) is designated as the poverty threshold. For an application of this approach in the Netherlands, see Hagenaars and De Vos (1988).

based budgets. It also argued that actual consumption levels are the best indicator of living standards and that overall levels of expenditure—rather than expenditure shares on specific items—represent the appropriate focus, given that consumers differ in their preferences and can and do adjust their spending patterns for price changes.

The committee recommended that a "prevailing living standard" be established as the median of after-tax expenditures for the reference family of two adults and two children (with the standard for other family types determined by means of an equivalence scale) and that the prevailing standard be updated annually with new expenditure data.[26] Three other standards would depend on the prevailing standard: the "social abundance standard" would be 50 percent above the prevailing standard; the "lower living standard" would be two-thirds of the prevailing standard; and the "social minimum standard" would be one-half the prevailing standard. To make more concrete to the public what levels of living these various standards represented, the committee recommended that breakdowns of expenditures for different family types be developed, corresponding to the total spending level for each standard. Furthermore, the committee recommended that, when possible, illustrations be provided of lists of goods and quantities that could be afforded within each expenditure category.

The social minimum standard for a two-adult/two-child family recommended by the committee for 1979 (representing one-half median after-tax expenditures) was $15,584 in 1992 dollars, or 110 percent of the official 1992 two-adult/two-child poverty threshold (Expert Committee on Family Budget Revisions, 1980:Table IV-1). For 1991, the social minimum standard would be $19,987 in 1992 dollars, or 140 percent of the official threshold (Bureau of the Census, 1993d:Table 708).[27]

Issues in Deriving Relative Thresholds

There are a number of issues in deriving relative poverty thresholds from data on family (or household) income (or expenditures) that make them somewhat less straightforward to calculate than might appear. One issue concerns the type of adjustment to make for family size in determining the threshold for the reference family (an equivalence scale is always used to determine thresholds for other family types). Sometimes 50 percent (or another percent) of median income of all families is used as the threshold for a reference four-person

---

[26] The level of the prevailing standard for the reference family as of 1979 was about 105 percent of the BLS intermediate budget for that year, indicating that the BLS expert budget was very close to the median level of spending (Expert Committee on Family Budget Revisions, 1980:Table IV-1).

[27] This 1991 figure represents one-half average expenditures of four-person consumer units. Data are not available on one-half median expenditures of two-adult/two-child families.

family (see, e.g., U.S. House of Representatives, 1985). This approach, however, is problematic for updating the thresholds over time because of changes
in household and family composition. Thus, because of declining family size
in the United States—from 3.67 people in 1960 to 3.17 people in 1992—the
real median income of all families (before taxes) increased by 38 percent over
the period 1960-1992, but the real median income of four-person families
increased by 50 percent over the same period.[28]

Another approach is to apply an equivalence scale to the income amounts
for families or households in order to develop a per capita equivalent income
for the reference family (see, e.g., O'Higgins and Jenkins, 1990; Wolfson and
Evans, 1989). This approach takes account of changing household or family
size over time but is sensitive to the particular equivalence scale used. Still
another approach is to pick a reference family type and base the reference
poverty threshold on the distribution of income for those families. A possible
drawback to this approach, depending on the data source, is limited sample
size because information is used for only one family type.

Another issue concerns the definition of income (or expenditures). Occasionally, income is defined in before-tax terms; more typically, an after-tax
definition is used, which appropriately reflects the fact that families face different tax burdens. Rarely, however, do relative thresholds take account of other
important differences in nondiscretionary expenditures or charges against income. Thus, families who must pay for child care or incur other work
expenses to earn income are in a different position from families that do not
have those expenses. Although it may seem odd to introduce specific components (e.g., work expenses) into a relative measure, not doing so will distort
the comparison of poverty rates among important groups. Similarly, in the
absence of national health insurance in the United States, it is important to
recognize significant differences among families in their outlays for medical
care. Finally, it is important to recognize the receipt of in-kind benefits by
some families and not others. Any or all of these adjustments can be made by
developing separate thresholds for particular types of families (e.g., working
families with and without children and nonworking families) or by developing
a disposable money and near-money income definition of family resources.

---

[28] Data for family size figures come from Bureau of the Census (1993d:Table 65); for median
family income from Bureau of the Census (1982:Table 16; 1993b:Table 13); for median four-
person family income from Vaughan (1993:Table 1) and Bureau of the Census (1993b:Table
13). Comparisons in the text are made with all dollar figures expressed in constant 1992 CPI-U
dollars; comparisons with constant CPI-U-X1 dollars would show greater increases, but the
same relationship between trends in family and four-person family income. Also note that
family (or household) size changes can move in the opposite direction. Thus, average family
size increased in the United States from 3.5 persons in 1950 to 3.7 persons in 1965 (Bureau of
the Census, 1975:41).

We argue (see below and Chapter 4) that the latter course is more feasible and understandable.

Behavior of Relative Thresholds Over Time

Vaughan (1993) constructed time series from 1947 to 1989 of median four-person family income before and after taxes. We extended the two series to 1992 from Census Bureau data, converted all figures into constant 1992 dollars by using the CPI-U, and divided them by two; see Table 2-3. The resulting estimates of one-half median before-tax and after-tax four-person family income are problematic in some respects. Thus, some years are missing from Vaughan's series; also, Vaughan's procedures for estimating federal income and Social Security payroll taxes are rough.[29] Neither series takes account of in-kind income, although for defining poverty thresholds as a percentage of the median (as distinct from determining poverty status by comparing income to the thresholds), this is not such a problem—families at the median level do not generally receive such benefits as food stamps. In contrast, almost all two-adult/two-child families have one or more earners and hence pay taxes. Finally, neither series takes account of child care or other work expenses, which would have an effect on disposable income over time with the entry of more mothers into the work force.

Despite these problems, the two series provide some insights on the behavior of relative poverty thresholds over time. Table 2-3 shows that one-half median before-tax four-person family income increased over the period 1947-1992 in real terms from about $10,400 to about $22,300—an increase of 115 percent. The importance of taking taxes into account is evident in the fact that the estimated after-tax series increased only 86 percent over the same period. In relation to the official four-person family poverty threshold of $14,228 in 1992 dollars, both the before-tax and the after-tax series were considerably lower through about 1955, at about the same level through about 1965, and then well above that threshold thereafter. (The before-tax series

---

[29] Vaughan assumed that all four-person families represented a husband and wife filing jointly, with two dependents, with adjusted gross income equivalent to the observed before-tax median, all income from wage and salary earnings of only one worker, taking the standard deduction, and filing according to the tax law in effect in the particular year. For the years 1980-1986, he was able to use Census Bureau published estimates of after-tax income by before-tax income and household size, which are based on a detailed simulation of taxes (see, e.g., Bureau of the Census, 1988b). For 1989 he used unpublished estimates from the Census Bureau. Unfortunately, the Census Bureau's experimental income estimates, which exclude federal and state income tax and payroll tax from some resource definitions (see, e.g., Bureau of the Census, 1993a), are not helpful in estimating median after-tax income for four-person families. The estimates are not published by family size; also, the definitions are not clean in that other changes are made to income besides excluding taxes.

TABLE 2-3 Relative Poverty Thresholds for a Four-Person Family Derived as One-Half of Median Before-Tax and After-Tax Four-Person Family Income, 1947–1992, in Constant 1992 Dollars

| | One-Half Median Four-Person Family Income | | | |
| | Dollar Amount | | Percent of Official Threshold | |
Year	Before Taxes	After Taxes	Before Taxes	After Taxes
1947	10,356	9,695	72.8	68.1
1948	10,095	9,655	71.0	67.9
1949[a]	9,957	9,556	70.0	67.2
1950	10,697	10,106	75.2	71.0
1951	11,122	10,253	78.2	72.1
1952	11,576	10,530	81.4	74.0
1953[b]	11,631	10,567	81.7	74.3
1954[a,b]	12,431	11,258	87.4	79.1
1955	N.A.	N.A.	N.A.	N.A.
1956	N.A.	N.A.	N.A.	N.A.
1957	13,701	12,198	96.3	85.7
1958[a]	13,799	12,251	97.0	86.1
1959	14,633	12,866	102.8	90.4
1960	14,919	13,030	104.9	91.6
1961[a]	15,102	13,171	106.1	92.6
1962	15,693	13,635	110.3	95.8
1963	16,364	14,120	115.0	99.2
1964	16,945	14,858	119.1	104.4
1965	N.A.	N.A.	N.A.	N.A.
1966	18,059	15,660	126.9	110.1
1967	18,890	16,303	132.8	114.6
1968	N.A.	N.A.	N.A.	N.A.
1969	20,305	17,058	142.7	119.9
1970[a]	20,190	17,068	141.9	120.0
1971	20,137	17,238	141.5	121.2
1972	N.A.	N.A.	N.A.	N.A.
1973	21,661	18,236	152.2	128.2
1974	21,299	17,621	149.7	123.8
1975[a]	20,664	17,699	145.2	124.4
1976	21,347	17,807	150.0	125.2
1977	21,674	17,997	152.3	126.5
1978	21,978	18,098	154.5	127.2
1979	21,752	17,633	152.9	123.9
1980[a]	20,715	16,629	145.6	116.9
1981	20,277	15,991	142.5	112.4
1982[a]	20,078	15,975	141.1	112.3
1983	20,552	16,495	144.4	115.9
1984	20,995	16,768	147.6	117.9
1985	21,369	17,019	150.2	119.6
1986	22,220	17,626	156.2	123.9
1987	N.A.	N.A.	N.A.	N.A.
1988	N.A.	N.A.	N.A.	N.A.

TABLE 2-3   *Continued*

| | One-Half Median Four-Person Family Income | | | |
| | Dollar Amount | | Percent of Official Threshold | |
Year	Before Taxes	After Taxes	Before Taxes	After Taxes
1989	23,062	18,990	162.1	133.5
1990	22,249	N.A.	156.4	N.A.
1991[a]	22,174	N.A.	155.8	N.A.
1992	22,308	18,018	156.8	126.6

NOTES: Data for one-half median four-person family before-tax and after-tax income values for 1947-1989 derived from Vaughan (1993:Table 1); one-half median four-person family income before-tax values for 1990-1992 from Bureau of the Census (1993b:Table 13); one-half median four-person family income after-tax value for 1992 from the March 1993 CPS. All dollar values were converted to constant 1992 dollars using the CPI-U from Bureau of the Census (1993c:Table A-2); all percentages were calculated relative to the constant 1992 dollar value of $14,228 for the official two-adult/two-child poverty threshold (Bureau of the Census, 1993c:Table A).

[a]Year contained the low point of a recession as determined by the National Bureau of Economic Research (see Bureau of the Census, 1993b:B-1).

[b]Values estimated by Vaughan on the basis of the relationship between median income for families with two children and four-person families, 1947-1952 and 1955-1960.

went from 73% of the official threshold in 1947 to 157% of that threshold in 1992; the after-tax series went from 68% to 127% of the official threshold over the same period.)[30] These data indicate why the original 1963 threshold for a two-adult/two-child family was widely regarded as the right level for that time; such a figure, however, might well have been viewed as too high earlier in the post-World War II period, just as it has come under criticism by some as too low today.

Another clear finding is that relative thresholds are responsive to changes in the business cycle. In only one year over the entire period did the thresholds drop in *current* dollars (for the before-tax threshold in 1949). In *real* terms, however, they declined in most of the years that experienced recessionary conditions: for example, both the before-tax and the after-tax thresholds declined from 1979 to 1983, a period that included two recession years; they also declined during the most recent recession in 1990. In contrast, the before-tax and after-tax thresholds increased in real terms, sometimes to a considerable degree, in periods of economic growth.

---

[30] If the CPI-U-X1 is used to update the 1963 official threshold, then in 1992 the relative thresholds would exceed the official threshold by larger margins (the before-tax threshold would be about 171% and the after-tax threshold about 138% of the official threshold in 1992).

Again, there is no necessary relationship between a decline in the poverty threshold and a lower poverty rate or between an increase in the threshold and a higher rate (see Stephenson, 1977, on this point). Indeed, Wolfson and Evans (1989:52-53) found that poverty rates declined in Canada over the period 1967-1986, whether a relative updating method (based on adjusted median family income) or an absolute updating method (based on price inflation) was applied to the original LICOs. The decline was greater, however, for the absolute method. Also, during the recessionary conditions experienced in 1981-1986, poverty increased in Canada with either updating method, although the increase was greater for the absolute approach.[31]

If one believes that poverty thresholds must inevitably be adjusted for changes in real consumption, at least eventually, then a relative approach, which automatically updates the thresholds each year, has advantages. It will better preserve the continuity of time series over an approach that sporadically updates the thresholds. Nonetheless, the year-to-year variations in real terms exhibited by the relative poverty thresholds in Table 2-3 are disconcerting. To smooth out these variations, one suggestion is to develop the thresholds on a 3-year moving-average basis. Another suggestion, made by the Expert Committee on Family Budget Revisions (1980), is to take a "ratchet" approach, that is, to let the thresholds increase with real economic growth but not let them decline below the previous year's level in real terms.

SUBJECTIVE THRESHOLDS

An approach to defining poverty thresholds that has been the subject of considerable research, especially in Europe, makes use of public opinion data. Responses by samples of households to survey questions that ask for the minimum level of income or consumption needed by a certain type of household (or a household like theirs) to "get along" or to "make ends meet" are used to construct poverty thresholds, which are commonly labeled "subjective" thresholds.[32]

The subjective approach has the advantage that it obviates reliance on experts and relies instead on prevailing opinion in a society to set a poverty line for that society. There are many problems, however, in implementing a subjective approach, and the resulting thresholds must be interpreted with

---

[31] Similarly, Vaughan (1993:Table 1) estimated that the use of a subjective poverty threshold, which behaved in much the same manner over the post-World War II period as a relative threshold, would have produced a similar time trend of poverty rates as the official threshold. With the subjective threshold, poverty rates declined through the mid-1970s and then rose somewhat; poverty rates with the official threshold showed a similar but more pronounced decline followed by a similar but less pronounced increase.

[32] This label is unfortunate, given that all types of thresholds involve subjective elements.

caution. Research has found that subjective poverty thresholds vary significantly with the type of question and other differences in methodology. In the Netherlands, Flik and Van Praag (1991) developed estimates for several subjective poverty thresholds that varied by more than 200 percent. Some variation may be appropriate, to the extent that different questions carry different meanings, but research has also found significant variation with small modifications in question wording (see below). In general, little is known about how respondents interpret the questions—for example, whether they exclude taxes or include in-kind benefits in their responses.

Another problem is that estimates are often based on small sample sizes, which carry large standard errors. Although the standard errors can be reduced by increasing the sample size, the responses also often show wide variation around the mean. For example, a question in the 1993 General Social Survey about the weekly amount of a poverty line for a two-adult/two-child reference family (see below) elicited responses that averaged $341 per week, but they varied from as low as $25 to as high as $1,500 per week. The standard deviation was $167, or 49 percent of the mean—a high variation. (The range excludes two clear outlying responses of $5,000 and $7,000 per week.) Because of these characteristics of survey responses, it may be difficult to set an actual threshold using them with any confidence.

A quite different problem might arise if survey responses are known to be used to set official poverty thresholds: respondents might give different answers because of knowledge that the poverty line affects eligibility levels in a number of government assistance programs. More broadly, subjective responses may reveal more about underlying differences in expectations and current circumstances than about relative needs. For example, O'Hare et al. (1990) found that Hispanics gave answers to a question about the poverty line that were substantially lower than the answers of other groups. This result may have occurred simply because this group is constrained in income and consequently has lower expectations.

Research Findings

There has been extensive work on the development of subjective poverty thresholds, particularly by analysts in Europe (see, e.g., Flik and Van Praag, 1991; Goedhart et al., 1977; Hagenaars, 1986; Hagenaars and de Vos, 1988; Hagenaars and Van Praag, 1985; Van Praag, 1968; Van Praag, Dubnoff, and Van der Sar, 1988; Van Praag, Goedhart, and Kapteyn, 1980).[33] Analysts have sometimes used a single question on minimum income: "What do you consider an absolute minimum net income for a household such as yours?"

---

[33] Maritato (1992) provides a detailed review of the literature on subjective poverty measurement in Europe, Canada, and the United States.

Sometimes they have used a question evaluating income at multiple levels: "Under our conditions, I would call a net household income per week [or month or year] of about x very bad, bad, insufficient, sufficient, good, very good." One method uses a minimum income question together with a question on whether the household can, with its current income, make ends meet "with great difficulty, with difficulty, with some difficulty, rather easily, easily, or very easily." Analysts have also used different econometric techniques to estimate subjective poverty thresholds (or thresholds at various levels, including a poverty level and higher levels) from the survey responses. Typically, the methods try to take account of the influence of family size and the respondent's own income on these responses. Sometimes the estimation uses the data from only a subset of respondents, such as those who report that they can only make ends meet with their own income with some difficulty.

Work on subjective measures of poverty has also been done in the United States and Canada (see, e.g., Colasanto, Kapteyn, and Van der Gaag, 1984; Danziger et al., 1984; De Vos and Garner, 1991; Kilpatrick, 1973; Michalos, 1989; Morissette and Poulin, 1991; Poulin, 1988; Rainwater, 1974, 1992; Vaughan, 1993). The questions used in some of these studies asked respondents about the income needed for families similar to theirs to "make ends meet." But different question wordings have been used. For example, the question used by De Vos and Garner (1991) asked specifically about income needed before deductions, while the one used by Colasanto, Kapteyn, and Van der Gaag (1984) asked about after-tax income. The question used by Danziger et al. (1984) did not specify whether respondents were to answer in before-tax or in after-tax terms.

Although the variations in question wording were minor, the resulting estimated thresholds differ substantially.[34] De Vos and Garner (1991) estimated a poverty threshold (1982 CEX data) of $32,530 in 1992 dollars, or 229 percent of the official 1992 two-adult/two-child poverty threshold. Danziger et al. (1984) estimated a four-person family poverty threshold (with 1980 data from the 1979 Income Survey Development Program Research Panel) of $24,680 in 1992 dollars, or 173 percent of the official 1992 threshold. In contrast, Colasanto, Kapteyn, and Van der Gaag (1984) (with data from the 1981 Wisconsin Basic Needs Study) estimated a four-person family subjective threshold of only $12,160 in 1992 dollars, or 85 percent of the official 1992 threshold. The question analyzed by Colasanto, Kapteyn, and Van der Gaag specifically asked about after-tax income; also, their data source was limited to a single state (Wisconsin).

It seems clear that a good deal more work is needed before the approach of using survey responses to derive poverty thresholds could be seriously considered for an official measure. If such responses were available over time

---

[34] There were also differences in estimation methodology.

on a consistent basis, however, they could provide useful information with which to evaluate the official methodology for updating the thresholds.

Behavior of Subjective Thresholds Over Time

In the United States there are data available with which to derive subjective thresholds on a reasonably consistent basis. The Gallup Poll has asked samples of adults the following question for most years between 1946 and 1989: "What is the smallest amount of money a family of four (husband, wife and two children) needs each week to get along in this community?" Vaughan (1993) assembled the results from the Gallup Poll and various other sources for years between 1947 and 1989, converting the average weekly amounts to average yearly amounts.[35]

At the request of the panel, Gallup included the same get-along question in its August 1992 poll, and we included the average weekly amount (converted to an annual basis) with Vaughan's numbers; see Table 2-4. The resulting time series indicates that the get-along amount has increased over time (in constant 1992 dollars): from a level of about the same as that of the official 1992 two-adult/two-child poverty threshold in the period 1947-1950 to well above that threshold subsequently, reaching 176 percent of the threshold by 1992. In other words, the Gallup get-along amount has increased with increases in real income. It also seems to clearly represent a higher level than a poverty standard (but still below median income). In this regard, the fact that the get-along amount and the official poverty threshold were about the same in the late 1940s suggests that the poverty line, which was viewed as about "right" when it was adopted in the 1960s, would have been viewed as too high earlier in the post-World War II period.

In 1989 the Gallup Poll asked the get-along question in May, and then in July-October asked separate samples of adults a question designed specifically to elicit poverty levels: "People who have income below a certain level can be considered poor. That level is called the 'poverty line.' What amount of weekly income would you use as a poverty line for a family of four (husband, wife, and two children) in this community?" Vaughan used the relationship between the average of the poverty responses and the average of the get-along responses in 1989 (the ratio of the two means was 71.8%) to construct a series of subjective poverty thresholds for the period 1947-1989 from the get-along data.

At the request of the panel, Gallup included the poverty question in its August 1992 poll; the average poverty amount was 62.8 percent of the

---

[35] For some years, only medians are readily available. Ordinarily, one would prefer medians to means; however, in the early years of the Gallup series, there is evidence of instability in the medians due to rounding of amounts by respondents. Also, median figures published by Gallup are limited to nonfarm households.

TABLE 2-4 Subjective Poverty Thresholds for a Four-Person Family Derived from Survey Data, 1947–1993, in Constant 1992 Dollars

| | Average of Responses to Survey Questions | | | |
| | Dollar Amount, Four-Person Family | | Percent of Official Threshold | |
Year	"Get-Along" Level	"Poverty" Level	"Get-Along" Level	"Poverty" Level
1947	14,785	10,620	103.9	74.6
1948	15,718	11,288	110.5	79.3
1949[a]	15,244	10,947	107.1	76.9
1950	14,525	10,432	102.1	73.3
1951	15,433	11,084	108.5	77.9
1952	17,069	12,256	120.0	86.1
1953	16,342	11,734	114.9	82.5
1954[a]	17,316	12,434	121.7	87.4
1955	N.A.	N.A.	N.A.	N.A.
1956	N.A.	N.A.	N.A.	N.A.
1957	19,412	13,945	136.4	98.0
1958[a]	20,744	14,894	145.8	104.7
1959	20,809	14,941	146.3	105.0
1960	20,097	14,433	141.2	101.3
1961[a]	20,308	14,584	142.7	102.5
1962	20,083	14,420	141.2	101.4
1963	19,844	14,250	139.5	100.2
1964	20,086	14,424	141.2	101.3
1965	N.A.	N.A.	N.A.	N.A.
1966	21,842	15,684	153.5	110.2
1967	24,246	17,411	170.4	122.4
1968	N.A.	N.A.	N.A.	N.A.
1969	23,457	16,844	164.9	118.4
1970[a]	23,692	17,013	166.5	119.6
1971	24,499	17,591	172.2	123.6
1972	N.A.	N.A.	N.A.	N.A.
1973	24,483	17,582	172.1	123.6
1974	25,009	17,960	175.8	126.2
1975[a]	21,833	15,678	153.5	110.2
1976	23,976	17,218	168.5	121.0
1977	23,958	17,204	168.4	120.9
1978	24,505	17,597	172.2	123.7
1979	24,520	17,607	172.3	123.8
1980[a]	22,135	15,895	155.6	111.7
1981	24,400	17,522	171.5	123.2
1982[a]	22,983	16,505	161.5	116.0
1983	23,073	16,569	162.2	116.5
1984	23,452	16,841	164.8	118.4
1985	23,663	16,992	166.3	119.4
1986	24,230	17,399	170.3	122.3
1987	N.A.	N.A.	N.A.	N.A.
1988	N.A.	N.A.	N.A.	N.A.

TABLE 2-4 *Continued*

| | Average of Responses to Survey Questions | | | |
| | Dollar Amount, Four-Person Family | | Percent of Official Threshold | |
Year	"Get-Along" Level	"Poverty" Level	"Get-Along" Level	"Poverty" Level
1989	24,653	17,703	173.3	124.4
1990	N.A.	N.A.	N.A.	N.A.
1991[a]	N.A.	N.A.	N.A.	N.A.
1992	25,028	15,714	175.9	110.4
1993	N.A.	17,228	N.A.	121.1

NOTES: "Get-along" levels for 1947-1989 are from Gallup Poll data assembled by Vaughan (1993:Table 1). Get-along amounts for most years are mean weekly responses, annualized on the basis of a 52-week, 364-day year. Get-along amounts for 1970, 1973, 1975, 1977, and 1980 are median amounts for persons in nonfarm households. See Vaughan (1993) for more details on sources. "Poverty" levels for 1947–1989 are from Vaughan (1993:Table 1), derived by assuming a constant relationship of the poverty amount to the get-along amount of 71.8 percent. (This level was observed in 1989, when, in addition to asking one sample the get-along question, the Gallup Poll asked separate samples a question on the poverty level; see O'Hare, 1990, and O'Hare et al., 1990:18.) See text for wording of the get-along and poverty questions.

Get-along and poverty levels for 1992 are from Gallup Poll questions administered to the same sample of persons (sample size of 901); amounts are annualized mean weekly responses (derived from tabulations provided to the panel). The poverty level for 1993 is from the General Social Survey (sample size of 1,385) of the National Opinion Research Center; amounts are annualized mean weekly responses (derived from tabulations provided to the panel, excluding two outliers).

All dollar values were converted to constant 1992 dollars using the CPI-U from Bureau of the Census (1993c:Table A-2); all percentages were calculated relative to the constant 1992 dollar value of $14,228 for the official two-adult/two-child poverty threshold (Bureau of the Census, 1993c:Table A).

[a]Year contained the low point of a recession as determined by the National Bureau of Economic Research (see Bureau of the Census, 1993b:B-1).

average get-along amount in that survey. Because the two questions were administered to the same respondents in 1992 (instead of to different samples as in 1989), the lower ratio in 1992 may stem from the influence of respondents' get-along answers, elicited first, on their poverty answers. Most recently, in 1993, also at our request, the General Social Survey administered the poverty question (but not the get-along question).[36] Table 2-4 includes the

---

[36] The General Social Survey also included the poverty question for a family of three and a question on the minimum amount needed specifically for food. The Wisconsin Survey (a national telephone survey) also included both the get-along and the poverty questions in 1992 to the same respondents. The Wisconsin data are not strictly comparable, however, as the questions pertained to monthly rather than weekly amounts. Also, the sample size was very small—only 528 responses.

average weekly amounts (converted to an annual basis) for 1992 and 1993 with Vaughan's poverty numbers for 1947-1989.

The sample sizes are small in each year and, at least partly for this reason, the year-to-year changes in the estimated Gallup poverty level (and similarly in the get-along level) show considerable variation. Nonetheless, some clear patterns emerge. Most striking, the estimated poverty level from the Gallup Poll data shows about the same relationship to the official poverty threshold as does one-half the median after-tax four-person family income (compare with Table 2-3). Both of these series were below the official threshold through 1955, about the same as the official threshold through about 1965, and then above the official threshold.

It seems clear that subjective poverty thresholds respond to changes in real income or consumption, both up and down. For example, one can see dips in the Gallup get-along and poverty levels in real terms in periods of recession from the data in Table 2-4. One major question for poverty analysts is the time-series elasticity of subjective poverty thresholds with respect to changes in median income or consumption. If the elasticity is 1 or very close to 1 (i.e., if a percentage change in the threshold series is the same as the percentage change in the income series), one could argue for a strictly relative approach to updating poverty thresholds. If the elasticity is somewhat less than 1, one might prefer an updating method somewhere between a completely relative and an absolute approach.

Vaughan (1993:42) estimated the elasticity of the Gallup get-along series for 1947-1989 with respect to median after-tax four-person family income as 0.80 (using constant 1967 dollars and only the years for which means rather than medians were available). Not surprisingly, because of generally increasing taxes over the post-World War II period, Vaughan's estimate of the elasticity of the get-along series with respect to median *before-tax* four-person family income is lower, 0.65. With respect to average family income, Rainwater (1992) estimated the elasticity as 1.0 for the get-along series through 1986.[37] Maritato (1992), in a review of get-along responses in Canada over the period 1973-1985 presented in Michalos (1989), estimated the elasticity with respect to family income (whether mean or median) as 0.70.

CONCLUSIONS

We draw several conclusions from our review of alternative concepts that could be used to derive and update poverty thresholds for the United States. First, it is clear that all approaches involve judgments—whether in choosing a

---

[37] One reason for Rainwater's result may be his use of current dollars. If the elasticity is truly less than 1 and the correct regression is in real terms, then the estimated coefficient will be biased toward 1 if current dollars are used. Maritato also used current dollars.

particular distribution (e.g., income or expenditures and from which data set) and a particular cutoff point for a relative poverty threshold (it is only by convention that 50% of the median is the common cutoff); in choosing a particular question wording and estimation method (e.g., using the full set or a subset of respondents) for deriving a subjective poverty threshold from survey data; or in deriving the specifications for an expert budget. As a result, poverty thresholds developed by different applications of a particular approach (e.g., by different experts), as well as by different approaches, differ.

Second, it is clear that all concepts have large elements of relativity in them. In developing a poverty standard, some reference is invariably made to the living conditions of the particular time and place. Consequently, poverty thresholds constructed at different times tend to reflect real changes in consumption. This is true, by definition, of relative thresholds. And there is strong evidence that survey responses about poverty or minimum income levels are also relative to time and place: the time-series elasticities of subjective responses with respect to median income are high (although not 1.0).[38] Finally, on close inspection, it turns out that expert budgets—at the time of their development—are also relative. And while the practice is to update an expert budget for price changes until it is replaced by a new standard, the new standard typically takes account of the real changes in income or consumption since the old standard was set. For example, the post-World War II BLS family budgets, which were revised at about 10-year intervals, each time mirrored median levels of expenditure.

Table 2-5, which includes thresholds developed by several approaches, illustrates both of these points. Columns 1 and 2 list thresholds developed around 1980 and 1990, respectively (in 1992 dollars). The thresholds listed in each column vary, indicating the effects of different judgments about concepts, methods, and data. The thresholds also show relativity to time and place: for most thresholds for which comparable estimates are available for around 1980 and around 1990 (excluding the thresholds that are updated simply for price changes), the value (in 1992 dollars) increases from the earlier to the later year. (See also Table 2-1, which shows the large increases in real terms in the value of thresholds developed by the Orshansky multiplier method and those specified as 50 percent of median income over the period 1950 to 1992.)

Given the evidence of relativity in the way in which poverty thresholds are commonly derived, we conclude that the key point for consideration is not whether to treat poverty thresholds as absolute or relative, but, rather,

---

[38] In various countries, cross-sectional elasticities of respondents' answers about minimum income with respect to their own income have been estimated at 0.40 to 0.60 (see Maritato, 1992:Table 1), indicating that respondents in better-off societies will tend to set a higher poverty line than respondents in less wealthy countries.

TABLE 2-5   Examples of Poverty Thresholds for Four-Person Families Set by Various Methods for Years Around 1980 and 1990, in Constant 1992 Dollars

Type and Source of Threshold	Thresholds Set for Years Around 1980	Thresholds Set for Years Around 1990
Expert Budget Thresholds		
Official (Orshansky 1963 threshold indexed by CPI-U)	14,228	14,228
Orshansky 1963 threshold indexed by CPI-U-X1	13,082	13,082
Orshansky food multiplier developed from CEX data	16,163 (1980)	20,659 (1991)
Ruggles housing multiplier	21,331 (1980)	21,640 (1992)
Weinberg/Lamas food/housing multiplier—25th percentile	N.A.	20,267 (1989)
Weinberg/Lamas food/housing multiplier—35th percentile	N.A.	21,790 (1989)
BLS lower level budget	19,587 (1981)	N.A.
Renwick budget[a]	N.A.	17,600 (1992)
Schwarz and Volgy budget	N.A.	18,983 (1990)
Relative Thresholds		
Vaughan one-half median before-tax four-person family income	20,715 (1980)	22,308 (1992)
Vaughan one-half median after-tax four-person family income	16,629 (1980)	18,018 (1992)
Expert Committee on Family Budget Revisions social minimum	15,584 (1979)	19,987 (1991)[b]
Subjective Thresholds		
Vaughan "poverty"	15,895 (1980)	17,703 (1989)
General Social Survey "poverty"	N.A.	17,228 (1993)
Colasanto et al.	12,160 (1981)	N.A.
Danziger et al.[c]	24,680 (1980)	N.A.
De Vos and Garner[d]	32,530 (1982)	N.A.

SOURCE: See Tables 2-1, 2-2, 2-3, 2-4, and text.

NOTE: All thresholds are after-tax unless otherwise noted; dates in parentheses are the year for which the threshold was developed; all amounts are expressed in constant 1992 dollars using the CPI-U (except the second one, as noted).

[a]Renwick threshold calculated as weighted average of thresholds for two-adult/two-child families with one earner and two earners. (Weighting assumes that 75% of two-adult/two-child families have two earners and that one-third of those pay for day care.)

[b]Calculated as one-half average (rather than median) expenditures of four-person consumer units.

[c]Survey question did not specify whether respondents were to indicate minimum income level before or after taxes.

[d]Survey question asked respondents to indicate minimum income level before taxes.

how often to update them for real changes in living standards. We believe there are advantages to an automatic updating method over an approach that updates the thresholds at sporadic intervals. We also conclude that it is time to reconsider the current U.S. thresholds, which have been maintained in absolute terms for more than 30 years and rest on survey data that are almost 40 years old. We recommend a new concept and procedure for updating the U.S. poverty thresholds; however, given the element of judgment involved, we do not recommend an initial threshold for a two-adult/two-child family.

In considering concepts for a poverty threshold, we identified some attractive features of Orshansky's original multiplier method (and that of other expert budgets), in particular, the reference to specific needs (e.g., food). This feature produces poverty thresholds that have a normative cast, which we believe is likely to be more attractive to policy makers and the public than are thresholds developed by a purely relative approach (e.g., one-half median after-tax adjusted family income). But, in practice, the Orshansky multiplier approach is little different from a purely relative approach because the multiplier that is applied to the food budget (and essentially drives the thresholds) includes all spending—on luxuries as well as necessities—by the average family.

We believe a preferable approach is one that updates the thresholds in a conservative or quasi-relative manner—one that drives the thresholds by changes in spending on necessities that pertain to a concept of poverty rather than by changes in spending on all kinds of consumption. We also believe the bundle of necessities should include more than just food. However, to try to develop a detailed list seems an exercise in futility and likely to raise needless controversy. A good compromise, we concluded, is to specify a bundle of food, clothing, and shelter (including utilities) and apply a small, fixed multiple for other needed spending, such as personal care, household supplies, and non-work-related transportation.

Everyone agrees that food, clothing, and shelter are necessary goods and services (although the level of each that is needed is a matter of debate). These categories are evident in society's thinking about the needs of the poor, as evidenced in homeless shelters, soup kitchens, and winter clothing drives. The food, clothing, and shelter bundle also constitutes a large share of spending for the average family—45 percent in 1991 of total after-tax expenditures by four-person consumer units (Bureau of the Census, 1993d:Table 708). Most important, historically these items have behaved like necessities: that is, their combined elasticity with respect to total expenditures has been less than 1.0 (we estimate that elasticity at about 0.65 over the period 1959-1991).[39]

---

[39] This estimate is derived from data in the National Income and Product Accounts (NIPA) for 1959–1991, the log of personal consumption expenditures on the sum of food, clothing and shoes, housing, fuel oil and coal, and electricity and gas regressed on the log of total personal

More broadly, the basic concept—food, clothing, and shelter plus a little more— is as easy to understand as the original concept of food times a multiplier.

On the basis of the historical evidence, to update the poverty thresholds for real changes in expenditures on food, clothing, and shelter times a small, fixed multiple means that they will track real changes in total consumption but in a conservative manner. That is, the percentage changes in the thresholds will lag somewhat behind the percentage changes in total expenditures and so will lag somewhat behind the change in a purely relative measure, such as one-half median income (or the Orshansky approach). We find justification for a conservative approach to updating the thresholds from the behavior of subjective thresholds over time, which clearly move with real growth in living standards (hence, outstripping inflation), but on a less than 1-for-1 basis (most estimates range from 0.65 to 0.80). This conservative approach may also be more acceptable to policy makers and the public than making a complete switch from the absolute procedure used to update the official thresholds over the past 30 years to a purely relative procedure.

Although we propose to relate the U.S. poverty thresholds to specific goods (food, clothing, and shelter), we do not propose to have the budget levels for these goods set on the basis of expert standards (e.g., for a certain type of diet or dwelling). We believe it is preferable to turn directly to actual expenditure data as the basis for setting the levels. This approach makes explicit both the judgment and the relativity that are inherent in all of the methods for deriving poverty thresholds that we have reviewed (including expert budgets). Also, with this approach it is more feasible to implement changes on an annual basis than would be an approach of having experts review the budget levels every year.

Finally, we conclude that important socioeconomic changes, such as the increase in the number of mothers who work outside the home, make it imperative to address an issue that has received relatively little attention in the debate over poverty thresholds: how to adjust them for differences in family circumstances. Poverty analysts have given considerable attention to how to adjust the thresholds for family size and composition differences and some attention to how to adjust them for cost-of-living differences among geographic areas (see Chapter 3). Almost universally, it is agreed that poverty thresholds should be specified in after-tax terms, recognizing that families differ in tax burdens and hence in their disposable income (although the current U.S. poverty measure does not correspondingly define family income

---

consumption expenditures minus expenditures for medical care, with all amounts in constant 1987 dollars (see Council of Economic Advisers, 1992:Table B-12). The reason for subtracting medical care expenditures is that the NIPA includes payments by insurance as well as out-of-pocket expenditures. A similarly derived estimate of the elasticity of food with respect to total expenditures minus medical care is 0.33.

in after-tax terms for comparison with the thresholds).[40] However, there are only a few examples of efforts to develop poverty thresholds that consider the different needs of working parents and workers generally in comparison with nonworkers or the variations in people's health care needs (Renwick and Bergmann, 1993, is an exception). Yet if these different needs (e.g., of working parents for child care in order to earn income) are not recognized, the poverty measure will not appropriately describe the differences in poverty among important population groups.

We propose to deal with these kinds of circumstances by subtracting such expenses as child care from family resources (see Chapter 4). The implication for the discussion here is that the proposed threshold concept is not quite the same as the concepts reviewed above. The proposed budget includes such categories as food that apply to all family types, as do all budgets, but most other budgets explicitly or implicitly include an average for such expenses as child care for which the need varies across otherwise similar types of families. This difference in the proposed concept must be considered, along with the real increase in consumption that has occurred since the early 1960s, when evaluating the level of the current threshold and whether it is appropriate for the United States today.

IMPLEMENTING THE PROPOSED APPROACH

To implement the proposed concept and updating procedure for the reference family poverty threshold is straightforward once the values of two parameters have been specified: (1) a percentage of median expenditures by two-adult/two-child families on the sum of food, clothing, and shelter (including utilities); and (2) a multiplier to apply to the amount for food, clothing, and shelter so as to add a small fraction for other needed spending. As a hypothetical example, suppose that median expenditures on food, clothing, and shelter by two-adult/two-child families are $15,500 in year T and $15,650 in year $T + 1$ (in constant dollars), for a real increase of 1 percent. Also suppose that, for deriving the reference family poverty threshold, the percentage of the median is specified as 80 percent and the multiplier as 1.20. Then, the initial threshold in year T is $[0.80(15,500) \times 1.20]$, or $14,880 and the threshold in year $T + 1$ is $[0.80(15,650) \times 1.20]$, or $15,024—also a real increase of 1 percent. By assuming, as has occurred historically, that total spending increased by more than 1 percent between year T and $T + 1$, then the reference family poverty threshold would have been updated in real terms in a quasi-relative rather than in a completely relative manner.

The recommended procedure is somewhat more complicated than the

---

[40] The appropriateness of using after-tax income data was recognized when the official thresholds were originally developed, but such data were not available at the time.

illustration because, in order to increase the sample size and also to smooth out year-to-year changes in the threshold and lag them behind changes in real consumption, we recommend that the calculations for each year be performed with the average of CEX data for the previous 3 years. Also, to express each year's reference family threshold in current dollars, it will be necessary to make an appropriate price adjustment to the CEX data. One way to do this is to convert the dollar amounts on each of the 3 years of CEX data files into current dollars by means of the CPI before calculating the threshold. Finally, after each year's reference family threshold is determined, the thresholds for other family types and areas of the country should be calculated by using the recommended equivalence scale and cost-of-housing index (see Chapter 3).

Setting the Initial Threshold

We do not recommend a value for the initial reference family threshold on which to base a new official poverty statistics series with the recommended poverty measure. However, we do reach a conclusion about a range for the initial reference family threshold that we believe is reasonable. Our conclusion is informed by analysis of consumer expenditure data, consideration of the values of other thresholds developed in recent years on the basis of alternative concepts, and our judgment.

Analysis of 1989-1991 CEX Data

We analyzed data from the interview survey component of the 1989-1991 CEX to help us form a judgment about a reasonable level for the initial reference family threshold under the proposed concept. Importantly, as part of this process, we gained experience with the data and how best to use them for calculating each year's reference family threshold.

The CEX, under its current design, is a continuing survey with two components—the Interview Survey and the Diary Survey. The Interview Survey includes a sample of about 5,000 consumer units, who are interviewed at 3-month intervals for a year.[41] Data are collected on most but not all categories of expenditures. The Diary Survey, which obtains 2-week diaries of all expenses incurred during the period from about 6,000 consumer units, is used to supplement the Interview Survey data for expenditures that are not collected or not adequately reported in that survey. Because the two compo-

---

[41] Each quarter the Interview Survey includes an added number of consumer units (about 1,800), who are given an initial interview to bound their later responses. BLS defines consumer units in a manner that is similar to but not quite the same as the Census Bureau definition of families and unrelated individuals (see Appendix B for a description of the CEX).

nents include different samples, it is only possible to use the Interview Survey for the kind of microlevel analysis that we required.[42]

BLS prepared a large number of tabulations for us from the 1991 Interview Survey and the 1989-1991 surveys combined. For processing convenience and to meet our timetable, these tabulations treated each quarterly interview falling within a calendar year as a separate observation, inflating the amounts by four to obtain annual figures. This procedure increases sample size because it uses all of the available data and not just the data for consumer units who responded to all interviews within a year.[43] For actual use in updating the reference family poverty threshold, however, we believe it would be preferable to aggregate quarterly amounts for those units with complete data, making an appropriate adjustment to the weights to account for other units.

The Basic Bundle   We began our analysis by looking at the distribution of expenditures on the basic bundle of food, clothing, and shelter (including utilities). BLS arrayed consumer units by their expenditures on these four categories, separately and combined, and, in each instance, determined the dollar values corresponding to the spending level for every 5 percent of units, from the lowest 5 percent to the highest 5 percent.

In examining spending patterns on food, clothing, and shelter, we found it convenient to look at the distribution in terms of the dollar values that demarcated every 5th percentile of the distribution. However, for purposes of calculating the reference family poverty threshold, whatever percentile value is chosen must be reexpressed as a percentage of median expenditures on food, clothing, and shelter for the same reason that relative thresholds are expressed as a percentage of median income or expenditures rather than as a percentile value. That is, if the thresholds are expressed as, say, the 25th or 30th percentile of income or expenditures, then, by definition, 25 or 30 percent of families are always poor; however, if the thresholds are expressed as, say, 40, 50, or 60 percent of median income or expenditures, then changes that affect the distribution of income or expenditures below the median can increase or decrease the poverty rate. As an example, a recession could move some families in the lower half of the income distribution from above to below 50 percent of the median, so that the poverty rate increased whether median income itself stayed the same or fell. Conversely, an income assistance program could move families from below to above 50 percent of median income, so that the poverty rate decreased whether median income stayed the same or

---

[42] The Interview Survey is adequate to use by itself for the categories in the basic bundle. BLS estimates that the Interview Survey obtains about the same aggregate amount of expenditures on food as the Diary Survey, and the Interview Survey is used exclusively by BLS for estimates of expenditures on clothing, shelter, and utilities.

[43] The effective sample size is not as large as the number of quarterly observations, however, because many of these observations are from the same consumer units and hence are correlated.

rose. Similarly, the food, clothing, and shelter component of the reference family poverty threshold under the proposed concept must be expressed as a percentage of median expenditures on these categories.

In the BLS tabulations, "food" included expenditures on food purchased for home use and away from home, excluding nonfood items purchased at grocery stores and alcohol. "Clothing" included expenditures on all kinds of apparel as well as sewing materials. "Shelter" included rent and, for owners, payments on mortgage interest (but not principal), taxes, and maintenance and repair. (The shelter variable for home owners was defined in this way for processing convenience; a preferable definition would include actual outlays for mortgage payments, taxes, insurance, and maintenance and repairs, together with an imputed amount for the estimated rental value of the home net of such outlays. Such a definition would treat homeowners with low or no mortgage payments in a comparable manner with other homeowners and renters.) "Utilities" included such fuels as natural gas and electricity, telephone, and such public services as water and sewer.

Values for every 5th percentile were determined for two-adult/two-child consumer units and selected other family types. Values were also determined by arraying the data for all types of units and converting each unit's expenditures into the equivalent of a two-adult/two-child unit by means of an equivalence scale. For this exercise, two variations of the proposed equivalence scale were used, one with a scale economy factor of 0.65 and the other with a scale economy factor of 0.75, each applied to the number of equivalent adults (the proposed scale treats children under 18 as 0.70 of an adult; see Chapter 3).

On the basis of these tabulations, we concluded that it is preferable to work with the expenditure values that result from arraying the *sum* of each consumer unit's expenditures on food, clothing, shelter, and utilities, constructed from 3 years' worth of data. We had originally liked the idea of building up a budget by taking values from the separate arrays for each of these expenditures. The budget-building approach, however, encounters the problem of zero expenditures on more detailed items, especially using quarterly observations, so we recommend using the sum of these items, which is more robust.

We also concluded that it is preferable to use the array for a single reference family type—two-adult/two-child families—even though this procedure considerably reduces the sample size in comparison with the procedure of converting each consumer unit's expenditures to an amount equivalent to a two-adult/two-child family. (The sample size reduction for the 1989-1991 CEX is from 61,385 quarterly observations for all consumer units to 5,485 observations for two-adult/two-child families.)

The use of different equivalence scales produces somewhat different percentile values: for example, median expenditures on the sum of food, clothing, and shelter differed by $800 between the two scales that we applied.

More important, changes over time in family composition, such as a continued decline in family size, could change the poverty thresholds in different ways depending on the choice of scale. Yet there is no agreement in the research community on the best form of an equivalence scale. Hence, we believe it is preferable to develop the expenditure array for the same family type each year. In this regard, while the sample size for two-adult/two-child families is adequate for this purpose when 3 years' worth of CEX data are pooled, it would clearly be advantageous to have a larger size for the survey.

The final set of percentile values (for each 5% of units) that we examined was derived from arraying the annualized expenditures of two-adult/two-child consumer units on the sum of food, clothing, shelter, and utilities for the period 1989-1991; see Table 2-6, which also shows each percentile value as a percentage of the median. In 1992 dollars, the median value is $15,344.[44]

The designation of a percentile value for food, clothing, and shelter—which, when expressed as a constant percentage of the median, will drive the poverty thresholds in future years—is obviously a matter of judgment. We do not recommend a specific value or even a range; we do, however, conclude that a reasonable range for the food, clothing, and shelter component of the reference family threshold would be from the 30th to the 35th percentile, or from 78 to 83 percent of the median. In 1992 dollars, this range is from $11,950 to $12,719.

What would these amounts buy? Illustratively, a family at the 30th percentile might spend the following: $355 per month or $4,260 annually for food, which is the value of the Thrifty Food Plan for a four-person family; $545 per month or about $6,550 per year for rent and utilities (including telephone) for a two-bedroom apartment, which is the fair market rent in 1992 for such units that is the basis of federal housing assistance; and $95 per month ($24 per family member) or $1,140 per year for clothing. The total per year for a family at the 30th percentile is $11,950. A family at the 35th percentile would spend an extra $64 per month on food, clothing, and shelter, or an extra $770 per year, for a total of $12,720.

For comparison, the following are the allotments in two recently developed expert budgets for a two-adult/two-child family (in 1992 dollars):

• Renwick (1993a): $420 per month or $5,040 per year for food (the value of the Low-Cost Food Plan, which Renwick used instead of the Thrifty Food Plan—the latter was designed for temporary or emergency use and has never been updated in real terms); $428 per month or $5,136 for housing

---

[44] The 1989-1991 CEX data originally supplied to us were in nominal dollars. We converted the data to constant 1992 dollars by applying the weighted average of the price increases for 1989-1992, 1990-1992, and 1991-1992. A preferable procedure is to adjust the data for each year to the dollars of the year for which the threshold is being calculated before producing the expenditure array.

TABLE 2-6 Percentile Values of Expenditures on the Panel's Basic Bundle by Two-Adult/Two-Child Families, 1989-1991 Consumer Expenditure Survey, in Constant 1992 Dollars, with Multiplier

	Basic Expenditures		Multiplier of Larger Bundle to Basic Bundle	
Percentile	Dollar Amount	Percent of Median	Definition 1[a]	Definition 2[b]
5th	7,041	45.9	1.18	1.20
10th	8,374	54.6	1.22	1.25
15th	9,275	60.4	1.21	1.23
20th	10,188	66.4	1.18	1.19
25th	11,100	72.3	1.18	1.20
30th	11,950	77.9	1.19	1.23
35th	12,719	82.9	1.20	1.26
40th	13,575	88.5	1.15	1.18
45th	14,389	93.8	1.16	1.21
50th (median)	15,344	100.0	1.14	1.17
55th	16,282	106.1	1.17	1.19
60th	17,277	112.6	1.15	1.18
65th	18,369	119.7	1.13	1.16
70th	19,627	127.9	1.15	1.20
75th	20,989	136.8	1.15	1.18
80th	22,521	146.8	1.15	1.18
85th	24,594	160.3	1.13	1.16
90th	27,580	179.7	1.14	1.17
95th	34,094	222.2	1.12	1.16
100th	114,942	749.1	1.09	1.13

NOTES: Data are from tabulations prepared by the Bureau of Labor Statistics from the Interview Survey component of the 1989-1991 Consumer Expenditure Survey; all amounts were converted to 1992 dollars by the CPI-U. The multipliers were derived from the average of families with expenditures on the basic bundle within the range from 2.5 percentiles below to 2.5 percentiles above each 5th percentile level (e.g., the multiplier for the 15th percentile value was derived from the average of families spending between the 12.5 and 17.5 percentiles on the basic bundle).

[a]Definition 1 for the multiplier defines the larger bundle of goods as the basic bundle (food, clothing, shelter, including utilities) plus personal care and one-half of total transportation costs.

[b]Definition 2 defines the larger bundle as the basic bundle plus personal care, education, reading materials, and one-half of total transportation costs.

(rent, utilities, and telephone, developed as the 25th percentile of the distribution of rents for all two-bedroom apartments); and $105 per month or $1,260 per year for clothing (developed by adjusting the clothing component of the BLS lower level budget for inflation)—for a total of $11,436 per year on these categories.

• Schwarz and Volgy (1992): $355 per month or $4,260 per year for food; $554 per month or $6,648 per year for rent, utilities, and telephone for

a two-bedroom apartment; and $90 per month or $1,080 per year for clothing—for a total of $11,988 per year on these categories.

The total amounts for both Renwick (1993a) and Schwarz and Volgy
(1992)—$11,436 and $11,988—are similar to the value of $11,950 for the
30th percentile of food, clothing, and shelter expenditures from the CEX.
The sum of the larger food and clothing allowances in Renwick and the larger
housing allowance in Schwarz and Volgy is $12,948, which is higher than the
value of $12,719 for the 35th percentile of food, clothing, and shelter expen-
ditures from the CEX.

The Multiplier   We then considered the multiplier to be applied to the
food, clothing, and shelter component of the poverty threshold so as to allow
a small fraction for other needed expenditures. BLS developed tabulations for
us, from the 1989-1991 CEX Interview Survey, of the ratio of a broader
bundle of expenditures to expenditures on the basic bundle. (The multipliers
were calculated for families spending around each 5th percentile level on food,
clothing, and shelter, from the lowest 5th to the highest 5th.)   For our
purpose, the definition of the broader bundle always excluded costs that we
propose be deducted from family resources instead of included in the thresholds (e.g., child care and out-of-pocket medical care expenditures; see Chapter 4). We also excluded some other costs in order to implement our recommendation for a small fixed multiple applied to a larger basic budget.

The Interview Survey may seem ill-suited for constructing a multiplier
because it excludes such items as household cleaning supplies and some types
of personal care items that one might think should be included in a poverty
budget (e.g., shampoo and soap). (These items are picked up in the Diary
Survey of the CEX, which we could not analyze.) But our purpose was not
to mimic the type of detailed budget-building exercise followed by BLS in the
Family Budgets Program or more recently by Renwick and Bergmann (1993)
and Schwarz and Volgy (1992). Rather, we wanted to get a rough idea of
what could constitute a fairly lean multiplier applied to a larger budget for
food, clothing, and shelter.

With the available Interview Survey data, we looked at several alternative
definitions of a broader bundle, including a definition (1) that included the
basic bundle plus personal care items and one-half of total transportation costs,
and a definition (2) that included the basic bundle plus personal care items,
education expenses, reading materials, and one-half of total transportation
costs. We arbitrarily chose to exclude one-half of transportation costs because
the Interview Survey does not distinguish between work expenses, which we
propose to deduct from resources, and personal transportation for errands,
vacations, etc.[45] Our calculations showed that multipliers for two-adult/two-

---

[45] In fact, it appears that the federal statistical system does not anywhere provide information
on the allocation by families of transportation costs for work and nonwork uses. One estimate

child families at or below the median level of expenditures on the basic bundle varied from 1.14 to 1.22 for the first definition and from 1.17 to 1.26 for the second definition (see Table 2-6). We concluded that a reasonable range for the multiplier to apply to the food, clothing, and shelter component of the reference family poverty threshold is 1.15 to 1.25. If the amount for food, clothing, and shelter is $11,950-$12,720 per year (in 1992 dollars), then a multiplier in the range of 1.15-1.25 will provide an added $1,790-$3,180 per year, or about $150-$265 per month, for all other consumption.[46]

For comparison, the implicit multipliers on food, clothing, and shelter in some expert poverty budgets for two-adult/two-child families (after excluding those expenditures that we propose to deduct from resources) range from 1.14 to 1.30:

• 1.14, covering personal care, household supplies, and non-work-related transportation (Renwick, 1993a);
• 1.29, covering personal care, household furnishings and operations, non-work-related transportation, reading, recreation, alcohol, tobacco, education, and miscellaneous (Bureau of Labor Statistics, 1982:Table 1);[47] and
• 1.30, covering personal care, household supplies, non-work-related transportation, and such incidentals as newspapers, stamps, stationery (Schwarz and Volgy, 1992).

The Basic Bundle and Multiplier Together On the basis of our review of CEX data, we concluded that a reasonable range for the initial poverty threshold for a two-adult/two-child family is $13,700 to $15,900 (in 1992 dollars). The lower end of this range is the value of the 30th percentile of expenditures on food, clothing, and shelter (or 78% of the median) times 1.15; the upper end of the range is the value of the 35th percentile of expenditures on food, clothing, and shelter (or 83% of the median) times 1.25 (both rounded to the nearest $100).

Of course, it would be possible to obtain an initial reference family threshold within the same range with a higher (lower) value for food, clothing, and shelter and a lower (higher) value of the multiplier. We cannot claim scientific backing for the ranges of values that we conclude are reasonable for these two parameters, or for the range for the initial poverty threshold itself. We can point to the reasonableness of the ranges we suggest both in terms of

---

prepared for us by the Energy Information Administration, based on automobile and truck usage only, suggests that the allocation might be one-third work and two-thirds nonwork uses (letter from Lynda T. Carlson to the panel, 1994).

[46] The amount for the 1.15 multiplier in Chapter 1 is shown as $1,750 instead of $1,790 per year because that is the amount when the lower end of the suggested range is rounded down to the nearest $100.

[47] This estimate of the multiplier is for the BLS lower level budget, which was about two-thirds of the intermediate budget and not intended to represent a poverty level.

what these amounts would buy and in comparison with other thresholds (see below).

However, it should be clear that building a poverty threshold on food, clothing, and shelter plus a little more does not imply that families must spend their income accordingly. Families may spend less on food, clothing, and shelter than implied in the poverty threshold and not necessarily be poor. They may, for example, grow some of their own food or make some of their own clothing in order to increase their available income for other spending. They are poor only if their total income (net of nondiscretionary expenses) is below the poverty line. Conversely, families may spend more on food, clothing, and shelter than implied in the poverty threshold and yet still be poor if their net income falls below the poverty line. The proposed threshold concept is not intended to mandate a spending pattern for low-income people but to lead to an initial threshold that is reasonable for purposes of deriving poverty statistics. More important, that concept is intended to provide a method for updating the initial threshold that takes account of real increases in consumption for basic necessities—food, clothing, and shelter—that pertain to an economic measure of poverty.

Comparison with Other Thresholds

The range of $13,700-$15,900 that we concluded is reasonable for the initial reference family threshold is 96-112 percent of the official 1992 two-adult/two-child threshold of $14,228. The range is lower than other recently developed thresholds (see column 2 of Table 2-5, above). It would appear that it does not represent much, if any, updating of the current threshold for real increases in living standards.

However, the proposed threshold concept differs from most of the concepts we reviewed by treating some kinds of expenses as deductions from resources rather than including them in the threshold (not only taxes, but also other work expenses and out-of-pocket medical care expenses). To get a better sense of how the range of $13,700-$15,900 relates to other thresholds, we sought a way to convert the current threshold and recently developed thresholds to the proposed budget concept. Data limitations made it difficult to carry out such a conversion, but we developed a procedure that provides a rough approximation.

For our analysis of the effects of the proposed measure compared with the current measure (see Chapter 5), we added estimates to the March 1993 CPS of each family's spending on child care and other work-related expenses and out-of-pocket medical care expenses (including health insurance premiums). We estimated the average combined deductions for two-adult/two-child families with after-tax income around the median (using families from 7.5 percentiles below to 7.5 percentiles above the median to increase the sample size).

The ratio of this average to median after-tax income for two–adult/two–child families was 0.84. We then applied this ratio to other thresholds to convert them, approximately, to the proposed budget concept (see Table 1-4 in Chapter 1). For the thresholds developed by Renwick (1993a) and Schwarz and Volgy (1992), we made the conversion by inspecting their budgets. We note that the ratios of the "as converted" to the "as developed" amounts in Table 1-4 for the Renwick and Schwarz and Volgy budgets are 0.74 and 0.82, respectively. These ratios are lower than the ratio we calculated because their budgets assume that every two–adult/two–child family spends the maximum allowance for such items as work expenses.

The official 1992 threshold, before conversion to the proposed budget concept, is $14,228, and the range of other thresholds shown in Table 1-4 is $17,200 to $21,800 (rounded to the nearest $100). After conversion, the official threshold is $12,000, and the estimated range of other thresholds is $13,100 to $18,300, or 9 to 53 percent higher than the official threshold. The Renwick budget of $13,100 is an outlier at the low end of the range; four other thresholds (two subjective thresholds, a relative threshold expressed as one-half median after-tax income of four-person families, and the Schwarz and Volgy budget) are clustered between $14,400 and $15,600; two other thresholds (the relative threshold recommended by the Expert Committee on Family Budget Revisions and the lower of the two Weinberg and Lamas multiplier thresholds) are between $16,800 and $17,100; and three other thresholds (variations of the multiplier method that make use of expenditure data) are between $17,400 and $18,300. In comparison, the range that we conclude is reasonable, $13,700-$15,900, is 14 to 33 higher than the official threshold and falls within but toward the lower end of the estimated range of other thresholds.[48] Thus, it represents a conservative updating in real terms of the current threshold, consistent with our recommendation.

Analysis Over Time

The most important aspect of the proposed threshold concept is not so much the threshold that it produces for a designated start-up year, but how it moves that initial threshold over time. Our intent was to recommend a concept and procedure that would update the initial reference family poverty threshold for changes in real consumption but in a conservative manner.

Unfortunately, there is no good times series with which to evaluate the likely behavior of the proposed procedure. The National Income and Product

---

[48] The range of 13,700–$15,900 is 37–42 percent of median before-tax income for two-adult/two-child families in 1992 and 45–53 percent of median after-tax income converted as described in the text to the proposed threshold concept. We do not have an exact estimate of the range as a percentage of disposable income defined with all of the adjustments that we recommend (see Chapter 4).

Accounts (NIPA) estimates of personal consumption expenditures (PCE) suggest, as we noted above, that the procedure would work as intended: we estimated the elasticity of the basic bundle with respect to total consumption minus medical care as 0.65. Indeed, we briefly considered the use of the PCE estimates (specifically, the change each year in real expenditures on the basic bundle) to update the initial reference family poverty threshold. The PCE estimates are not suitable for this purpose, however, for two major reasons: they include expenditures by nonprofit institutions as well as households, and while they can be adjusted for population growth, they cannot be adjusted for changes in family size over time.

Thus, we turned back to the CEX. The current continuing CEX was initiated in 1980. Consumer expenditure surveys were also conducted in 1972-1973 and 1960-1961 (and at intervals of about 10-15 years back to the turn of the century). The design of the surveys was not the same over time; also, there is evidence of some deterioration in the reporting of expenditures in the CEX in comparison with the NIPA (see, e.g., Gieseman, 1987; Slesnick, 1991a). With so few data points and those of doubtful comparability, it is very difficult to construct a historical time series with which to evaluate the proposed updating procedure.

To get a very rough estimate of what a poverty threshold developed with the proposed procedure would look like now in comparison with the one actually developed for 1963, we first adjusted median 1991 CEX expenditures on the bundle of food, clothing, and shelter to correct for the greater extent of underreporting (vis-à-vis the NIPA) in that year than was observed in the 1960-1961 CEX. We then calculated the ratio of median expenditures on the basic bundle by two-adult/two-child families in the 2 years (with data supplied by BLS) and applied this ratio to $14,228, the official poverty threshold as of 1963 in 1992 dollars.[49] The result was a poverty threshold of $16,152 in 1992 dollars, representing an increase of 14 percent in the thresholds over the period. This increase compares to a 21 to 24 percent increase in Vaughan's subjective thresholds over about the same period (1963-1993 or 1963-1989; see Table 2-4).[50]

For the period 1980-1991, BLS provided us with a comparable time series from the CEX (although data for 1986 are missing because of tape storage

---

[49] For want of an alternative, we picked the official threshold, which enjoyed widespread support as the right level for 1963, even though the proposed concept—unlike the original concept—treats some expenses as deductions from family resources. We did not believe it appropriate for this exercise to use the ratio of 0.84 to convert the official threshold to the proposed concept because the spending level on such expenses as child care and out-of-pocket medical care would have differed in 1963 from the level in 1992.

[50] The increase over the period 1963–1992 was only 10 percent, but the 1992 subjective poverty line is from a Gallup Poll in which the same respondents were asked the get-along question followed by the poverty question. In contrast, the poverty questions in 1989 and 1993 were administered to respondents who were not also asked the get-along question.

TABLE 2-7 Poverty Thresholds Developed Under Panel's Proposed
Procedure, in Constant 1992 Dollars

| | Single-Year Thresholds | | 3-Year Moving Averages | |
Year	Dollar Amount	Percent of Official Threshold	Dollar Amount	Percent of Official Threshold
1980	14,228	100.0	N.A.	N.A.
1981	14,227	100.0	N.A.	N.A.
1982	14,537	102.2	N.A.	N.A.
1983	14,739	103.6	14,331	100.7
1984	14,374	101.0	14,501	101.9
1985	15,246	107.2	14,550	102.3
1986	N.A.	N.A.	14,786	103.9
1987	14,649	103.0	14,809	104.1
1988	15,134	106.4	14,946	105.0
1989	14,899	104.7	14,892	104.7
1990	15,026	105.6	14,894	104.7
1991	15,219	107.0	15,020	105.6
1992	N.A.	N.A.	15,048	105.8

NOTES: Data are from tabulations of the CEX Interview Survey for years 1980-1985 and 1987–1991 provided to the panel by the Bureau of Labor Statistics. Single-year thresholds were constructed by applying the year-to-year change in median expenditures on the sum of food, clothing, and shelter (including utilities) by two-adult/two-child families to the starting threshold of $14,228 (the official threshold in 1992 dollars).

Because data are not available for 1986, the 3-year moving-average figure for 1987 is the average of 1985 and 1984; that for 1988 is the average of 1985 and 1987; and that for 1989 is the average of 1987 and 1988. Otherwise, moving-average thresholds are the average of the single-year thresholds for the 3 prior years. Data for 1982–1983 apply to urban families only.

problems, and the CEX interviews in 1982-1983 included only urban families because of budget cuts). We needed a starting point for this series and, for want of a better choice, pegged it at the official poverty line. The thresholds produced under the proposed procedure, when using a single year's worth of data, move somewhat erratically, with a small overall increase of 7 percent in real terms between 1980 and 1991; see Table 2-7.[51] By comparison, Vaughan's subjective poverty thresholds increased by 8-11 percent over the same period (1980-1993 or 1980-1989; see Table 2-4), and relative thresholds expressed as one-half median after-tax four-person family income increased by 8-14 percent over the same period (1980-1993 or 1980-1989; see Table 2-3).

The variations in the thresholds we calculated are likely due in part to

---

[51] Again, because we picked an arbitrary starting point, we updated the thresholds by applying the ratio of the medians for each pair of years, rather than using a percentage of the median times a multiplier.

small sample sizes for two-adult/two-child consumer units in single years of the CEX. Also, it appears that the thresholds are not as responsive to economic ups and downs as are relative and subjective thresholds reviewed above (see Tables 2-3 and 2-4). A reason may be that people at or below the median alter their consumption of other items in response to economic ups and downs before they alter their consumption of the basic bundle of food, clothing, and shelter.

Our last calculation was to smooth the thresholds for 1980-1991 by constructing 3-year moving averages for 1983-1992 (see Table 2-7). The smoothed series behaves quite reasonably, increasing slowly but steadily over the period by about 5 percent in real terms.

Further Evaluation

We strongly believe that the principles underlying the proposed threshold concept and updating procedure are an improvement over both the original concept (food times a large, changing multiplier) and that concept as actually implemented (adjusting the thresholds only for price changes). The proposed concept, in contrast, updates the thresholds for real changes in consumption of a bundle of necessities rather than of all goods and services. The concept also retains a normative cast, with its emphasis on food, clothing, and shelter (plus a little more).

We are reasonably confident that the CEX data for implementing the proposed concept and updating procedure will produce thresholds that behave in the intended manner. However, we would obviously have preferred to have a longer time series with which to evaluate the likely behavior of the thresholds. We also would have liked to assess the effects of some methodological improvements that we believe should be made in using the CEX data (e.g., construct annual estimates for each consumer unit, use imputed rent for homeowner shelter expenditures). Finally, we believe that it is very important to improve the underlying data—for example, expanding the sample size of the CEX and reducing the extent of underreporting would make more robust the estimates needed to update the poverty thresholds. More generally, the United States would benefit from improvements in data on consumer expenditures, savings, and wealth, which are needed for many important purposes, including the measurement of poverty (see Chapter 5).

One concern with using a continuing survey to update the poverty thresholds is the effects that changes in data quality or other aspects of the survey may have on estimates of the required parameters over time. This concern applies to the proposed concept, which relies on 3 years' worth of CEX data to update each year's reference family poverty threshold. (It also applies to relative concepts that peg the thresholds at, say, one-half median adjusted family income or expenditures, and to subjective concepts that make use of

survey responses about the poverty line or minimum income.)[52] In the case of
the proposed concept, a change in the quality of reporting of expenditures,
whether an improvement or a deterioration in reporting, could alter the time
series of poverty thresholds even though the underlying phenomena (i.e., real
expenditures on food, clothing, and shelter) had not changed. The possibility
of changes in the thresholds occurring as artifacts of fluctuations in reporting
or other changes to the underlying CEX data will necessitate careful monitoring of the year-to-year consistency in the survey,

A second concern with the proposed concept is how the poverty thresholds behave as the economy moves through the business cycle. To facilitate
evaluating the thresholds that are developed by the proposed procedure and
their implications for poverty rates, it will be important to generate another,
unofficial set of thresholds and rates based on them for some time. This other
set should represent an initial set of thresholds (developed as we have outlined
for the reference family and adjusted appropriately for different types of families and areas of the country) that are updated for price changes rather than for
real changes in basic consumption. We believe that tying the thresholds to
changes in consumption of the basic necessities of food, clothing, and shelter,
together with the use of 3 years' worth of data to develop each year's reference
family threshold, will moderate the sensitivity of the thresholds to changes in
the business cycle. However, another unofficial set of thresholds that are
updated simply for price changes will ensure that important information is
available with which to assess the behavior of the official thresholds at the next
regularly scheduled review of the poverty measure.

---

[52] Although not as obvious, the same concern applies to the current concept, which maintains
the thresholds unchanged in real terms through an inflation adjustment that is based on a
continuing survey of consumer prices. However, the survey that is used to estimate the year-
to-year change in the CPI is more robust than the CEX. There is a similar concern with the
estimation of family resources for comparison with the thresholds, however they are updated:
thus, changes in the quality of income reporting or other aspects of the March CPS could affect
the time series of poverty rates under the current measure.

Adjusting Poverty Thresholds

3

The previous chapter focused on the derivation of a poverty threshold for a reference family of two adults and two children. A poverty threshold that is appropriate for this type of family, however, may not be appropriate for another type of family: a single person obviously needs less money than a family of four, and a family of eight needs more money. These differences are recognized in the current poverty measure, which uses different thresholds for different family types. And even for a given family type, the amount of money needed to stay above the poverty threshold will likely be different in a large city than in a small town, and it may also differ by region of the country. There is therefore an argument for adjusting the thresholds, not only for family size, but also for place of residence. This kind of adjustment is not made in the official poverty thresholds. In this chapter, we consider these adjustments and present our recommended procedures for adjusting the reference family threshold. We first discuss adjustments by family type and then by geographic area of residence.

ADJUSTMENTS BY FAMILY TYPE

The Concept of an Equivalence Scale

Equivalence scales are measures of the relative costs of living of families of different sizes and compositions that are otherwise similar. For example, if a family of two adults can live as well as a family of two adults and two children while spending only two-thirds as much, then relative to the reference family of two adults and two children, the equivalence scale value for a two–adult family is two-thirds. For the purpose of poverty measurement, the use of an equivalence scale is to scale up or down the threshold for the reference family to provide corresponding thresholds for other family types.

The concept underlying such a scale appears straightforward and is similar in spirit to a standard cost-of-living index number. If it costs twice as much at one time to maintain a given standard of living as it did at an earlier date, then one needs twice as much money to reach the equivalent standard of living. The idea of an equivalence scale is the same, but instead of comparing two different sets of prices, one compares two different family types. In spite of this apparent simplicity, a precise characterization of equivalence scales is elusive, and the many scales proposed in the literature differ not only by the usual margin of empirical uncertainty, but also in their underlying conception: different authors are not always measuring the same thing. As a result, it is possible to find a wide range of scales, which have very different implications for the total number of people in poverty as well as for the distribution of poverty among families of different types. Depending on the scale used, the poverty rate can be substantially higher or lower, and the demographic composition of those considered poor can change dramatically.

Overview and Recommendation

One simple method of adjusting the reference family threshold by family type is to scale it in proportion to the number of people in a family. In the language of "equivalence scales," a single person would need one-quarter as much as a family of four, a married couple without children one-half as much as a family of four, and a family of eight twice as much as a family of four. Most people, including the members of the panel, regard this as an extreme position, since it makes no allowance for the fact that children are different from adults, nor for the economies of scale possible for larger families by sharing kitchens, bathrooms, and bedrooms or by buying products in bulk. This straight proportion rule clearly understates the needs of small families relative to large ones, and, hence, it will overestimate the number of poor people in large families relative to those in small families.

The opposite extreme is to make no adjustments for family type and to apply the basic poverty threshold to all families irrespective of size or composition. This "zero" adjustment for family size is as unpalatable as is the straight proportion adjustment of multiplying the threshold by family size. It assumes that one adult needs as much as a two-adult/two-child family and also that a four-adult family or a family of two adults and three or more children needs no more than the two-adult/two-child family. There is widespread agreement that the appropriate adjustment lies somewhere between the two extremes; however, there is much less agreement on exactly how much to adjust the threshold for children relative to adults or how to measure economies of scale for larger households.

We have reviewed the adjustments for family type that are embodied in the official poverty thresholds, as well as those that are implicit in other government programs. We have also considered numerous other proposals in the literature, including those that use empirical analysis in an attempt to establish an objective adjustment on the basis of comparing the behavior of families of different types. Although the empirical evidence helps determine the limits of what makes sense, there is no objective procedure for measuring the different needs for different family types. As with the determination of the reference family poverty threshold itself, for which empirical evidence can inform but not prescribe what is fundamentally a social or political judgment, so with the adjustments for different family types. Thus, similarly, we have opted for a procedure that, while taking into account the empirical evidence and previous experience, recognizes that the decision is based on judgment and seeks to make the process as transparent as possible.

Our recommended procedure follows from our conclusion that the equivalence scale implicit in the official poverty thresholds is problematic and should be replaced. We say "implicit" because the official thresholds were developed separately for each family type rather than by the application of a formal scale to a reference family threshold. The basis for the official thresholds was a set of estimates of different food requirements for adults and children of various ages in families of different sizes. The assumptions underlying the differences are questionable, as is the assumption that differences in food needs adequately capture differences in needs for housing and other goods. One particularly questionable assumption is that people aged 65 and older need less to eat and so should have lower poverty thresholds than younger people; this assumption underlies the official thresholds for unrelated individuals and members of two-person families. Also, the implicit scale (which can be calculated by comparing the differences among the official thresholds for various family types) exhibits a number of irregularities and anomalies: for example, the second child in a family adds more costs than the first child.

We propose that poverty thresholds for different family types be developed by applying an explicit scale to the reference family poverty threshold. The scale should distinguish the needs of children under 18 and adults but not make other distinctions by age; the scale should also recognize economies of scale for larger families. A scale of this type is the following:

$$\text{scale value} = (A + PK)^F,$$

where A is the number of adults in the family, K is the number of children, each of whom is treated as a proportion P of an adult, and F is the scale economy factor. The formula calculates the number of adult equivalents ($A + PK$) and raises the result to a power F that reflects economies of scale for larger families. We recommend values for both P and F near 0.70; to be specific, we recommend setting P at 0.70 (i.e., each child is treated as 70% of an adult) and

F in the range of 0.65 to 0.75. To calculate the actual thresholds, the ratio of the scale value from the formula for each family type to the value for the reference family type is applied to the reference family threshold.

> **RECOMMENDATION 3.1. The four-person (two adult/two child) poverty threshold should be adjusted for other family types by means of an equivalence scale that reflects differences in consumption by adults and children under 18 and economies of scale for larger families. A scale that meets these criteria is the following: children under 18 are treated as consuming 70 percent as much as adults on average; economies of scale are computed by taking the number of adult equivalents in a family (i.e., the number of adults plus 0.70 times the number of children), and then by raising this number to a power of from 0.65 to 0.75.**

To explain the basis for our recommendation, we review types of equivalence scales, including the scale inherent in the official thresholds. In the discussion, we present our reasons for recommending that children be treated as needing 70 percent as much, on average, as adults, and for suggesting a range of 0.65 to 0.75 for the factor used to adjust for economies of scale for larger families.

The Current Equivalence Scale

During the 1960s, when there was keen interest in developing a poverty measure for the United States, one widely cited measure did not employ an equivalence scale. The 1964 report of the Council of Economic Advisers (CEA) set the poverty line for 1962 at $3,000 for a family (of any size) and $1,500 for unrelated individuals. It is hard to defend the proposition that a family of five can live as cheaply as a family of two, and although some might argue that parents who have chosen to have larger families should not be regarded as poor simply because of that choice, the same can hardly be said of the children, who played no part in their parents' decision. If one is to construct a sensible measure of poverty, some equivalence scale must be used.

Mollie Orshansky, working at the Social Security Administration in the early 1960s, developed the poverty measure that was ultimately adopted for official use. Her central poverty threshold for a family of four was about the same as the CEA family threshold of $3,000, but she developed a whole range of thresholds that took family size and composition into account (Orshansky, 1963, 1965a). She thereby defined an equivalence scale, not directly, but by constructing a set of thresholds for different family types. Orshansky's thresholds were derived from looking at food budgets, and the equivalence scale that is implicit in them is a consequence of her judgments about needs for food and other goods.

The underpinning for Orshansky's thresholds was the U.S. Department of

Agriculture (USDA) Economy Food Plan, which provided the estimated cost of a minimally adequate diet for adults and children of various ages and for families of different sizes. (The latter estimates reflect assumptions about economies of scale on food; see Peterkin et al., 1983.) Orshansky's food budgets were based on the USDA estimates, coupled with assumptions about the ages of the children in each size and type of family. She developed separate budgets for families on the basis of the sex of the family head, the family size, the number of family members under the age of 18, and, for one- and two-person units, the age of the family head (under age 65 or 65 and older).

According to the 1955 Household Food Consumption Survey, the average family of three or more spent approximately one-third of its after-tax money income on food. On the basis of this evidence, Orshansky created thresholds for families of three or more by multiplying her estimated food costs by three. She examined families of two separately, however, on the grounds that smaller families are less able to take advantage of economies of scale and so must absorb higher per capita fixed costs. The average family of two spent 27 percent of its income on food, so the multiplier for families of this size was set at 3.70 (1.00/0.27). Without using a food plan and a multiplier, she set thresholds for unrelated individuals, characterized by sex and age, at 80 percent of the corresponding threshold for two-person families.[1] This figure implies that two adults can live as well as one person on 125 percent as much income (1.0/0.8). Finally, she took 70 percent of her thresholds as the thresholds for farm families.

In 1969 the Bureau of the Budget adopted Orshansky's thresholds (and thereby her equivalence scale) for the official measure of poverty, with the modification that the farm thresholds were raised from 70 to 85 percent of the nonfarm thresholds. In 1981 the nonfarm thresholds were applied also to farm families; the thresholds for families headed by women and men were averaged; and the largest family size category for the thresholds was raised from families of seven or more to families of nine or more. With the exception of these fairly minor changes, the current equivalence scale comes directly from Orshansky's original work. Because of the way it was constructed, the scale has as many categories as the official poverty thresholds and is thus quite detailed. (There are 48 categories at present, reduced from 124 categories prior to 1981.) Most presentations summarize it using weighted averages: see Table 3-1, which expresses the weighted average thresholds for families of size two to size seven relative to the threshold for a single adult under age 65.

A key point to note is the essential arbitrariness of the equivalence scale

---

[1] Unrelated individuals aged 15 and older are treated as separate one-person "families" in the U.S. poverty measure. Some of them live alone in their own households, but others live with other people not related to them (e.g., they may board with a family or live with one or more unrelated roommates).

TABLE 3-1   Equivalence Scale Implicit in Official Weighted Average
Poverty Thresholds for 1992

Family Size	Scale Value Relative to a Single Adult (Under Age 65)	Increment in the Scale for Each Added Family Member (Relative to Single Adult Under Age 65)[a]
One person under age 65	1.000	0.00
One person aged 65 or over	0.922	−0.08
Two persons, head aged 65 or over	1.163	+0.16[b]
Two persons, head under age 65	1.294	+0.29
Three persons	1.533	+0.24
Four persons	1.964	+0.43
Six persons	2.273	+0.31
Six persons	2.622	+0.35
Seven persons	2.958	+0.34

SOURCE: Bureau of the Census (1993c:Table A).

[a]The values in this column represent the marginal effect of adding one more person to a
family. For example, the figure of 0.24 for a three-person family category is the added amount
for the third person, computed as the difference between the aggregate scale values in the first
column for three-person families and two-person families relative to the scale value for a single
adult.

[b]The value shown is for the increment in the scale for the second person in an elderly family
relative to a single adult under age 65. The increment in the scale for a second person in an
elderly family relative to a single adult aged 65 or over is 0.24—the difference between the scale
values of 1.163 and 0.922.

that underlies the current poverty measure. Even if one accepts the scientific
validity of the Economy Food Plan—itself a controversial matter since the
plan is based on a compromise between expert nutritional advice and actual
behavior—the derivation of the thresholds, and hence the equivalence scale,
rests on a chain of ad hoc adjustments. The scientific basis for them is elusive
or controversial, and, consequently, the scale is largely arbitrary.

   There are numerous specific criticisms of the current scale, that is, of the
way in which the poverty thresholds vary across family types. For example, it
seems unlikely that economies of scale in food are similar to those for other
goods, especially given the presumption that many economies of scale operate
through housing (see Nelson, 1993; Orshansky, 1968a). This criticism was
especially pertinent for the pre-1981 thresholds for farm and nonfarm families,
in which farm families, because they spend less on food on average than
nonfarm families, had lower thresholds. This distinction would make sense
only if less is also needed for all necessities other than food, such as clothing
and shelter, something for which there is no clear evidence. Although the
farm-nonfarm distinction no longer exists, a similar situation occurs for elderly

individuals living in one- and two-person units who have somewhat lower thresholds than do the nonelderly because they are assumed to need less food.

There are also a number of disturbing irregularities in the current scale. If there are economies of scale as family size increases, then the increment in the scale for an additional person should be lower for larger families. Yet as Ruggles (1990:66) has pointed out, this is not true of the current scale: on a weighted average basis relative to a single adult (as seen in Table 3-1), a second person in a family adds 0.29 to the scale, a third person adds only 0.24, a fourth person adds 0.43, and a fifth person adds 0.31. In some cases, single-parent families have higher thresholds than married-couple families of the same size, implying that children cost more than adults in certain size families. As one example, the child in a two-person single-parent family adds more to the family's costs than does the spouse in a married-couple family: see Figure 3-1, which graphs—separately for married-couple and single-parent families—the increment in the scale for each added family member relative to a single

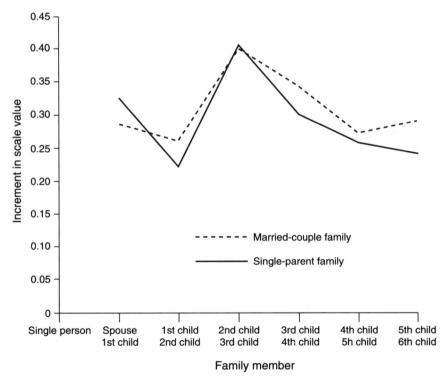

FIGURE 3-1 Equivalence scale implicit in the current poverty thresholds: increment for each added family member (relative to a scale value of 1.00 for a single adult under age 65). SOURCE: Data from Bureau of the Census (1993c:Table A).

adult under age 65. These irregularities come in part from the assumptions that Orshansky had to make about the ages of children in families when using the food plans.

We believe that these sorts of difficulties are always likely to be present in any method that is based on the construction of "ideal" or "expert" budgets for different family types, whether the budgets derive from food, as in Orshansky's procedure, or from a wider basket of goods as, for example, proposed by Ruggles (1990) and implemented by Renwick (1993a, 1993b).[2] Expert poverty budgets are inevitably the result of families' actual spending patterns and a series of adjustments that reflect judgments about what a low-income family "ought" to purchase. Because these budgets are always at least somewhat arbitrary, they impart no legitimacy to the equivalence scales that are implicit within them. We prefer a more direct approach that recognizes the arbitrariness by setting an equivalence scale formula directly and transparently and then using it to scale the threshold for a reference family type to derive poverty thresholds for other family types.

Alternative Equivalence Scales

Although there is wide agreement that different family types should have different poverty thresholds, that children have different needs from adults, and that larger households can benefit from economies of scale by sharing some items of consumption, there is little agreement about how the differences should be measured, and there is a wide range of scales in the literature. This section discusses some of these scales, as well as their conceptual and empirical basis.

Programmatic Equivalence Scales

In addition to the scale implicit in the official poverty thresholds, there are a number of other scales embodied in government programs or official pronouncements; see Table 3-2. The Bureau of Labor Statistics (BLS) estimated its own scale for the Family Budgets Program.[3] For this program, BLS estimated higher, intermediate, and lower budgets for two types of reference families: (1) a four-person family living in an urban area and comprising a husband aged 38 and employed full-time, a homemaker wife (no age speci-

---

[2] Renwick (1993b:Table 6) presents budgets for single-parent families of size two to size seven, consisting of separately developed estimates (including assumptions about scale economies) for food, housing, household operations, health care, transportation, clothing, and personal care. One key assumption that shapes her implicit equivalence scale is that a parent needs her or his own bedroom and that only two children can share a bedroom.

[3] BLS last respecified the family budgets for 1966-1967 and last published them, updated for price changes, for 1981.

TABLE 3-2 Selected Alternative Equivalence Scales: Increment in the Scale Value for a Spouse and Each Added Child (Relative to a Scale Value of 1.00 for a Single-Adult Family)

Source or Type of Scale	Family Size				
	2	3	4	5	6
Per capita	1.00	1.00	1.00	1.00	1.00
Official U.S. poverty thresholds[a]	0.29	0.26	0.40	0.35	0.27
Bureau of Labor Statistics Family Budgets Program[b]	0.67	0.61	0.50	0.50	0.56
U.S. Department of Agriculture (food only)[c,d]	0.83	0.80	0.70	0.63	0.80
Organization for Economic Cooperation and Development[e]	0.70	0.50	0.50	0.50	0.50
Canadian low-income cut-offs (LICOs) (1986 base)[f]	0.36	0.37	0.26	0.18	N.A.
Lazear-Michael (1980a)[g]	0.06	0.24	0.18	0.22	N.A.
Lazear-Michael (1988)[h]	1.00	0.40	0.40	0.40	0.40
Jorgenson-Slesnik[i]	0.76	0.60	0.73	0.34	1.28
Van der Gaag and Smolensky[j]	0.45	0.10	0.17	0.10	0.09
Income Survey Development Program (ISDP)[k]	0.47	0.18	0.16	0.13	0.11
Rainwater (1990)[c,l]	0.26	0.18	0.15	0.12	0.11
Statistics Canada[c,m]	0.17	0.27	0.23	0.00	N.A.

NOTE: Add values across, plus 1.00 for the first adult, to obtain the scale value for a particular size family.

[a]Calculated from the thresholds for a married-couple family of the specified family size compared to the threshold for an unrelated individual under age 65 (Bureau of the Census, 1993c:Table A).

[b]Derived on the basis of Engel curves and food shares. The scale values shown are for a family in which the head is aged 35–54 (in Sherwood, 1977:Table 7).

[c]Scale values do not distinguish between adults and children.

[d]Derived by adding the costs of individual food plans and adjusting for household economies of scale in the use of food (Peterkin et al., 1983:15).

[e]Derived on the basis that a second adult adds 70 percent to the single adult's budget and each child adds another 50 percent (Organization for Economic Cooperation and Development, 1982).

[f]Derived using a method similar to the iso-prop method (in Wolfson and Evans, 1989:55); see text.

[g]Derived using a variant of the Barten model.

[h]Derived using a variant of the Rothbarth model; see text.

[i]Derived using a variant of the Barten model, which also distinguishes by the age, race, and sex of the houshold head, geographic region, and farm-nonfarm residence. The scale values shown are for a family headed by a nonfarm white male between the ages of 25 and 34 and living in the Northeast (in Jorgenson and Slesnik, 1987:Table 2).

[j]A subjective scale applying to households in which the head is under age 65 (in Danziger et al., 1984:Table 2).

continued on next page

TABLE 3-2   *Continued*

[k]A subjective scale applying to households in which the head is under age 65, derived from the 1979 ISDP Research Panel by estimating the log of the answer to a survey question regressed on the log of income, the log of family size, and the age and sex of the family head (in Danziger et al., 1984:Table 2).

[l]A subjective scale derived from Gallup Poll data on the amount needed to get along by estimating the log of the annualized get-along income amount regressed on the log of income, the log of family size, and the respondent's age (Rainwater, 1990:19).

[m]A subjective scale based on 1986 data (in Wolfson and Evans, 1989:55).

fied), a girl of 8, and a boy of 13; and (2) a retired couple aged 65 or older, in reasonably good health and living independently. BLS developed an equivalence scale to adjust these budgets for other family types, by applying the Engel methodology (discussed below) to data from the 1960-1961 Consumer Expenditure Survey (CEX). The key assumption of this methodology is that families spending an equal proportion of income on food have attained an equivalent level of living.

The USDA also developed its own equivalence scale to determine adjustments to its food plans for the economies of scale of larger families. (The food plans themselves were constructed for adults and children of different sexes and ages.) The resulting scale values, applied to the cost of the Thrifty Food Plan for a reference family of four persons (husband and wife aged 20-54 and two children aged 6-8 and 9-11) are used in setting benefit levels in the Food Stamp Program. (The Thrifty Food Plan is the successor to the Economy Food Plan that formed the basis of the original poverty thresholds.) The USDA scale was originally developed in 1962 and revised in 1975 on the basis of data from a 1965 survey of food consumption of nonfarm households (Kerr and Peterkin, 1975). The scale has not been changed since 1975 because, according to an evaluation study (Greger, 1985:26), "the superiority of alternate adjustment factors was not clear." The USDA scale, which applies to food consumption only, is more generous for larger families than the BLS scale, which, in turn, is more generous than the scale implicit in the official poverty thresholds (see Table 3-2).

Other organizations have dealt with the equivalence scale issue by proposing simple formulas, in the same general spirit as our own recommendation. Most notably, the Organization for Economic Cooperation and Development (OECD) (1982) has used an administratively convenient scale in which the first adult counts as 1.0, an additional adult counts as 0.7, and children count as 0.5 of an adult (see O'Higgins and Jenkins, 1990, for an application of the OECD poverty measure). Although there is no explicit recognition of economies of scale in these numbers, they are built into the scale, most obviously in the "discount" for the second adult.

An even simpler scale underlies the poverty guidelines, which were originally developed by the Office of Economic Opportunity and are issued annually by the U.S. Department of Health and Human Services (see Burke, 1993:Table 12) and used to determine eligibility for many government assistance programs (see Chapter 7). They are constructed by smoothing the official thresholds for different size families: the resulting implicit equivalence scale counts the first adult as 1.0 and each additional adult or child as 0.35.

Behavioral Scales

Simple weighting schemes, like the OECD or our own recommendation, have the obvious merit of transparency, but they take no account of actual behavior except insofar as their plausibility is anchored in everyday experience. For at least a century, economists and others have tried to provide a more solid foundation for equivalence scales, analyzing patterns of household behavior in an attempt to measure the differential needs of adults and children, as well as economies of scale. At its simplest, one might attempt to measure the costs of children by looking at family budgets and identifying how much a poor family spends on such child-related expenditure items as food, clothing, and education. There are many such attempts in the literature: see, for example, Dublin and Lotka (1946), who wanted to calculate the "money value of a man" and needed to deduct the cost of bringing him to maturity; more recently, Lindert (1978) wanted to use child costs to predict fertility.

The fundamental problem with such attempts is that adding children to a family without adding additional resources can only cause the family to rearrange its purchases. If a family spends more on child goods, it must spend less on something else. Consequently, a complete accounting of the "additional" expenditures associated with children would lead to the inevitable conclusion that children cost nothing. Although the children come with needs, which cause additional expenditures on some goods, those needs are paid for out of the same resources, which makes the family as a whole worse off, causing a reduction in expenditures in other goods. If one is going to calculate the cost of the children from the data, one must compare families of different types but at the same level of living. That is, in order to calculate measures of the cost of the children, or, indeed, of the extent of household economies of scale, one must have some procedure for knowing when two families of different types are equally well off; only in that way will a comparison of their expenditure patterns reveal what is the cost of the children or the extent of economies of scale.

These arguments suggest that in order to calculate the equivalence scale by comparing expenditure patterns, one needs to know the equivalence scale to start with, so that one can be sure of comparing two households at the same level of well-being. If so, there is essentially no hope of using behavior to calibrate the scales, a result that has been formally demonstrated by Pollak and Wales (1979). Although calculating the cost of a change in family size may appear to be analogous to the problem of calculating the money needed to compensate for a price change—something that is routinely done in applied economics—the two problems are not the same. In the case of a price increase, one can observe how much a family consumes and so get a good idea of how much a price increase will cost it. But when a child is added to a family, one does not know how much the child consumes (or how much the parents alter their own consumption accordingly) and so cannot price out its cost.

The situation is not quite hopeless. If one can devise a general rule that indicates when households of different compositions are equally well off, one can use it to calculate the scale. The discussion above showed that such a rule cannot be deduced from the data. In principle, postulating such a rule is not very different from picking a set of arbitrary but plausible values to constitute an equivalence scale, but it is easier to propose and defend a single rule than a whole set of scale values. The use of a single principle guarantees that the scale values for different family types are internally consistent, unlike the scale values implicit in the current official poverty thresholds. In the next two subsections, we discuss two different rules for determining when households are equally well off and the procedures for calculating equivalence scale values that are associated with each. (See Table 3-2 for examples of scales developed by these rules.)

The Engel and Iso-Prop Methods   The most famous of the procedures for determining equivalence scales dates back to the work of Ernst Engel and uses the share of a family budget devoted to food as an indicator of living standards (E. Engel, 1895). Engel's Law, that the share of food expenditure in the budget declines as people become better off, is one of the earliest and most widely confirmed empirical generalizations in economics. It is also true that, at the same level of income or total expenditure, households with more children spend a larger share of their budget on food. Engel went beyond these two empirical facts to assert that the share of food in the budget correctly indicates the standard of living across families of different types. If one accepts this assertion, one has a simple and easily applied rule for detecting which of two families is better off, even when the families have different compositions. If the food share for two families is the same—that is, if they are on the same food "iso-prop" curve—they are equally well off. Hence, all one needs to do to calculate the cost of an additional family member is to calculate how much must be added to the budget to restore the family's food share to its original value.

Figure 3-2, which shows the relationship between the food share and family income for two families, illustrates how Engel's procedure works. Line

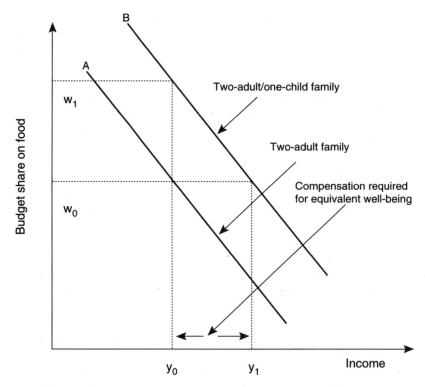

FIGURE 3-2 Engel method for equivalence scales. (See text for discussion.)

A is for a two-adult family, and line B is for that family with the addition of a child. Line B is higher at all levels of income: that is, more is spent on food at all income levels. In the original situation, the small family has income y_0 and food share w_0, which rises to w_1 after the addition of the child. According to Engel, this family is restored to its original standard of living when its food share returns to its original value. This would happen if the family's income was increased to y_1, or if the family received some compensation equivalent to $y_1 - y_0$. The equivalence scale value for a two-adult/one-child family relative to a two-person family is given by the ratio of y_1 to y_0.

In practice, the Engel method would be implemented, not diagrammatically, but by fitting an Engel curve in which food expenditures—or the share of expenditures on food—is linked to income and family characteristics. The estimated equation can then be used to calculate what increase in income is equivalent to an additional family member (of various types), and the equivalence scale values are calculated exactly as above. The example was cast in terms of two parents having their first child, but so long as one is prepared to accept Engel's basic assertion that food shares indicate welfare, the method can be used to compare any family type with any other family type and so to produce a complete set of equivalence scale values. This method will presumably also capture any economies of scale so long as they are reflected in the food share, as they must be if the Engel assertion is correct.

It is also possible to extend the Engel method beyond the share of food to the share of other necessities; this iso-prop approach was introduced by Watts (1967; see also Seneca and Taussig, 1971) and underlies the Canadian low-income cut-offs (LICOs) (see Wolfson and Evans, 1989). When goods other than food are included, the assumption is that the share of those goods indicates family welfare. Hence, the procedure will work in the same way as does Engel's, provided that the share falls with income (because the goods are necessities) and rises with family size.

The Engel method and its iso-prop variants are only as good as the basic assumption that the food (or other necessity) share correctly indicates family welfare, which can be argued. Even if Engel's Law is correct, and even if larger families spend a larger share of their budget on food, there is no automatic implication that the food share is a valid indicator of the standard of living. Engel's Law says that richer families have lower food shares, so that, among families of the same composition, it makes sense to argue that families with higher food shares are poorer than families with lower food shares, which is no more than a restatement of the law. Larger families spend a larger share on food, as do poorer families, but it does not follow that larger families spend more on food because they are poorer or that one can measure how much poorer they are by calculating the income drop that would have produced the same effect.

Nicholson (1976) has convincingly argued that the food share is a poor indicator of the standard of living. Consider again a married couple who have their first child, and suppose for the purposes of the argument that one has managed to calculate the correct compensation and that the appropriate amount has been paid to the family. What will happen? The parents have been fully compensated and so are expected to spend, out of their share of family resources, the same fraction on food as they did before the birth of the child. But a child consumes mostly food and clothing, so this fully compensated family actually spends a larger share of its total budget on food. According to Engel, the family is worse off than it was before because its food share is higher, and it must be paid more to compensate it for the cost of the child. By this argument, the compensation calculated according to the Engel method assigns too large a cost to children. Nicholson's argument is a persuasive one, and we do not believe that the food (or necessities) share should be used to calculate equivalence scale values.

The Rothbarth and Other Methods   Instead of using food share, Rothbarth (1943) used expenditures on adult goods as an indicator of the standard of living, if not of the whole family, at least of its adult members. Using the same example of a married couple with a child, the argument is that the child brings needs but no resources and that those needs can be met only by making cuts elsewhere in the budget. If one can find some goods that children do not consume—alcohol, tobacco, and adult clothing being the most obvious and frequently used examples—their consumption should decline when a child is added to the family. The decline is caused by the diversion of income to the child, so that if one can calculate the reduction in income that would produce that same decline, one has calculated the amount of income diverted to the child, and, thus, its cost.

The mechanics of the procedure are similar to those of the Engel method and are illustrated in Figure 3-3. Again, there is curve A for the original family and curve B for the larger family containing the child, but now they slope upwards, since expenditure on adult goods is assumed to rise with income. And it is the lower curve, curve B, that is associated with the larger family because expenditures on adult goods are cut to make room for the additional expenses associated with the child. The original family with income y_0 spends a_0 on adult goods, which is reduced to a_1 in the presence of the child. If income is increased to y_1 from y_0, the original level of expenditure on adult goods is restored, and, according to Rothbarth, so are the living standards of the parents. The difference $y_1 - y_0$ is therefore the cost of the child, and the ratio of y_1 to y_0 is the equivalence scale value for the two family types.

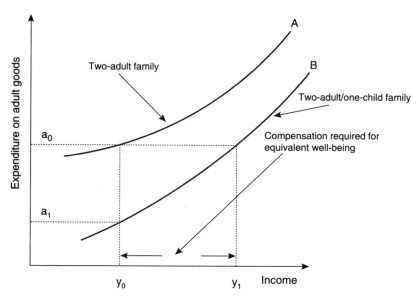

FIGURE 3-3 Rothbarth method for equivalence scales. (See text for discussion.)

   The Rothbarth procedure does not suppose that adults derive welfare only from adult goods: adults and children share in the household expenditures on most goods—including food and shelter. The adult goods are special because they are not consumed by children, so that for them one observes the consequences of the resource diversion to the child uncontaminated by the additional expenditures generated by the child. The decline in expenditures in adult goods shows, not the decline in the living standards of the parents, but the amount of money that the parents have diverted to the child, which is the information needed.

   It is possible to raise objections to the Rothbarth procedure, just as it was possible to object to the Engel procedure. In particular, although children do not consume adult goods, their presence may alter their parents' tastes for adult goods. For example, prospective mothers are advised neither to smoke nor to consume alcohol during pregnancy. Similarly, the presence of a child or children in the household is likely to change the way the parents spend their leisure time and "spare" cash. As a result, it may be difficult or impossible to find pure adult goods—goods for which family consumption is not directly affected by the presence of children. Rothbarth's method is also confined to measuring the cost of children; it makes no contribution to measuring the cost of additional adults or the size of economies of scale. These objections, although real, are a good deal less fundamental than Nicholson's criticism of the Engel method (see Deaton and Muellbauer, 1986, for further discussion). Rothbarth's method, or closely related variants, has been used in the United States by a number of researchers (see, e.g., Lazear and Michael, 1988).

   Most of the several other methods for estimating equivalence scales that have been discussed in the literature in economics and econometrics (see Deaton and Muellbauer, 1980:Ch.8, and Browning, 1992, for reviews) are more ambitious than either the Engel or the Rothbarth procedures in that they attempt to measure the differential needs of adults and children on a commodity-by-commodity basis. They are also a good deal more complex than either the Rothbarth or the Engel methods, and, consequently, are much more difficult to interpret. In many cases, it is difficult to know what fundamental assumption is driving the results. For Engel, the food share indicates welfare, and for Rothbarth, adult goods indicate adult welfare, and it is these "identifying" assumptions that allow one to derive the scale. For the more complex schemes, the identifying assumptions are far from clear, which means that it is difficult to know exactly what is being measured or whether the concept is a sensible one.

Subjective Scales

If it is accepted that equivalence scales are based more on their plausibility than on empirical evidence, there is much to be said for simply asking people what the scale should be. This has been done in a number of social surveys by asking respondents how much they would need to just avoid poverty and then linking the results to variations in family size.

The 1979 Income Survey Development Program (ISDP) Research Panel asked the following question: "Living where you do now and meeting the expenses you consider necessary, what would be the very smallest income you (and your family) would need to make ends meet?" The answers were converted to a logarithmic scale and regressed on the logarithm of family after-tax income, the logarithm of family size, and the age and gender of the head of the family. The coefficients from this equation were then used to predict an income that yielded a consistent level of well-being for families of different sizes and composition. The equivalence scale was created by dividing the predicted income for any size family by the predicted income for the reference family (Danziger et al., 1984); see Table 3-2.

Rainwater (1990:Table 5) analyzed Gallup Poll data on the "smallest amount of money a family of four needs each week to get along in this community," regressing the logarithm of the annualized amounts on the logarithm of income, the logarithm of family size, and the respondent's age. With one exception (the increment in the scale value for two-person families), the Rainwater and ISDP scales are remarkably similar considering the different questions, samples, and estimated equations (see Table 3-2). Statistics Canada, however, found that such scales are typically sensitive both to question wording and to the model estimated (Wolfson and Evans, 1989:41).

Subjective scales are attractive because they ask the opinion of the same people for whom the scales are devised. But it does appear that the precise question wording may affect answers, and people may take their "wants" into account as well as their needs. The scales often do not consistently decrease with each additional household member (see Table 3-2). These inconsistencies may reflect general difficulties with answers to subjective questions: respondents are being asked about topics that may be far from their everyday experience and to which they may never have given serious thought. And interviewers do not have any way of cross-checking absurd or nonsensical responses (see Bradbury, 1989, on problems with subjective equivalence scales).

Recommended Procedure

We do not believe that any of the published methods for adjusting poverty thresholds provide a fully defensible rationale for calculating the kind of equivalence scale that is needed for different family types. But we do believe that the poverty line must be adjusted for differences in family sizes and composition; we also believe that some correction is better than no correction; and we believe that it is possible to do better than scaling in proportion to the number of people in the family.

Our recommended procedure recognizes the differences between adults and children and allows for economies of scale so that the cost per adult equivalent falls as the number of adult equivalents rises. We explicitly recognize the arbitrariness that is inherent in all scales. We have selected a set of scale values for which internal consistency is guaranteed by their derivation from a single rule, but for which ultimate support comes from their transparency and plausibility. At the same time, we have tried to check that the scale values are at least roughly consistent with the Rothbarth procedure as applied to data from the CEX, because the Rothbarth method is the most defensible of existing methods.

We recognize that our proposed equivalence scale is crude and makes no allowance for the effects of relative prices, location, or variations in scale values that may relate to the level of living of the family. Nor does our procedure anchor economies of scale to the particular commodities—primarily housing—that generate them. However, we note that several of the adjustments that might conceivably be made through an equivalence scale (such as for child care or commuting expenses) are made on the resource side of the poverty measure, rather than to the thresholds, and are thus taken into account (see Chapter 4). But many omitted issues are left for future research, and we regard our recommendation as no more than a sensible way that is a clear improvement on current practice.

Our recommended equivalence scale—as well as the relationship to other equivalence scales—can be described through the use of the general formula introduced above (for a family with A adults and K children):

$$\text{scale value} = (A + PK)^F.$$

Both parameters P and F lie between 0 and 1.0. If P is set to 1.0, children and adults are assumed to consume the same amount at the poverty line. If F is set to 0, household economies of scale are assumed (unrealistically) to be so large that the scale values are unity for all family types, and the poverty line will be the same for all; a family of four would need only as much as a single individual. If F is set to 1.0. no economies of scale are assumed. Setting both F and P equal to 1.0 gives the per capita result in Table 3-2.

Ruggles (1990:77) recommends using the square root of family size as an equivalence scale short of extensive revisions in the current scale and, in conversation with the panel, Harold Watts also endorsed this approach. This proposal is a special case of the formula, in which P is unity and F is 0.5:

$$\text{scale value} = (A + K)^{0.5}.$$

Ruggles argues that setting F to 0.5 maintains the overall elasticity of the Orshansky scales while smoothing out some of the irregularities. Entering this recommendation into our general equation makes obvious the fact that the relationship of child to adult consumption is not directly addressed, although since large families tend to contain a larger proportion of children, the economies of scale that come from the square root rule are coincidentally picking up the distinction between adults and children. The alternative is (as we propose) to make F larger and to compensate by setting K to less than 1.0, thus explicitly recognizing the distinction between pure economies of scale and family composition. Since we consider the needs of, say, five adult family members living together to be greater than the needs of a family of two adults and three children, we prefer our formula to that suggested by Ruggles.

The OECD equivalence scale (Organization for Economic Cooperation and Development, 1982) sets a single adult to be 1.0, each additional adult to be 0.7, and each child to be 0.5. This rule can be written in the same general way:

$$\text{scale value} = [1.0 + 0.7(A{-}1) + 0.5K]^{1.0}.$$

In this case, there is no adjustment for economies of scale beyond the family composition adjustment for the second and additional adults. A third adult adds as much to household needs as does a second or fourth adult. The OECD scale, in contrast to the square-root rule, puts all of the adjustment on adult and child differences, without an explicit recognition of economies of scale except for the difference between the first and second adult. In fact, the OECD scale can be well approximated by ignoring the distinction between adults and children and between the first and second adult and simply raising family size to the power of 0.72 (see Buhmann et al., 1988).

Betson and Michael (1993) provide estimates of the parameters in the general formula from work of Betson (1990), who estimated the cost of children by using the Rothbarth method and data from the 1980-1986 CEX; see Table 3-3. Betson (1990) reported the estimated percentages of total expenditures devoted to children (see first column of Table 3-3) and the proportional cost of children in one- and two-parent families (see second column of Table 3-3). For example, two parents with a child are estimated to spend 24 percent of their budget on their child and hence would need 31 percent more income than a childless couple to be equally well off. The estimates presented in Table 3-3 cannot be directly interpreted in terms of the relationship between the consumption needs of children relative to adults (P) nor the scale economy factor (F). To select which two parameters would best fit the information contained in Table 3-3, Betson and Michael (1993) chose the parameters that minimized the sum of squared deviations of the observed proportional costs of children (the five values in the second column of Table 3-3) from the fitted proportional costs of children expressed in terms of the panel's recommended equivalence scale formula:

$$\frac{\text{scale value } (A,K)}{\text{scale value } (A,0)} = \left(\frac{A + PK}{A}\right)^{F}.$$

TABLE 3-3   Estimates of the Cost of Children (Using Rothbarth Method)

Family Type	Percent of Family Budget Spent on Children (P)	Scale Value of the Family Type $[1/(1-P)]^a$
Single-Parent Family		
One child	0.307	1.443
Two children	0.496	1.984
Two-Parent Family		
One child	0.237	1.311
Two children	0.354	1.548
Three children	0.407	1.686

SOURCE: From Betson and Michael (1993); Betson (1990).

^{a}The scale value in column 2 is derived as the inverse of 1 minus the estimate in column 1. Scale values for children in a single-parent family are expressed relative to a value of 1.00 for a single-adult family; scale values for children in a two-parent family are expressed relative to a value of 1.00 for a two-adult family.

The fitted parameters using these estimates are

$$\text{scale value} = (A + 0.70K)^{0.762}.$$

Thus, Betson and Michael's work suggests a scale in which children are treated as 0.70 of an adult and in which the number of adult equivalents is raised to a power of 0.76 to account for scale economies for larger families.

We recommend a scale in which children are treated as 0.70 of an adult (as in the Betson and Michael results) and in which the number of adult equivalents in the family is raised to a power in the range of 0.65 to 0.75 (similar to, but not exactly the same as, the Betson and Michael results). The high value of our recommended range represents the Betson and Michael result of 0.76 rounded down to 0.75. The low value of the range is suggested because this value does not make such a large difference for the poverty threshold for single-person families (compared with the official threshold—see below).

We believe that the general form of the proposed scale satisfies two critical criteria: it recognizes the differences between children and adults and adjusts for scale economies with increasing family size in a consistent manner. In addition, it is easy to explain and implement. Finally, the use of a scale formula of this type acknowledges the inevitable arbitrariness in adjusting the poverty thresholds for different family circumstances rather than disguising it in opaque econometric analysis.

Figure 3-4 shows the current scale, the square-root proposal, the proposed scale with scale economy factors of 0.65 and 0.75, and the OECD scale.

In comparing these scales, one can see that the current scale generally assumes the greatest economies of scale as family size increases while the OECD scale assumes the least economies of scale. (An exception is the square-root proposal, which assumes greater economies of scale for families of size five or larger.) We rejected the current scale because, as shown above, it is inconsistent across family types. Also, in our opinion, it assumes economies of scale that are too large for large families and for families of two in comparison with one-person families. The square-root proposal is an improvement but ignores the differences between adults and children and is even less generous to large

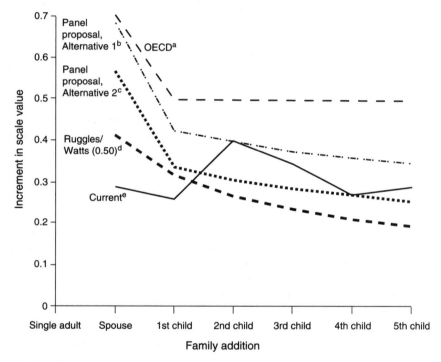

FIGURE 3-4 Alternative equivalence scales: increment for each added family member (relative to a scale value of 1.00 for a single adult). [a]The OECD scale adds 0.70 for each added adult and 0.50 for each child. [b]Each child is treated as 0.70 of an adult, and the number of adult equivalents in the family is raised to a power of 0.75. [c]Each child is treated as 0.70 of an adult, and the number of adult equivalents in the family is raised to a power of 0.65. [d]Suggested by Ruggles (1990) and Watts (in conversation with the panel): each child is treated as the equivalent of an adult, and the number of people in the family is raised to a power of 0.50. [e]The current scale is calculated by converting the 1992 threshold for each family type to the 1992 threshold for an unrelated individual under age 65; the threshold for two adults is the one in which the head is under age 65.

families. At the other extreme, the OECD method is straightforward and easy to use, but, in our opinion, it assumes economies of scale that are too small across the family size distribution. The range of scale economy factors that we recommend (0.65 to 0.75) produces results that are between the extremes and more consistent across family size.[4]

It is because the choice of an equivalence scale cannot avoid arbitrariness that we suggest a range for the scale economy factor, F. Judgment is also involved in setting the parameter P for the proportionate needs of children relative to adults, and we could have suggested a range for P as well as for F. However, it becomes difficult to grasp the implications of alternative equivalence scales across the family size distribution if both parameters are varied. Moreover, the two parameters are, as we have discussed, not independent. Thus, if P is set at 1.0, implying no difference between the needs of children and adults, then it is appropriate to set F closer to zero (as in the square-root proposal), because F then accounts both for economies of scale in the strict sense and also for the fact that larger families include more children. If, however, as we propose, children are assumed to need less than adults, then it is appropriate to raise F closer to a value of 1.0, although how much closer is, to repeat, a matter of judgment. For these reasons, we recommend a value of 0.70 for P and a range for F of 0.65 to 0.75, which is consistent with the value for P.

In reaching a judgment on the specific form of the equivalence scale for implementation, it will be important to consider the implications of a particular value of F in relation to the current scale. Although one wants to improve on that scale, there is an argument for making a choice that does not represent a great departure from the current implicit scale for particular population groups. In this regard, we note the importance of applying the scale to the poverty threshold for the reference family of two adults and two children rather than to the threshold for a one-person family. Because the current scale assumes such great scale economies in moving from one-person to two-person families, it is clear that the use of almost any other scale, including those that we propose, will produce significantly higher thresholds for two-person and larger families. The only exception, again, is the square-root proposal, which will produce larger thresholds for small families but smaller thresholds for large families than the current scale.

---

[4] The low-income measure recently adopted on an experimental basis by Statistics Canada to supplement the low-income cut-offs uses an equivalence scale formula to adjust the reference threshold for a one-person family. The formula treats each added adult in the family as 0.40 of the first adult and each added child under age 16 as 0.30 of the first adult, with one exception: in a single-parent family, the first child is treated as 0.40 of the adult (see Statistics Canada, 1991:172-173). This scale gives results similar to the square-root proposal for families of size one to size five and results similar to our proposal with a 0.65 scale economy factor for larger families.

TABLE 3-4 Alternative Equivalence Scales, with Scale Values Expressed Relative to a Value of 1.00 for a Family of Two Adults and Two Children

Family Type	Type of Scale				
	Current Official[a]	0.50 Scale Economy Factor[b]	0.65 Scale Economy Factor[c]	0.75 Scale Economy Factor[d]	OECD[e]
One-person family[f]	0.513	0.500	0.451	0.399	0.370
Married couple	0.660	0.707	0.708	0.672	0.630
Plus one child	0.794	0.866	0.861	0.841	0.815
Plus two children	1.000	1.000	1.000	1.000	1.000
Plus three children	1.177	1.118	1.130	1.151	1.185
Plus four children	1.318	1.225	1.251	1.295	1.370
Plus five children	1.476	1.323	1.367	1.434	1.556

[a]The current scale is calculated by expressing the official 1992 threshold for each family type as a multiple of the 1992 threshold for a family of two adults and two children; the thresholds for unrelated individuals and two-adult families are those for people under age 65.

[b]Suggested by Ruggles (1990) and Watts (in conversation with the panel): each child is treated as the equivalent of an adult, and the number of people in the family is raised to a power of 0.50. The resulting scale value for each family type is converted to a ratio of the scale value for two-adult/two-child families.

[c]Each child is treated as 0.70 of an adult, and the number of adult equivalents in the family is raised to a power of 0.65. The resulting scale value for each family type is converted to a ratio of the scale value for two-adult/two-child families.

[d]Each child is treated as 0.70 of an adult, and the number of adult equivalents in the family is raised to a power of 0.75. The resulting scale value for each family type is converted to a ratio of the scale value for two-adult/two-child families.

[e]The OECD scale adds 0.70 for each added adult and 0.50 for each child. The resulting scale value for each family type is converted to a ratio of the scale value for two-adult/two-child families.

[f]Includes people living alone and with others in a household not related to them.

By applying the proposed scale to the threshold for the reference two-adult/two-child family, the differences from the current scale are reduced for families in most size categories; see Table 3-4 and Figure 3-5. Specifically, for a given value of the reference family threshold, the proposed scale with a scale economy factor of 0.75 produces very similar thresholds as the current scale for all family size categories except for one-person families, for which it produces a threshold value that is less than 80 percent of that produced by the current scale. The proposed scale with a scale economy factor of 0.65 produces thresholds that are reasonably close to the official thresholds for all categories—somewhat lower for one-person families and families of five to seven members and somewhat higher for families of two and three members. In our analysis with March CPS data (see Chapter 5), we explore the implications of the choice of a scale economy factor on poverty rates for families of different sizes and other population groups.

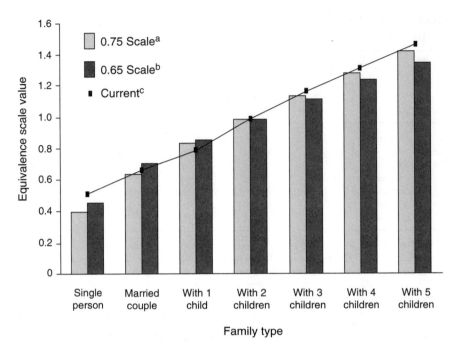

FIGURE 3-5 Current and proposed equivalence scales expressed relative to a value of 1.00 for a family of two adults and two children. [a]Each child is treated as 0.70 of an adult, and the number of adult equivalents in the family is raised to a power of 0.75. The resulting scale value for each family type is converted to a ratio of the scale value for two-adult/two-child families. [b]Each child is treated as 0.70 of an adult, and the number of adult equivalents in the family is raised to a power of 0.65. The resulting scale value for each family type is converted to a ratio of the scale value for two-adult/two-child families. [c]The current scale is calculated by converting the official 1992 threshold for each family type to the 1992 threshold for a family of two adults and two children; the thresholds for unrelated individuals and two-adult families are those for people under age 65.

ADJUSTMENTS BY GEOGRAPHIC AREA

Overview and Recommendations

There is wide agreement that it is desirable to adjust poverty thresholds for differences in prices. Indeed, the current official thresholds are regularly updated for changes in the Consumer Price Index (CPI) to keep them constant in real terms. However, no adjustment has been made for spatial differences in prices, not because the adjustment is necessarily undesirable in principle, but because of the practical difficulties of adequately measuring those differences. There are no geographic area cost-of-living indexes that correspond to the CPI: BLS produces price indexes for a limited number of metropolitan areas, but not for rural areas. Moreover, the BLS indexes are designed to allow comparison of differences in price inflation across areas; they do not permit comparison of price *levels* across areas.

Yet there has been a substantial amount of empirical research on the issue, and we believe that it is important to make at least a partial adjustment for geographic cost-of-living variations. At this stage of knowledge, we recommend that the adjustment be made for the housing component of the poverty thresholds. Research indicates that housing (including utilities) is the item for which prices vary most across the country, and considerable effort has been devoted to estimating interarea housing cost indexes. We believe that data available from the decennial census will support an adequate adjustment for housing cost differences, which we recommend be implemented by size of metropolitan area within nine regions of the country. We recommend research on ways to update the housing cost index values for intercensal years. And we recommend further research, not only on geographic variations in housing prices, but also on cost-of-living differences more generally. Such research should be linked to the priority of improving the U.S. database on household consumption (see Chapter 5).

RECOMMENDATION 3.2. **The poverty thresholds should be adjusted for differences in the cost of housing across geographic areas of the country. Available data from the decennial census permit the development of a reasonable cost-of-housing index for nine regions and, within each region, for several population size categories of metropolitan areas. The index should be applied to the housing portion of the poverty thresholds.**

RECOMMENDATION 3.3. **Appropriate agencies should conduct research to determine methods that could be used to update the geographic housing cost component of the poverty thresholds between the decennial censuses.**

RECOMMENDATION 3.4. **Appropriate agencies should conduct research to improve the estimation of geographic cost-of living differences in housing as well as other components of the poverty budget. Agencies should consider improvements to data series, such as the BLS area price indexes, that have the potential to support improved estimates of cost-of-living differences.**

Feasibility and Desirability

The feasibility and desirability of adjusting the poverty thresholds for geographic cost-of-living differences has been the topic of repeated discussion and analysis for a long time. A principal impediment to making any such adjustment has been the lack of adequate data, although there are also conceptual and measurement issues to resolve.

Some analysts have argued against the whole idea of adjusting the poverty thresholds for area price differences on the grounds that such differences are likely to be offset by income differences and, hence, do not represent real differences in life quality. Indeed, the available data suggest that areas with higher prices are also areas with higher income levels: for example, a cost-of-housing index that we calculated for states correlates highly with state median family income.[5] Economic theory suggests that, over the long run, measures of "quality of life" (taking into account both prices and wage levels) will equalize across areas because people will continually migrate to the more pleasant areas, causing prices to rise and wages to fall (see Bloomquist, Berger, and Hoehn, 1988; Roback, 1982; and Rosen, 1979).

The counterargument, with which we agree (see Ruggles, 1990), is that poverty is not measuring the "quality of life" in broad terms, but minimum levels of need. As such, the poverty thresholds should be higher in areas with higher prices—even if average incomes are also higher. Also, many spells of poverty are short (see Chapter 6), which argues for geographic adjustments of the poverty thresholds because families cannot be expected to quickly change location when they experience a decline in income (see Renwick and Bergmann, 1993, on this point).

Given that one wants to adjust the poverty thresholds for geographic price differences, the question is how to do it. It is sometimes suggested that interarea differences in income or wages be used as a proxy for interarea price differences. As noted above, there is a high correlation between area income levels and area price levels; however, income and wages are affected by factors other than prices, and it seems preferable to work toward measuring price differences directly.[6] One approach is to measure what it costs in different locations to purchase a fixed market basket of goods, that is, to develop a fixed-weight interarea price index. Under this approach, the same consumption items are included in the market basket for all areas of the country, and the same weight or fraction of the market basket is assigned to each item (e.g., vehicle purchases or winter clothing).

Another approach is to price different market baskets in different areas under the assumption that needs differ across areas. For example, the market

---

[5] The rank-order correlation is .893, computed using Spearman's r. We estimated state cost-of-housing indexes for analysis of differences among states in eligibility and benefit standards for the Aid to Families with Dependent Children (AFDC) program (see Chapter 8).

[6] The use of interarea differences in income levels could overestimate differences in price levels: for example, the variation in state median family income is wider than the variation that we calculated in a state cost-of-housing index adjusted for the share of housing in the proposed poverty budget; see Table 8-4 in Chapter 8.

basket might include more winter clothing or home heating fuel in colder than in warmer climate areas, or the market basket might give a higher weight to vehicle purchase and maintenance costs in rural and other areas that lack public transportation. Such an approach seems to make intuitive sense; however, its implementation quickly leads to a host of difficult and hard-to-defend judgments. For example, higher air conditioning costs in warmer areas may offset lower heating costs; or, car owners in rural areas may get better gasoline mileage that lowers their vehicle use costs.

Even harder to develop and justify are the use of different market baskets that reflect consumption differences across regions that are not explained by such factors as climate differences. For example, on the basis of observed interregional differences in food consumption patterns, the BLS Family Budgets Program gave higher weight to less expensive foods—such as lard and pork—and lower weights to more expensive foods—such as butter and beef—in the budgets for areas in the South relative to the North (see Expert Committee on Family Budget Revisions, 1980; Sherwood, 1975, 1977). Although people in different regions may have different tastes for foods (or other items), it seems dubious to thereby conclude that such differences should be reflected in the market basket for pricing. To do so is to assume that Northerners "require" a more expensive diet than Southerners, or, alternatively, to assume that consumers would be equally satisfied with any one of the market baskets that is priced. We conclude that the fixed-weight type of interarea price index is preferable to an approach that attempts to specify "needed" or "appropriate" differences in area market baskets.

In this regard, the Expert Committee on Family Budget Revisions (1980:Chap. VII) recommended that a fixed-weight interarea price index be developed for the BLS family budgets and that the market baskets themselves not vary by area. The Committee found that people trade off housing and transportation costs so that the total for these two items does not vary importantly by region or city size; hence, the Committee recommended against interarea differences in the transportation component of the budget. The Committee also argued that regional differences in food consumption should not be used to develop different food budgets by region. Finally, the Committee suggested that, while estimates could be developed of additional expenditures for utilities and clothing needed for different climates, these estimates should not be reflected in the budgets themselves but rather in tabulations by area of the gross income needed to support the standard budget plus any climate allowance plus state and local taxes.[7]

---

[7] The Committee initially attempted to estimate area budgets representing equivalent levels of living by trying to find total expenditure levels that were consistent with average spending patterns and with spending enough on food to purchase the USDA Moderate Food Plan; however, the analysis failed to turn up consistent or robust findings.

The use of a fixed-weight interarea price index avoids the difficult problems of specifying differing regional market baskets, but many formidable definitional and measurement issues remain. One conceptual issue concerns the specification of the market basket for the purpose of adjusting the poverty thresholds: whether to use a basket with items and weights based on the expenditure patterns of typical families, as is done for the Consumer Price Index, or a basket that reflects the spending patterns of families at lower expenditure levels. We believe that a reasonable approach would link the market basket to spending patterns of families with expenditures somewhat below the median.

If one assumes that an appropriate market basket is specified, the next set of problems concerns data and measurement. In order to have an adequate fixed-weight interarea price index, the sample of prices must be large enough in each area for reliable estimation, and consistent definitions must be applied for all of the items that are priced (e.g., the same type and quality of new car or winter coat must be priced in the same type of sales outlet in each area).

Research Findings on Price Differences

Given all of the difficulties noted above, one might be tempted to give up on the task of developing an interarea price index for use in adjusting the poverty thresholds. Arguing for a continued effort to develop a reasonable approach is the evidence we have—admittedly imperfect—of important price differentials across areas.

As of fall 1981, the last year for which BLS published the family budgets, the relative cost of the lower consumption budget for a family of four, for urban areas in the 48 contiguous states, varied from about 113 percent of the national average in the San Francisco-Oakland and Seattle-Everett metropolitan areas to 91 percent of the average in nonmetropolitan urban areas of the South (Bureau of Labor Statistics, 1982:Table 4).[8] In general, relative costs were higher in metropolitan than in nonmetropolitan areas and in the West and Northeast than in the South.

As noted above, a problem with the BLS interarea price index for the Family Budgets Program is that it reflected varying market baskets across regions. Sherwood (1975:Table 1) compared the BLS index with a fixed-weight interarea index for the intermediate (or "standard") budget for fall 1973. He found the same general patterns; however, the relative cost of the standard budget in the South was not quite as low or that in the Northeast quite as high with the fixed-weight index as with the BLS index.

BLS has continued to publish consumer price indexes for regions, popu-

---

[8] Relative costs in Alaska and Hawaii were 146 and 126 percent, respectively, of the national average.

lation size classes of metropolitan areas, and the largest metropolitan areas. However, these indexes can properly be used only to compare rates of change in prices across areas—not price levels—because the data come from a probability sample of prices that is designed to produce the national CPI, and so there is no particular consistency across areas in items that are priced. Trends in price changes across areas over the past decade do suggest, however, that the regional and size-of-place price differentials measured in the old Family Budgets Program still persist and, indeed, may have increased. Thus, from 1983 (when the index in each region equaled 100) to 1992, prices increased by 47 percent in the Northeast and 42 percent in the West, compared with 36-37 percent in the Midwest and South (Bureau of the Census, 1993d:Table 761).

ACCRA (formerly the American Chamber of Commerce Researchers Association) publishes a fixed-weight interarea price index that in 1992 covered 300 metropolitan areas across the country.[9] The market basket applies to a "midmanagement" rather than poverty budget standard, but the relative cost patterns across areas are similar to those cited for the BLS Family Budgets Program index, although with an even wider dispersion. (In this regard, the BLS index for the higher budget showed similar patterns but somewhat more dispersion than the index for the lower budget.) Some higher cost areas in 1992 according to the ACCRA (1992:Table 1) index were New York City with an index value of 214 (relative to 100 for all areas), Boston with an index value of 137, and Los Angeles-Long Beach with an index value of 130; some lower cost areas were such small urban places as Moultrie, Georgia, with an index value of 87 and Kennett, Missouri, with an index value of 83.

Recently, economists at BLS have been reanalyzing the price data that are collected for the CPI for the 30 largest metropolitan areas, Anchorage and Honolulu, and samples of smaller metropolitan areas. In all, price data are collected in 85 geographic areas, most of which are grouped together (for publication) by region and city size class. The object of the reanalysis has been to develop a fixed-weight interarea price index that can be used to compare relative costs across areas, rather than just relative rates of change in prices (Kokoski, 1991; Kokoski, Cardiff, and Moulton, 1992, 1994). The approach uses hedonic regression methods (see below) to determine the contribution of geographic location to the prices of various items.

The BLS research is still in progress, and, for purposes of adjusting the poverty thresholds, it would be necessary to expand the price sample to cover rural as well as urban areas and to increase the sample size in urban areas to improve reliability. Nonetheless, the research is very promising. Moreover, the findings to date suggest an interim approach that would be an improve-

---

[9] Participating Chambers of Commerce price items for the index according to standards set by ACCRA.

ment over not adjusting the poverty thresholds at all for geographic price difference—to adjust the thresholds for differences in the cost of housing.

Overall, using BLS price data for the period July 1988-June 1989, Kokoski, Cardiff, and Moulton (1992) found little variation in prices by geographic area for many components of the CPI. For example, the index values for food at home (which accounts for 10% of the CPI market basket) ranged from 93 to 107 (with the geometric mean of all areas in the sample equal to 100). This range of values excludes Anchorage and Honolulu, for which the food-at-home index values were 126 and 139, respectively. However, for some categories of expenditures, Anchorage and Honolulu did not have higher costs than other areas. Index values for the category of private transportation commodities, which account for 16 percent of the CPI market basket (and include new and used vehicles, gasoline and oil, coolant and fluids, and automobile parts and equipment), ranged from 91 to 105. Greater variation was observed for clothing (index values of 67 to 154) and professional medical services (index values of 62 to 147), but these items account for relatively small proportions of the CPI market basket (6% and 3%, respectively). The component with the largest variation was shelter, with index values from 52 to 183. Utilities also showed considerable variation, with index values from 57 to 152. Together, these two components account for 33 percent of the CPI market basket (25% for shelter and 8% for utilities).

The 1976 Poverty Studies Task Force (Economic Research Service, 1976) reported the same finding as in the BLS research—that interarea price differences are greater for housing (including utilities) than for other commodities.[10] These results, coupled with the fact that housing is such a large component of spending, led us to look for a methodology that could provide a reasonable basis for adjusting the poverty thresholds for interarea housing cost differences. We found that considerable analytical effort has been expended to develop estimates of geographic differences in housing costs; the chief methodological challenge has been to devise methods that estimate differences in prices per se and not differences in the characteristics or quality of the housing being priced.

Estimating Geographic Variations in Housing Costs

Several methodologies have been used to estimate geographic housing cost differences, including:

• the methods used by the U.S. Department of Housing and Urban Development (HUD) to calculate fair market rents for metropolitan areas and nonmetropolitan counties;

---

[10] The 1976 study recommended against adjusting the poverty thresholds for geographic price differences because of the lack of adequate data.

- the methods used for the BLS Family Budgets Program; and
- hedonic regression methods, which attempt to isolate the contribution of individual characteristics of the housing unit to its price (geographic location is included as an independent variable of the regression in order to capture the effect of location controlling for all other characteristics of the unit).

HUD Fair Market Rents

For the administration of rental housing subsidies, HUD has developed a set of fair market rents, which vary by geographic location. Fair market rents are estimated annually for 2,416 counties that are outside metropolitan areas and all 341 U.S. metropolitan areas (Office of Policy Development and Research, 1992a).

Fair market rents are defined to equal gross rent (including utilities) at the 45th percentile of the rent distribution of standard quality rental housing units. HUD uses one of three data sources to make "base-year" estimates: (1) the American Housing Survey (AHS) provides estimates for 44 of the largest metropolitan areas, which include one-half of the nation's rental housing stock; (2) the decennial census; and (3) local random digit dialing telephone surveys. The base-year estimates are updated by using the shelter component of the local area CPI, where available, or estimates of price changes developed by the telephone surveys for HUD regions.

For fair market rents derived from AHS data, the sample for estimating the 45th percentile value for each bedroom size category consists of units occupied by recent movers, excluding public housing units, newly built units, noncash rental units, and units that lack certain characteristics indicative of housing quality. For rents derived from decennial census data, the sample for estimating the 45th percentile value is somewhat more heterogeneous because it is not possible to exclude public housing units, and there is less information with which to determine housing quality.

In 1989, the index values for HUD fair market rents for two-bedroom standard rental units relative to a U.S. average value of 1.00 ranged from 1.73 in San Francisco to 0.58 in nonmetropolitan areas of the Midwest. As expected, areas in the Northeast and the West had higher average rents than areas in the Midwest and the South. Areas in the Northeast and West also had higher rents relative to area median income than areas in the Midwest and the South (Kathryn Nelson, private communication).

There are some problems with the HUD fair market rents. First, they do not fully adjust for interarea differences in the quality of housing. Although all housing units sampled are said to be of "standard" quality, there may be a large variation within that category. Second, they are based on only one-third of the housing stock since only recent movers are surveyed. Rents for the other two-thirds may be lower as a result of a discount for long-term renters.

Finally, the rents in some areas are adjusted upwards because of legislative mandates.

At the same time, the methodology used to develop the fair market rents has advantages, chief among them that it is straightforward and can be applied to all areas of the country. Indeed, from the perspective of adjusting the poverty thresholds, there is an attraction to using the methodology with decennial census data. Although the census database is limited in content, it provides adequate sample sizes and an ability to estimate housing costs on a consistent basis for the entire nation (at least for the census year).

BLS Family Budgets Program

The BLS Family Budgets Program included an allowance for shelter costs in the intermediate budget that represented a weighted average of costs for a standard five-room rental unit, and a standard five- or six-room owned home that was purchased by the family 6 years prior to the budget reference date. The units that were priced met recommendations on essential household equipment, adequate utilities, and neighborhood location, originally made by the American Public Health Association and the U.S. Public Housing Administration (see Expert Committee on Family Budget Revisions, 1980). Weight variations between areas assumed varying quantities and types of fuel associated with climatic differences.

BLS developed shelter cost indexes for 40 metropolitan areas and the nonmetropolitan areas of the four census regions. Excluding Alaska and Hawaii, the BLS sample area with the highest shelter costs in 1973 was Boston, with an index value of 1.48; the area with the lowest shelter costs was Austin, with an index value of 0.68. When the measurement is limited to differences in *rental* costs, there was somewhat less dispersion in the index values across areas: in 1973 the BLS area with the highest rental costs was San Francisco, with an index of 1.44; the areas with the lowest rental costs were Austin and Baton Rouge, with indexes of 0.76 (Sherwood; 1975:14).

Like the HUD approach, the BLS approach to estimating shelter costs for the Family Budgets Program can be criticized for not controlling sufficiently for differences in the characteristics of the housing units for which cost data were obtained. Hence, it is likely that interarea price differences were affected by differences in quality, but, as Sherwood (1975) pointed out, how much variation is attributable to price differences and how much to quality differences is unknown. Also, it is not known whether the price differentials would have been the same for other specifications of units, such as larger or smaller units or homes purchased more recently than 6 years ago.

Rosen (1978) further criticized the BLS approach of specifying, a priori, a particular set of housing characteristics to use in developing interarea housing cost indexes. He argued that the BLS method ignores the possibility of factor substitutions in housing production across cities. Moreover, the units that were priced and used in the BLS calculation might not be representative of units in a given community; also, there might be systematic differences across cities in the characteristics that were excluded.

Hedonic Models

Many analysts have taken another approach to estimating the price effects of various housing characteristics, including the price effect of geographic location. This approach is to develop a hedonic regression pricing model that relates observed market prices of housing to the implicit prices of the characteristics of the unit. In other words, hedonic models are used to isolate the contribution of individual housing characteristics to the price of housing. Examples of hedonic models include those developed by:

- Gillingham (1975), who analyzed microdata on individual housing units in 10 cities drawn from the 1960-1961 Comprehensive Housing Unit Survey conducted by BLS together with data on neighborhood characteristics from the 1960 decennial census;
- Blackley, Follain, and Lee (1986), who analyzed data from the 1975 and 1978 Annual Housing Survey to calculate housing cost indexes for 34 metropolitan areas;
- Thibodeau (1989), who created housing price indexes for 60 metropolitan areas using Annual Housing Survey data for 1974-1983; and
- Kokoski, Cardiff, and Moulton (1992, 1994), who produced interarea price indexes for consumer goods and services (including housing) as of 1989 for 44 areas (32 large metropolitan areas and 12 other region and city size classifications), using the CPI database (see also Moulton, 1992).

Hedonic models are subject to a number of criticisms. Rosen (1978) objected that the choice of characteristics to include in any model is arbitrary. He also pointed out that the rank order of the indexes for cities or metropolitan areas usually depends on which city is used as the reference city (i.e., which city is assigned an index value of 1.0). Gillingham (1975) documented this phenomenon in his work. He and other analysts also estimated large standard errors for area-specific indexes; further, they found that the size of the standard error was affected by the specification of the bundle of characteristics included in the particular hedonic model.

Kokoski, Cardiff, and Moulton (1992, 1994) attempted to correct for some of the problems with hedonic models in their analysis, which used the BLS CPI database for selected metropolitan areas matched with neighborhood characteristics data from the decennial census. This database has the advantage of relatively large sample sizes for the areas covered. The authors regressed the natural logarithm of the price of shelter on characteristic variables. (Their

TABLE 3-5 Hedonic Model Price Indexes for Rent and Rental Equivalence, and Combined Multilateral Index, Selected Areas, July 1988–June 1989

Area or Population Size	Index for Renters	Index for Owners	Combined Index	Rank
Northeast				
New York City	1.216	1.877	1.818	2
New York-Connecticut suburbs	1.404	1.711	1.830	1
New Jersey suburbs	1.329	1.514	1.635	6
Philadelphia-Wilmington-Trenton	1.000	1.000	1.117	13
Boston-Lawrence-Salem	1.326	1.613	1.712	3
Pittsburgh-Beaver Valley	0.726	0.698	0.786	36
Buffalo-Niagara Falls	0.783	0.821	0.903	25
Areas of 500,000–1,200,000	0.987	0.952	1.068	15
Areas of 100,000–500,000	0.786	0.758	0.850	28
Areas under 100,000	0.802	0.912	0.982	21
Midwest				
Chicago-Gary-Lake County	1.004	1.034	1.143	12
Detroit-Ann Arbor	0.928	0.873	0.985	20
Cleveland-Akron-Lorain	0.758	0.753	0.839	30
Minneapolis-St. Paul	0.954	0.886	1.004	18
St. Louis-East St. Louis	0.740	0.729	0.812	33
Cincinnati-Hamilton	0.765	0.742	0.833	31
Kansas City, Mo.-Kan.	0.713	0.702	0.784	37
Milwaukee	0.887	0.892	0.993	19
Areas of 500,000–1,200,000	0.716	0.707	0.789	35
Areas of 100,000–500,000	0.667	0.651	0.729	40
Areas under 100,000	0.522	0.449	0.518	44
South				
Washington, D.C.	1.049	1.165	1.266	11
Dallas-Fort Worth	0.673	0.745	0.807	34
Houston-Galveston-Brazoria	0.555	0.639	0.685	41
Miami-Fort Lauderdale	0.939	0.905	1.020	17
Atlanta	0.794	0.868	0.945	23
Baltimore	0.861	0.954	1.035	16
Tampa-St. Petersburg-Clearwater	0.755	0.684	0.782	38
New Orleans	0.776	0.810	0.892	26
Areas of 500,000–1,200,000	0.682	0.704	0.778	39
Areas of 100,000–500,000	0.557	0.583	0.642	42
Areas under 100,000	0.551	0.516	0.585	43
West				
Los Angeles County	1.427	1.551	1.690	4
Greater Los Angeles	1.375	1.286	1.462	9
San Francisco-Oakland-San Jose	1.423	1.535	1.676	5
Seattle-Tacoma	0.927	0.976	1.073	14
San Diego	1.153	1.426	1.498	8
Denver-Boulder	0.758	0.898	0.959	22
Portland-Vancouver	0.858	0.830	0.935	24
Honolulu	1.184	1.470	1.550	7

TABLE 3-5 *Continued*

Area or Population Size	Index for Renters	Index for Owners	Combined Index	Rank
West—*continued*				
Anchorage	1.004	1.219	1.289	10
Areas of 500,000–1,200,000	0.705	0.803	0.863	27
Areas of 100,000–500,000	0.727	0.774	0.848	29
Areas under 100,000	0.718	0.742	0.820	32
Low index value	0.522	0.449	0.518	
Median index value	0.798	0.871	0.952	
High index value	1.427	1.877	1.830	

SOURCE: Kokoski, Cardiff, and Moulton (1992:Table 2.4).

NOTE: Areas are ordered within region by population size as of the 1990 census; rankings are assigned to the combined index values from 1 (highest cost) to 44 (lowest cost).

equations included some 33 attributes of housing units and neighborhoods.) They created bilateral interarea price indexes from the resulting antilogs of the estimated coefficients on the area dummy variables, and then created "multilateral" indexes from the bilateral indexes. The authors claim that the resulting multilateral indexes are independent of the choice of reference area and, hence, that the rankings for areas are stable.

The results obtained by Kokoski, Cardiff, and Moulton (1992) for July 1988–June 1989 tend to accord with common expectations about the location and magnitudes of high- and low-cost areas; see Table 3-5. The major cities in the Northeast (Boston and New York City) and the West (Los Angeles, San Francisco, and San Diego) have the highest shelter costs, with index values between 1.46 and 1.83. Washington, D.C., Philadelphia, and Chicago have mid-range index values, while other major cities in the Midwest (e.g., St. Louis, Cleveland) and the South (e.g., Houston and Dallas) have substantially lower shelter costs, with index values between 0.69 and 0.84. Small urban areas generally have lower shelter costs than larger metropolitan areas in the same region. Indexes for rent and owners' equivalent rent tend to be highly correlated. In areas in which rent control is important (e.g., New York, Los Angeles, and San Francisco), the index for owners' equivalent rent is substantially higher than the rent index.

Discussion

What can one conclude from the work to date to develop interarea housing cost indexes? Clearly, there are no easy answers to the question of how to develop a reliable index. Not only does the use of different methods yield different results, but researchers have also estimated differing index values for the same areas even when using similar methods and data (e.g., compare Blackley, Follain, and Lee, 1986, and Thibodeau, 1989). The work at BLS to extend and improve the hedonic methodology so that the results are more stable with respect to such factors as the choice of reference area or independent variables is very promising, but this effort is still developmental. Moreover, data problems remain: the data source with the largest sample size and coverage (the decennial census) has limited information on housing characteristics, while other data sources that are richer in content (the CPI database and the American Housing Survey) are smaller in size and restricted in the areas they cover.[11]

Yet despite all the methodological problems and uncertainties, it is clear that the cost of housing differs across geographic location. For example, HUD fair market rents differ significantly across areas even when they are adjusted for the median income of the area. Overall, we believe the findings support the importance of an adjustment of the poverty thresholds for geographic variations in housing costs.

Furthermore, despite the problems and uncertainties, the literature helps indicate the size of geographic area for which an adjustment would be feasible and appropriate. Data are not available with which to develop housing cost indexes for every city and town in the United States, but an adjustment for areas classified by population size within region would accord with findings that intraregional differences are highly correlated with population: larger cities or metropolitan areas within a region are more expensive than smaller areas. This pattern is evident in the results from Kokoski, Cardiff, and Moulton (1992, 1994), and in other studies as well (e.g., Thibodeau, 1989); Ruggles (1990) recommends an adjustment of this type.

Recommended Approach

At the current state of knowledge, we conclude that a feasible way to move toward a comprehensive interarea price index with which to adjust the poverty thresholds is first to develop an interarea price index for shelter. Not only are housing costs a large component of a poverty budget, but housing cost

---

[11] The national component of the American Housing Survey is conducted every two years and currently includes about 57,000 housing units; the sample is designed to produce national estimates, and the geographic identification made available to users is limited to four regions and central city-suburb and urban-rural classifications. The metropolitan component currently includes samples of about 5,000 housing units in each of 44 metropolitan areas; 11 areas are surveyed each year on a rotating cycle. The CPI database (described above) obtains price data for about 85 areas, most of which are combined for publication into size classes within each of four regions.

variations are also significant across areas, and there are data and methods available with which to develop a reasonable index. Such an index should take account of differences by region and size of place.

For constructing housing cost index values for the purpose of adjusting the poverty thresholds for all families, not just urban families or families in selected areas, we conclude that it is almost a necessity to turn to the decennial census, despite its limited data content. Given a decision to use census data, the HUD methodology for developing fair market rents has appeal. This methodology is subject to criticism because of its use of a limited number of characteristics to define a "standard" rental apartment unit for comparing rental costs across areas. But until more sophisticated methods are fully developed and, more important, improvements effected in the underlying database with which to apply these methods, the HUD methodology appears to offer a reasonable alternative that is easy to understand and straightforward to implement.

We implemented a modified version of the HUD approach with 1990 census data to determine whether we could develop interarea housing cost index values that accorded reasonably well with major findings in the literature.[12] We obtained a copy of an extract of 1990 census data for every U.S. county (originally prepared for HUD). This extract provided the distribution of rents for two-bedroom apartments that had complete plumbing facilities, kitchen facilities, and electricity and in which the occupant had moved in within the last 5 years. (Units for which no cash rent was paid or for which the rent covered one or more meals were excluded.)

Using these data, we first produced index values (relative to 1.0 for the nation as a whole) for each of the 341 metropolitan areas in the country and for nonmetropolitan areas within each state. Compared to the 32 metropolitan areas for which Kokoski, Cardiff, and Moulton (1992) also computed index values by using hedonic techniques with the CPI database, our index showed similar patterns, although less variation. For these 32 areas, our index values ranged from 1.67 to 0.88; the Kokoski, Cardiff, and Moulton values ranged from 1.83 to 0.69.[13] The rank–order correlation of our index values with those of Kokoski, Cardiff, and Moulton is very high (.897 computed using Spearman's *r*).

We next grouped the metropolitan areas into six population size categories within each of the nine census regions (divisions), aggregated the nonmetropolitan areas by region, and recomputed the index values. Following

---

[12] The modification was that, for reasons of feasibility and consistency of estimates across the nation, we used decennial census data exclusively rather than a combination of census, AHS, and random digit dialing survey data.

[13] One reason for the difference may be that our index values included utilities, which Kokoski, Cardiff, and Moulton found in a separate analysis varied somewhat less than shelter costs per se.

TABLE 3-6   Cost-of-Housing Index Values (Relative to 1.00 for the
United States as a Whole) by Region (Census Division) and Size of
Metropolitan Area

Region and Population Size	Index Value
New England (Connecticut, Maine, Massachusetts, New Hampshire, Rhode Island, Vermont)	
Nonmetropolitan areas	1.062
Metropolitan areas under 250,000	1.368
Metropolitan areas 250,000–500,000	1.290
Metropolitan areas 500,000–1,000,000	1.335
Metropolitan areas 1,000,000–2,500,000	1.321
Metropolitan areas 2,500,000 or more	1.475
Middle Atlantic (New Jersey, New York, Pennsylvania)	
Nonmetropolitan areas	0.797
Metropolitan areas under 250,000	0.771
Metropolitan areas 250,000–500,000	0.992
Metropolitan areas 500,000–1,000,000	1.045
Metropolitan areas 1,000,000–2,500,000	0.943
Metropolitan areas 2,500,000 or more	1.424
East North Central (Illinois, Indiana, Michigan, Ohio, Wisconsin)	
Nonmetropolitan areas	0.713
Metropolitan areas under 250,000	0.864
Metropolitan areas 250,000–500,000	0.906
Metropolitan areas 500,000–1,000,000	0.969
Metropolitan areas 1,000,000–2,500,000	0.988
Metropolitan areas 2,500,000 or more	1.133
West North Central (Iowa, Kansas, Minnesota, Missouri, Nebraska, North Dakota, South Dakota)	
Nonmetropolitan areas	0.630
Metropolitan areas under 250,000	0.817
Metropolitan areas 250,000–500,000	0.913
Metropolitan areas 500,000–1,000,000	0.956
Metropolitan areas 1,000,000–2,500,000	1.063
Metropolitan areas 2,500,000 or more	N.A.
South Atlantic (Delaware, District of Columbia, Florida, Georgia, Maryland, North Carolina, South Carolina, Virginia, West Virginia)	
Nonmetropolitan areas	0.713
Metropolitan areas under 250,000	0.873
Metropolitan areas 250,000–500,000	0.911
Metropolitan areas 500,000–1,000,000	1.016
Metropolitan areas 1,000,000–2,500,000	1.097
Metropolitan areas 2,500,000 or more	1.270
East South Central (Alabama, Kentucky, Mississippi, Tennessee)	
Nonmetropolitan areas	0.564
Metropolitan areas under 250,000	0.757
Metropolitan areas 250,000–500,000	0.852
Metropolitan areas 500,000–1,000,000	0.878

TABLE 3-6 *Continued*

Region and Population Size	Index Value
East South Central—*continued*	
Metropolitan areas 1,000,000–2,500,000	N.A.
Metropolitan areas 2,500,000 or more	N.A.
West South Central (Arkansas, Louisiana, Oklahoma, Texas)	
Nonmetropolitan areas	0.617
Metropolitan areas under 250,000	0.780
Metropolitan areas 250,000–500,000	0.797
Metropolitan areas 500,000–1,000,000	0.868
Metropolitan areas 1,000,000–2,500,000	0.914
Metropolitan areas 2,500,000 or more	1.011
Mountain (Arizona, Colorado, Idaho, Montana, Nevada, New Mexico, Utah, Wyoming)	
Nonmetropolitan areas	0.713
Metropolitan areas under 250,000	0.841
Metropolitan areas 250,000–500,000	0.946
Metropolitan areas 500,000–1,000,000	1.090
Metropolitan areas 1,000,000–2,500,000	1.006
Metropolitan areas 2,500,000 or more	N.A.
Pacific (Alaska, California, Hawaii, Oregon, Washington)	
Nonmetropolitan areas	0.891
Metropolitan areas under 250,000	0.978
Metropolitan areas 250,000–500,000	1.041
Metropolitan areas 500,000–1,000,000	1.063
Metropolitan areas 1,000,000–2,500,000	1.236
Metropolitan areas 2,500,000 or more	1.492
Low index value	0.564
Median index value	0.951
High index value	1.492

NOTE: Housing cost indexes calculated from 1990 census data on gross rent for two-bedroom apartments with specified characteristics; index values drawn from the 45th percentile of the gross rent distribution (see text).

N.A., Not applicable: no such areas in the region.

the HUD approach, the index values were based on the cost of housing at the 45th percentile of the value of the distribution for each area. The results of our calculations produced the expected findings of higher index values in the Northeast and West and higher index values for larger relative to smaller areas; see Table 3-6.

We further adjusted these index values for the estimated fraction of the poverty budget accounted for by housing (including utilities), which we set at 44 percent. In effect, we produced a fixed-weight interarea price index with two components—housing and all other goods and services—in which the price of other goods and services is assumed not to vary.[14] This adjustment narrowed the range of index values (and, hence, the range of poverty thresholds: for example, the adjusted index value for metropolitan areas with 2,500,000 or more population in New England dropped from 1.475 to 1.209; conversely, the adjusted index value for metropolitan areas with 250,000–500,000 population in the West South Central division rose from 0.797 to 0.911. Finally, we collapsed the index values for geographic areas smaller than 250,000 population because of restrictions on area identification in the surveys that are available for estimating poverty rates (the Current Population Survey and the Survey of Income and Program Participation). The final set of 41 index values that we used for our analysis of the likely effects of implementing our proposed poverty measure is provided in Table 5-3 in Chapter 5.[15]

Before deciding on a set of index values by metropolitan area size category within region, we looked at index values produced in the same manner for each of the 50 states and the District of Columbia. There has been interest expressed in adjusting the poverty thresholds for state cost-of-living differences for such purposes as allocating funds to disadvantaged school districts under the Elementary and Secondary Education Act.

To compare the set of state index values and our proposed set, we assumed that the index values we originally calculated for each of the 341 individual metropolitan areas and for the nonmetropolitan components of each state were the "truth."[16] We then determined what fraction of the population would be misclassified—relative to the individual metropolitan and nonmetropolitan area index values—by using a single index value for the nation as a whole or separate index values for the nine regions (divisions), for states, and for the proposed classification by metropolitan area population size category within region.[17]

We found that the use of the national index value of 1.0 (i.e., not adjust-

---

[14] The estimate of 44 percent comes from CEX tabulations of expenditures of two-adult/two-child families. We looked at families spending at the 35th percentile of the distribution on food, housing, and clothing, determined the share of housing of that total, and converted that share to a fraction of the total poverty budget, including food, housing, and clothing times a multiplier of 1.15. Clearly, one could derive somewhat different values of the fraction of housing in the budget, depending on the percentile or multiplier chosen.

[15] The figure of 41 index values represents nine regions (census divisions) by five size classes of metropolitan areas, minus four categories that have zero population: the West North Central, East South Central, and Mountain divisions lack any metropolitan areas larger than 2,500,000 population, and the East South Central division lacks any metropolitan areas of 1,000,000 to 2,500,000 population.

[16] In practice, however, we do not believe that it makes sense to develop such a large number of separate indexes for adjusting the poverty thresholds for several reasons: one is that there is a problem of small sample size for rental units with the specified characteristics in smaller metropolitan areas.

[17] The analysis was carried out using index values for the population size categories shown in Table 3-6 before any collapsing.

ing the poverty thresholds for cost-of-housing variations across areas) would result in 55 percent of the population having an index value that differed by more than 20 percent from its own metropolitan (or nonmetropolitan) area-specific index. The use of regional index values (for the nine census divisions) would result in 45 percent of the population having an index value that differed by more than 20 percent from its own area-specific index. The use of state index values would result in 33 percent of the population having an index value that differed by more than 20 percent from its own area-specific index. In contrast, the use of the proposed index values for metropolitan area size categories within regions would result in only 9 percent of the population having an index value that differed by more than 20 percent from its own area-specific index. In other words, a higher fraction of the population would be assigned a more accurate index value with our proposal than with a regional or state housing cost index. These results demonstrate the superiority of our proposal compared with the alternatives of adjusting solely for regional variations in the cost of housing or of adjusting for variations across states.[18]

The proposed procedure should not be viewed as the last word on the issue of adjusting poverty thresholds for area differences in the cost of living, but rather as a modest step in the right direction. The procedure only takes account of housing cost differences and, even for those differences, will assign index values to people in some areas that are considerably in error. The procedure also does not take account of housing cost variations *within* areas (e.g., differences in costs between central cities, suburbs, and exurbs of, say, large metropolitan areas). And it does not take account of special circumstances, such as significantly higher housing costs for areas in Alaska and Hawaii than are reflected in the index values for the Pacific region as a whole.[19] Finally, the proposed method is a crude instrument for attempting to measure housing price differences that do not also reflect quality differences. Nonetheless, within the constraints of available data, we believe that the proposed procedure is a significant improvement over the current situation of no adjustment. The methodology is understandable, operationally feasible, and produces results that conform well with other findings from research.

Updating the Housing Cost Index

The index values for cost-of-housing differences can readily be revised as necessary every 10 years as new decennial census data become available. How-

---

[18] For some purposes, it may still be desirable to use state index values to adjust poverty thresholds for differences in the cost of housing (or the cost of living generally). For example, this type of adjustment may make sense when the poverty thresholds are used as the need standard for such assistance programs as AFDC (see Chapter 8).

[19] It would certainly be possible to make some ad hoc adjustments to our index, but we did not believe it desirable for us to attempt such an effort.

ever, revising the index as infrequently as every 10 years could result in a blip in the poverty rates in many areas because of changing housing markets. For example, an area that was experiencing a housing "boom" at the time of one census could experience a housing "bust" at the next census and vice versa. It would be preferable to revise the index on a more frequent basis. Indeed, such a revision in the index values that we developed from 1990 census data would be desirable for the initial implementation of the proposed poverty measure.

HUD faces a similar need to update its fair market rents on a regular basis. To make annual adjustments, HUD uses data from several sources, (described above), including the American Housing Survey, local area CPI shelter cost indexes, and random digit dialing surveys. We encourage an assessment of the appropriateness of the HUD methods for updating the housing cost index values from the decennial census for use, in turn, in adjusting the poverty thresholds. We also encourage research on the usefulness and cost-effectiveness of other methods that could be considered.

Further Research

Obviously, the issue of how best to adjust poverty thresholds for geographic differences in the cost of housing and in the cost of living more broadly is an area for further research and development. We have argued that the proposed procedure for taking account of housing cost differences for metropolitan areas categorized by size of population within region represents an improvement over the current method of no adjustment at all. We have also noted the limitations of the procedure, which represents a step, but only a step, in the right direction.

We encourage appropriate agencies, such as BLS and HUD, to undertake research on improved methods for determining area price differences. Ideally, the research would include other goods besides housing and would consider such issues as the types of geographic areas (cities, counties, larger areas) for which an adjustment is feasible and appropriate. It would also address methodological issues, such as refinements to the hedonic regression models under development at BLS that appear so promising.

To effect much additional improvement in the methodology and the reliability of interarea price indexes, new data collection may be required. For example, expanding the sample for the American Housing Survey, which provides more detailed information on housing characteristics than the decennial census, would be one way to develop improved cost-of-housing indexes (whether using the proposed adaptation of the HUD methodology or hedonic methods). Even more broadly, expanding the BLS price samples for housing and other goods would be a way to develop comprehensive cost-of-living indexes that represent valid indicators of differences across areas in prices at a point in time and not just differences in the rate of price changes. However, these kinds of expanded data collection efforts would entail considerable cost. We believe it is worth investigating the cost-effectiveness of additional data collection, in terms of the expected improvements in the data for such purposes as adjusting the poverty thresholds.

In general, we believe that data related to consumer expenditures and prices need to be improved in the United States. Not only is the CPI database limited in sample size and area coverage, but the CEX, which is used to determine the CPI market basket, is very limited—in sample size and in other ways—for purposes of measuring and understanding poverty, consumption, and savings. We discuss issues of needed data improvements for poverty measurement, including improvements in the CEX, in Chapter 5. Before that discussion, in Chapter 4, we consider an appropriate definition of family resources to compare with the poverty thresholds for determination of poverty rates for the nation, geographic areas, and population groups.

Defining Resources

4

The determination of whether a family (or an individual) is in or out of poverty requires two pieces of information: a poverty threshold and an estimate of the family's economic resources. In the two preceding chapters, we examined thresholds and adjustments to them; in this chapter, we review definitions of family resources. We recommend a definition and analyze the elements that go into its derivation, considering for each the justification, methods and data for implementation, and needed research for improved implementation.

OVERVIEW AND RECOMMENDATION

The definition of family resources that has been used for determining poverty status in the United States ever since the current measure was adopted in the 1960s is annual gross money income. We believe this definition is seriously flawed and recommend a change: namely, that family resources be defined as disposable money and near-money income that is available for consumption of goods and services in the poverty budget.

A key to our recommendation is the principle of consistency between the resource definition and the threshold concept. That is, a defensible measure of poverty requires that resources and needs—the thresholds—be defined consistently. Hence, we approached the task of evaluating alternative family resource definitions by constant reference to the proposed concept for the poverty thresholds—namely, a budget for food, clothing, and shelter and a small additional amount for other needed consumption. For consistency with this budget concept, the definition of resources should include the value of near-money benefits, such as food stamps, that are available for consumption; it should exclude expenditures that are nondiscretionary and not available for consumption: out-of-pocket medical care expenditures (including health insurance premiums), income and payroll taxes, child care and other expenses that are necessary to earn income, and child support payments to another household. Instead of allowing for these kinds of expenses in the poverty budget, we propose, rather, to deduct them from resources for those families that incur them.

Even within the constraints imposed by our choice of a concept for the poverty thresholds, there are alternative ways to define family resources. We considered these from the perspective of two other criteria: that the definition be publicly acceptable and operationally feasible. Data limitations are a particularly important consideration for the family resource definition because of the costs of estimating resources for a large enough sample of the population from which to reliably determine the poverty rate for the nation as a whole and for various population groups. Indeed, data limitations will likely hinder the extent to which complete consistency between a threshold concept and a resource definition can be achieved in practice. Nonetheless, we stress the importance of striving for consistency.

In this respect, the current U.S. poverty measure has been deficient from the beginning. Most obviously, the poverty thresholds were derived from after-tax income data while resources were defined in before-tax terms. The reason for this discrepancy was that the data source for measuring poverty, the March income supplement to the Current Population Survey (CPS), did not obtain information that would readily allow families' taxes to be estimated.[1] Income and payroll taxes on the working poor were low when the poverty measure was developed, but they subsequently increased and, more recently, declined again. The official poverty statistics reflected none of these shifts in tax policy, although they affected the resources available to poor and near-poor families.

Other inconsistencies in the measure became apparent as society changed and new government programs were enacted. More mothers went to work outside their homes, thus incurring child care costs, yet the different needs of working and nonworking families were not reflected by modifying either the thresholds or the resource definition. In-kind benefit programs that provide such commodities as food and housing were small in scope when the current measure was developed but have increased enormously since then, yet the resource definition does not include their value.

---

[1] The CPS surveys 60,000 households each month with a series of questions that are used to determine the official monthly unemployment rate. The income supplement every March asks about sources of income for each adult household member for the previous calendar year (see Chapter 5 and Appendix B).

Since the current measure was adopted, data sources and procedures for estimating income have improved substantially. In 1980, the March CPS income questions were expanded, and questions were added about major in-kind benefits. In 1983, the Survey of Income and Program Participation (SIPP) was initiated to obtain more complete information on economic resources.[2] Also, methods were developed to adjust the March CPS income estimates in various ways (e.g., by subtracting taxes), and work is in progress on similar methods for SIPP. Yet, there has been no change in the data source or the definition of resources that is used to measure poverty.

Not only does the current poverty measure violate the consistency principle, but so does much work to date to investigate alternative measures. For example, the Census Bureau over the past decade has published a series of "experimental" poverty rate estimates from the March CPS: they are based on changes to the family resource definition but not on changes to the thresholds (see, e.g., Bureau of the Census, 1993a, 1995).[3] In some instances, this approach makes good sense: thus, the Census Bureau's estimates in which federal and state income taxes are subtracted from resources reflect a definition that is more consistent with the original threshold concept than is the current before-tax resource definition. In other instances, the changes to the resource definition are not consistent with the official thresholds. In particular, estimates by the Census Bureau (and others) in which the value of public and private health insurance benefits is added to families' resources violate the consistency principle. Since the official thresholds were first developed, medical care costs have escalated greatly, so it is inconsistent to add the value of health insurance benefits to resources without also increasing the thresholds.

The effect of just adding insurance values without also raising the thresholds is to ignore the added costs of staying out of poverty. It is also to assume that health insurance benefits are fungible (i.e., that they can be spent for other goods, such as food and housing) when this is not the case, except insofar as such benefits may free up other resources. Also, medical care costs vary significantly across the population, so that for appropriate comparisons of poverty among groups (e.g., the elderly versus younger people), it is not sufficient to increase the thresholds by an average amount for medical care.

---

[2] SIPP is a panel survey. Under the design used for the 1984–1993 panels, a new sample of 12,000–20,000 households was started each February and the members interviewed eight times at 4-month intervals, for a total of 32 months. Beginning in 1996, SIPP will be designed to have panels that last 48 months each and have larger samples of households (see Chapter 5 and Appendix B).

[3] The Census Bureau has been constrained in that Congress requested publication of estimates on the basis of alternative resource definitions (specifically, definitions that added the value of in-kind benefits), but the U.S. Office of Management and Budget did not change the thresholds.

We discuss these issues more fully in a later section of the chapter. Here we want to emphasize our principle of consistency between the definition of family resources and the threshold concept.

RECOMMENDATION 4.1. **In developing poverty statistics, any significant change in the definition of family resources should be accompanied by a consistent adjustment of the poverty thresholds.**

ALTERNATIVES FOR DEFINING RESOURCES

We considered three main alternatives to the current definition of family resources as gross money income. One alternative—the one we recommend—is to define resources as disposable money and near-money income. A second alternative, which is strongly advocated by a number of researchers, is to look at actual consumption or expenditures rather than income. A third alternative is a hybrid definition that adds to disposable income some kind of valuation of a family's asset holdings that could be used to finance consumption over a short period. This alternative is sometimes called a "crisis" definition of resources. Each alternative raises issues of determining the particular elements that comprise the definition—in a manner consistent with the threshold concept—and of determining appropriate and feasible methods and data sources for implementing each element.

Resources as Disposable Income

In comparing a definition of family resources as disposable money and near-money income with the current gross money income definition, it is clear that disposable income is preferable for measuring poverty in terms of satisfying the consistency principle. This conclusion holds whether the measurement uses the concept underlying the thresholds as originally defined or the concept that we propose.

The problem with the gross money income definition of family resources in relation to the threshold concept is that it is both too inclusive and not inclusive enough. Gross money income excludes the value of such in-kind benefits as food stamps, school meals, and public housing, yet these benefits support the types of consumption that were implicitly included in the originally developed poverty budget of food times three (and are included in the proposed poverty budget of food, clothing, shelter, and a little more). At the same time, gross money income does not exclude income and payroll taxes, but families have no choice in paying these taxes, and the money so spent cannot be used for consumption. Gross money income also does not exclude some other kinds of expenses that are not really discretionary and hence are not available for consumption of food, housing, and similar items. These expenses include out-of-pocket costs for medical care (including insurance premiums), expenses necessary to earn income (e.g., child care, commuting costs), and child support payments to another household.

By not taking account of taxes and other nondiscretionary expenses or the value of (nonmedical) in-kind benefits, the gross money income definition does not adequately characterize the extent of poverty overall or the extent of poverty among various population groups. Moreover, the gross money income definition cannot capture the effects on poverty of important government policy changes, some of which are designed explicitly to combat poverty. For example, the Earned Income Tax Credit (EITC), which operates as a type of negative income tax, was recently expanded with the explicit goal of eliminating (or greatly reducing) poverty for the working poor. Yet it cannot have any effect on the official poverty count because the current measure does not take account of either positive or negative taxes.

For example, prior to expansion of the EITC, a working family that paid taxes might have sufficiently low gross income to be classified as poor by the current measure. But if in the next year the family received a tax refund due to the expanded EITC that moved it above the poverty line, the current measure would still classify the family as poor. Another working family that paid taxes might have sufficiently high gross income to be classified as not poor under the current measure although its disposable income (after taxes) was below the poverty line. If in the next year the second family's taxes were offset by the EITC, both the current measure and a measure that uses a disposable income definition would classify the family as not poor. The current measure would show no change in the family's poverty status across the 2 years, but a measure using disposable income would show the family as poor in the first year and as having moved out of poverty in the second.

A disposable money and near-money income definition estimates the amount of resources a family actually has available for consumption. It includes the value of in-kind benefits that support consumption and excludes taxes and other nondiscretionary expenses that are not available for consumption. Such a definition provides a much better basis for comparing the extent of poverty across population groups—for example, distinguishing between working and nonworking families. It also provides a much better basis for identifying trends in poverty over time and the effects of public policy initiatives and societal changes on poverty trends.

Adjusting Income, Not Thresholds

Some analysts have proposed to attain a consistent poverty measure, not by changing the resource definition from gross to disposable income, but by constructing a larger array of thresholds: for example, higher thresholds for families with children in which the parents work than for other families with children, or higher thresholds for elderly people with higher expected out-of-pocket medical care costs.[4] We rejected this approach for a number of reasons.

Clearly, the poverty thresholds need to vary by family composition in order to represent (at least approximately) equivalent levels of need for such basic consumption items as food, clothing, and shelter. We have also argued that the thresholds should reflect the substantial differences that are evident in the cost of housing across geographic areas. However, proliferating the number of thresholds to account for other circumstances raises concerns of feasibility (as well as some concerns about presentation).

It would require a large number of added thresholds to properly account for the variations among families in their expected nondiscretionary expenses, such as out-of-pocket medical care costs, taxes, or work expenses. Not to account for such variations would be to assume that different kinds of families—e.g., families with different numbers of earners or families with or without members in poor health—face average costs when this is not the case. But the sample size of the Consumer Expenditure Survey (CEX), the basic source of data on spending, is too small to produce reliable estimates of all the needed thresholds. It might be possible to use other data sources to develop amounts for nondiscretionary expenses by which to adjust the basic thresholds derived from the CEX, but such an approach would be complicated and imprecise. A preferable approach, we believe, is for the survey that measures families' incomes to measure their actual nondiscretionary expenses at the same time. Depending on the scope of the income survey, some imputations from other data sources may be necessary to implement this approach (see below), but, overall, it seems more feasible to annually estimate disposable income than all the various thresholds.[5]

Another though less important problem with proliferating the number of thresholds concerns presentation: it would be difficult to have a reference threshold to use in public discussion of the poverty level. Thus, instead of citing the poverty line for a family of four, as is common practice, one would have to cite the poverty line for a family of four with, say, one earner—not nearly as intuitive a concept.

Still another less important problem is that, as Watts (1993) argues, the use of different thresholds for such characteristics as work status can distort com-

---

[4] Renwick and Bergmann (1993), for example, would use an income definition net of taxes and including values for in-kind benefits, but would account for out-of-pocket medical care costs, child care, and other work expenses in the thresholds rather than by adjusting income.

[5] Indeed, adjusting the thresholds rather than estimating disposable income does not wholly reduce the data demands on the income survey. For example, the income survey will need to ascertain such characteristics as health status of family members and whether the family pays child support in order to select the appropriate threshold for determining the family's poverty status.

parisons of the depth of poverty across population groups in relation to their basic consumption needs. Thus, whether child care or other work expenses are included in the thresholds or subtracted from income will not affect the poverty rate or the dollar size of the poverty gap. However, the relative importance of that gap, that is, the welfare ratio (the ratio of income to the poverty threshold), will be affected. Specifically, if the poverty thresholds are adjusted to include work expenses rather than deducting them from income, poor working families will appear relatively less poor than poor nonworking families with the same composition and dollar gap between income and needs. As Watts notes, however, one could argue that a poor working family is less well-off than a poor nonworking family with the same composition and gap between income and needs because of the greater demands on the working family's time (see Appendix C).

Recommendation

For a consistent measure of poverty with the proposed threshold concept, gross money income should be adjusted to obtain a disposable money and near-money income definition of family resources. Although there are issues of precisely how to define and estimate particular components of disposable income (e.g., whether and at what level to cap the deduction for child care expenditures by working parents), they do not affect the logic of the basic approach. The two other alternatives we considered (see below) also can satisfy the consistency principle; however, there are operational reasons and, in the case of the crisis definition, conceptual reasons to prefer the disposable income definition.

RECOMMENDATION 4.2. **The definition of family resources for comparison with the appropriate poverty threshold should be disposable money and near-money income. Specifically, resources should be calculated as follows:**

• **estimate gross money income from all public and private sources for a family or unrelated individual (which is income as defined in the current measure);**

• **add the value of near-money nonmedical in-kind benefits, such as food stamps, subsidized housing, school lunches, and home energy assistance;**

• **deduct out-of-pocket medical care expenditures, including health insurance premiums;**

• **deduct income taxes and Social Security payroll taxes;**

• **for families in which there is no nonworking parent, deduct actual child care costs, per week worked, not to exceed the earnings of the parent with the lower earnings or a cap that is adjusted annually for inflation;**

   • **for each working adult, deduct a flat amount per week worked (adjusted annually for inflation and not to exceed earnings) to account for work-related transportation and miscellaneous expenses; and**
   • **deduct child support payments from the income of the payer.**

In the remainder of this section, we review the major alternative family resource definitions and our reasons for deciding against them. In the rest of the chapter we develop in more detail the proposed definition of disposable money and near-money income. Although the definition meets the test of operational feasibility, the decision to adjust income rather than the thresholds does increase the data requirements for the survey that is used to determine families' poverty status. The March CPS does not collect all of the needed information for estimating disposable money and near-money income and, for various reasons, it is not likely to become better suited for this purpose in the future. SIPP currently obtains most of the needed information and, because it is designed as an income survey rather than as a supplement to a labor force survey, can readily be modified to provide an adequate database. We conclude (see Chapter 5) that SIPP should become the basis for the official poverty statistics in place of the March CPS.

Resources as Consumption or Expenditures

Many researchers argue that it is preferable, for a combination of theoretical and empirical reasons, to look at what families actually consume or spend rather than at their income in order to determine their poverty status (see, e.g., Cutler and Katz, 1991, 1992; Jorgenson and Slesnick, 1987; Mayer and Jencks, 1993; Slesnick, 1991a, 1991b). A basic premise of this view is that families and individuals derive material well-being from the actual consumption of goods and services rather than from the receipt of income per se; hence, it is appropriate to estimate their consumption directly.

To "estimate consumption" does not usually mean to inspect people's clothes or what they actually eat but, rather, to estimate what they spend on such items. Researchers in the field define consumption as a subset of families' total expenditures, excluding taxes, contributions to pension funds (which represent savings), and, often, gifts, and including expenditures made with assistance from in-kind benefit programs, such as food stamps. The data source for estimating consumption or expenditures is the CEX.[6]

---

[6] The CEX has two components—the Diary Survey and the Interview Survey. Researchers typically develop consumption-based measures of poverty from the Interview Survey, which provides detailed information on expenditures each quarter for about 5,000 "consumer units" (see Appendix B).

Rationale

One argument that is often made for consumption (or expenditures) as the resource definition rather than income is that consumption is a better estimate of families' long-term or "permanent" income. Thus, Friedman's (1957) permanent income hypothesis suggests that current income is comprised of a permanent component and a transitory component. Families with low levels of current income are disproportionately comprised of families with temporary income reductions. If consumption is based on permanent income and not on transitory income, families with negative "income shocks" will have consumption levels that are high relative to their income levels because they expect their long-term income to be higher, on average, than their current income. Consequently, they "dissave" in order to smooth consumption and thereby material well-being: for example, they may liquidate their savings accounts or borrow on their credit cards. Such families may be income-poor but able to maintain a constant standard of living through dissaving. The reverse will be true of high-income families, who will have consumption levels that are low relative to their income levels and positive savings.

Modigliani and Brumberg's (1954) closely related life-cycle model of behavior assumes that current consumption is equal to average lifetime resources. Thus, younger families, by borrowing, and older families, by spending down assets, tend to exhibit high consumption-to-income ratios, while middle-aged families with the highest earnings potential tend to exhibit relatively low consumption-to-income ratios. Again, it is supposed that families smooth consumption and well-being on the basis of wealth and on expected earnings by saving and dissaving at various points during their life cycles.

We note that it is not necessary to accept all of these arguments in order to support a consumption definition of resources. Thus, one need not accept the life-cycle model or the view that what is wanted is a measure of long-term or permanent income. One could simply believe it is preferable to estimate a family's actual consumption rather than the consumption that it could potentially achieve from its available income.

Another point that is often made in support of using consumption or expenditures rather than income as the resource definition is that income is poorly measured. Those making this argument can cite the known under-reporting of asset income (and other sources) in the March CPS, the likelihood that income earned "off the books" or illegally is not reported at all, and the fact that self-employed people who report business losses are often able to take sufficient cash out of their business to sustain their own standard of living.

Implications

Consumption and income definitions of resources have somewhat different implications for who is counted as poor. A consumption resource definition will include in the poverty count people who are income-rich but consumption-poor, that is, people who choose to spend at levels below the poverty threshold when they actually have incomes above that level. Some of these people may contract their spending because they foresee a drop in their income in the future, while others may simply opt for a low standard of living. In contrast, an income resource definition will exclude people from the poverty count who have an adequate income during the measurement period, whether they spend it or not.

At the same time, a consumption resource definition will exclude from the poverty count people who are income-poor (e.g., because they lost a job) but who sustain their consumption at a level above the poverty threshold by such means as borrowing from relatives or charging to the limit on their credit cards. In contrast, an income definition will count such people as poor.[7] This statement applies both to the current gross money income definition and to the proposed disposable money and near-money income definition.[8]

What one thinks of the contrasting ways in which consumption and income resource definitions treat people who are income-rich but consumption-poor and people who are in the reverse situation depends on one's view of the meaning and purpose of a poverty measure. One view is that the poverty measure should reflect the *actual level* of material well-being or consumption in the society (in terms of the number of people above the threshold), regardless of how that well-being is attained. Another view is that the poverty measure should reflect people's *ability* to obtain a level of material well-being above the threshold through the use of their own income and related resources. Some with this view would go farther to say that the members of a society have a *right* to be able to consume above the poverty level without having to resort to such means as begging, unsecured borrowing, stealing, or losing their homes. (For a discussion of the two perspectives, one emphasizing people's actual consumption levels and the other their ability to consume at a level above poverty from their own income, see Atkinson, 1989.)

In a somewhat different vein, a focus on current income (e.g., income available to families over a period such as a year) accords with the view that there is policy interest in measures of relatively short-term economic distress

---

[7] As currently implemented, an income definition will also count as poor self-employed people who have business losses in accounting terms but nonetheless have adequate cash flows from their businesses for their own needs. However, it is not necessary to estimate self-employment income in business accounting terms, and, in fact, SIPP obtains reports of cash drawn out of businesses.

[8] A crisis definition that adds asset values to income will similarly count some of the income-poor as not poor. It may even more closely resemble a consumption definition in this respect if it also includes credit card and overdraft limits.

among the population. This viewpoint would reject the notion that it is preferable to estimate permanent or life-cycle income. Furthermore, its proponents would argue that including amounts in income that are obtained by such means as charging to the limit on one's credit cards distorts the purpose of the poverty measure as a timely policy indicator of the possible need for public or private action to alleviate economic distress (see, e.g., Ruggles, 1990). Thus, a consumption resource definition is likely to lag behind other indicators of economic distress because of all the steps that families can take to sustain their consumption. In contrast, an income resource definition will include income-poor families who may be reaching the end of their ability to sustain their consumption through such means as unsecured borrowing. Hence, it may prove more useful as a warning signal to policy makers.

Assessment

On the fundamental question of whether to base the definition of family resources for the poverty measure on income or consumption, we believe that there are merits to the conceptual arguments on both sides of the debate. On balance, many members of the panel find more compelling the arguments in favor of a consumption definition that attempts to assess actual levels of material well-being. However, in the United States today, adequate data with which to implement a consumption-based resource definition for use in the official poverty measure are not available.

Although the federal government sponsors several comprehensive large-scale income surveys, the only regular consumption survey is the Consumer Expenditure Survey. Although the CEX had its beginnings nearly a century ago, it was conducted only every 10-15 years until 1980, when an annual survey began. The sample size of the CEX is significantly smaller than the sample size of the major income surveys, and the delay between collection and release is longer for consumption data than for income data.

The CEX is currently intended to support the periodic respecification of the market basket for the Consumer Price Index (CPI) and, more generally, to provide information on expenditure patterns. Its design—which features two separate surveys, one focused on larger and more regular expenditures and the other on smaller items—does not readily permit the development of a comprehensive resource estimate for individual families, which is essential for poverty measurement.[9] The CEX questionnaire is very detailed and complex, and response rates for the survey, which have averaged about 85 percent since 1980, are significantly lower than response rates for the major income surveys. Studies of data quality in the CEX have documented serious recall and other

---

[9] The CEX also does not readily support development of annual resource estimates (see Appendix B).

kinds of reporting errors. It would require a large commitment of funding to expand and improve the CEX to the point that it could be used for the ongoing measurement of poverty for both the total population and various groups.

Of course, income surveys also have reporting problems, and, indeed, many studies using a consumption or expenditure resource definition have found lower poverty rates than those using an income definition. One reason for the differences is that consumption exhibits less variation across families than does income. As a consequence, and since average consumption and average income are close to one another, the poverty rate will usually be lower with a consumption definition than with an income definition. Another reason for the differences is that the comparisons have not used the best available income data. Poverty measures constructed with CEX income data are much higher, and those constructed with March CPS income data are somewhat higher, than those obtained from CEX expenditure data. However, poverty measures constructed with SIPP income data are almost as low as those obtained from CEX expenditure data (see Chapter 5), largely because of improved reporting of many sources of income in SIPP for lower income people, compared with either the March CPS or the CEX (see Appendix B).

We conclude that the measurement of poverty in the United States must continue, at least for some years, to be based on an income definition of resources. As discussed further in Chapter 5, we urge work on improving the CEX so that it would be possible to consider seriously the use of a consumption- or expenditure-based definition of family resources for measuring poverty in the future.

Finally, we note that if a consumption-based resource definition is adopted for the poverty measure at some future time, there will still be the need for consistency between the resource definition and the threshold concept. As an example, with the proposed threshold concept, the consistency principle would require that work expenses not be considered as part of families' consumption, just as they are excluded from disposable income. The CEX, as currently designed, can produce consumption estimates that make most of the adjustments that we recommend to the resource definition for consistency with the proposed threshold concept. Thus, the CEX obtains information on most types of in-kind benefits, taxes, out-of-pocket medical care expenses, child care costs, and child support payments. However, commuting costs cannot be separated from other transportation expenses, and imputations are required for subsidized housing.

A Crisis Definition of Resources

In addition to their current income, many families have some cash on hand, and some families may have available one or more assets (e.g., savings accounts, bonds, stocks, automobiles, real property) that can be converted to cash to support current consumption. Also, some families receive lump sums during a year (e.g., realized capital gains, gifts, inheritances) that could be used for consumption purposes. By definition, assets are stocks, and income is a flow, so adding the two is not appropriate. (Similarly, by definition, lump sums represent transfers of capital not income.) Also, income includes income flows from assets (interests, rents, dividends), as well as from earnings and transfers.

However, some analysts have argued that the resource definition for poverty measurement should add to income the values for asset holdings of at least some types. Thus, David and Fitzgerald (1987) propose a crisis definition that would include regular income plus the value of financial assets that are readily converted to cash (e.g., savings accounts).[10] They argue that it is particularly important to include asset values for poverty measures that pertain to short periods (e.g., 1 or 4 months) because many people with short spells of low income may not be in a crisis situation so long as they have assets on which to draw. In fact, the major public assistance programs that have short accounting periods typically limit the amount of assets that applicants can hold and still be eligible for benefits. For example, Aid to Families with Dependent Children (AFDC) and food stamps pay benefits to people who experienced an income drop as recently as a month ago only if their "countable" assets are below a certain limit.

The argument is less compelling to include asset values for poverty measures that pertain to periods of a year (like the current measure) or longer. If one takes a longer term view of poverty and with an income definition, a poor person is someone who has insufficient income from assets and other sources with which to support consumption at an adequate level over an indefinite period. If one instead adds assets in by some method and counts them as spendable, one is taking a short-term view because the assets can only ameliorate the poverty temporarily.

Methodological and Measurement Issues

There are several possible methods for implementing a crisis definition of resources, which adds the value of assets or lump sum amounts to income (see Ruggles, 1990:Chap. 7). (Under any of these methods, to avoid double counting, reported income from assets must first be subtracted from resources.) One approach is to use a simple cutoff, as in AFDC and other assistance programs: that is, to stipulate that families, by definition, are not poor if they have more than a certain level of assets. The limit in assistance programs is

---

[10] They would exclude income from assets (e.g., interest) to avoid double counting.

generally in the range of $1,000-$3,000 for financial assets, and participants are usually also allowed to have a home, furnishings, and an inexpensive car. These limits may be too low for a poverty measure that is calculated on a basis longer than the 1-month accounting period used in such programs as AFDC.

Another approach is to convert assets to an annuity and add the annuity value to income.[11] This approach is appealing for the elderly poor who are out of the work force and hence have little prospect of moving out of poverty. It makes little sense to assume that they should use up their assets all at once, rather than stretching out the amount that they could realize by an annuity. However, the annuitization approach may understate the potential contribution of assets for other people. The contrasting approach is to assume that people will draw on the full value of their assets; however, this method may overstate the contribution of assets by assuming their easy convertibility to cash.

In addition to methodological issues in valuing assets, there are substantial estimation problems. It is difficult to obtain accurate reporting of asset values (and asset incomes) in household surveys. The March CPS asks about savings interest, dividends, and net rental income, but not about the underlying asset values, which would have to be imputed by using an assumed rate of return. Moreover, nonresponse rates to the asset income questions in the March CPS are high. SIPP obtains extensive information on both asset income and asset holdings; for most types of assets, income amounts are ascertained every 4 months and value amounts once a year. Nonresponse rates to yes–no questions in SIPP on asset ownership are low, but nonresponse rates to the income and value questions are high (although not as high as in some other surveys).[12]

Implications

Some work has been done by the Census Bureau and others to evaluate the effect of including the value of one or more types of assets in the resource definition for measuring poverty. David and Fitzgerald (1987:Table 4) compared a crisis measure of poverty to the current measure, using data from the 1984 SIPP panel: the crisis measure added to money income the capitalized value of reported interest from the prior interview. They assumed a 6 percent

---

[11] Moon (1977) used the annuitization approach (developed originally by Weisbrod and Hansen, 1968) in measuring the economic well-being of the elderly poor.

[12] Recently, the Health and Retirement Study, a panel survey of people ages 51 to 61, achieved more complete reporting of asset values by a technique called "bracketing," in which holders of an asset who don't know or refuse to provide a value are asked if the value is above a certain amount; if yes, whether it is above another (higher) amount, and so on. High rates of response are obtained by this method, although the response categories are very broad—for example, less than $1,000, $1,000 to $10,000, $10,000 to $50,000, $50,000 or more (Juster and Suzman, 1993:16-20).

interest rate and, to avoid double counting, they excluded interest amounts from income. When poverty status was determined on a monthly basis, the crisis poverty rate was 3 percentage points (21%) lower than the official rate; when the determination was made using a 4-month accounting period, the crisis rate was 2 percentage points (14%) lower than the official rate. However, when the determination was made on an annual basis, the crisis rate was only 1 percentage point (8%) lower than the official rate. David and Fitzgerald (1987:Table 7) found that the addition of the capitalized value of stocks and rental property made little difference, as very few families with money incomes below the poverty level reported such assets. Ruggles (1990:151) confirms that relatively few income-poor families have assets: in 1984-1985, 88 percent had less than $1,000 in financial assets, and only 7 percent had more than $3,000 in such assets.

The Census Bureau has developed estimates of the effects on the poverty rate of adding to income an estimated value for (net) realized capital gains and an estimated annuity value for home equity (net of property taxes). These estimates rely on complicated imputation procedures using data from other sources and numerous assumptions (see Bureau of the Census, 1993a:Apps. B,C), so the results should be viewed solely as illustrative. Nonetheless, they provide a rough sense of the implications for the poverty rate. In general, including realized capital gains has almost no effect, even for the elderly;[13] however, including an annuity value for home equity has a substantial impact, particularly for the elderly. Thus, in 1992 (Bureau of the Census, 1993a:Table 2), the inclusion of home equity value would have reduced the aggregate poverty rate by about 1 percentage point (from 14.5 to 13.0%) and the poverty rate for the elderly by almost 4 percentage points (from 12.9 to 9.0%).

Assessment

In general, we do not believe that it is appropriate to include asset values as part of family resources for purposes of the official poverty measure, for both conceptual and practical reasons. As noted above, to count assets as spendable is to take a short-term view of poverty. The year-long accounting period for the poverty measure, which we recommend retaining, argues for an income

---

[13] The Census Bureau's estimates of realized capital gains, derived from its federal income tax simulation model, take account of losses as well. From an asset accounting viewpoint, this approach is correct. From the viewpoint of a crisis definition of resources, one could argue that the actual cash received from a sale of an asset is what should be added to regular money income, even if that amount represents a loss in terms of the original asset value. In any case, the Census Bureau's current ability to simulate capital gains with any degree of accuracy for individual families is very limited: the simulation uses Internal Revenue Service (IRS) data on probabilities of incurring capital gains and the mean amounts by categories of adjusted gross income, type of return, and age of tax filer.

definition of resources rather than a definition that includes asset values. In addition, it is difficult to obtain accurate estimates of asset values in household surveys. Finally, as a practical matter, very few people who are income-poor on an annual basis have financial or other assets, with the exception of housing.[14]

We do recognize, however, that for some purposes, it may be desirable to have companion measures of poverty that take account of at least some types of assets. Thus, although we propose that the official poverty measure continue to be based on annual data, we believe it would be useful to develop measures for shorter and longer time periods as well (see Chapter 6). Measures for shorter periods (e.g., 4 months) may be more useful than annual measures to evaluate how effectively government assistance programs with short accounting periods target benefits to needy people. For consistency with program rules, short-term poverty measures would need to include financial asset values. In fact, it is likely easier, using SIPP data, to develop short-term measures that add asset values to income than to develop such measures on an annual basis. Fewer changes in family composition are likely to occur in a short time period and, hence, there will be less difficulty in attributing the asset values measured at the beginning of the accounting period to the appropriate family unit.

Finally, we support research and development to improve the reporting and valuation of assets for such purposes as estimating the distribution of wealth in relation to the distribution of income. The economic poverty measure is just one important indicator of economic deprivation and well-being; other indicators are important to develop, both in their own right and to provide an added perspective through cross-tabulation with the poverty measure.

PROPOSED RESOURCE DEFINITION

The rest of this chapter details the components of the proposed definition of family resources.

Money Income

The proposed definition of disposable money and near-money income begins with gross money income as defined for the current poverty measure. In the March CPS, money income is the sum of about 30-odd sources that are identified separately in that survey—including, for example, wages, net self-employment income, Social Security, private pensions, cash public assistance,

---

[14] See the discussion below of adding imputed net rent to the income of homeowners. This approach, which we urge be developed, treats housing as an in-kind benefit rather than an asset.

child support, alimony, interest on savings accounts, and dividends. SIPP asks about more than 60 separate sources of money income (see Appendix B).

Nonmedical In-Kind Benefits

Both the concept that underlay the original official poverty thresholds and the concept that we propose represent budgets for family consumption needs. Given such a concept, the resource definition should add to money income the value of near-money in-kind benefits that are intended to support consumption. Indeed, there is virtually unanimous support in the research community for this position: see, for example, the comments of Ellwood and Summers (1985), Blinder (1985), and Rees (1985) at a Conference on the Measurement of Noncash Benefits sponsored by the Census Bureau.

At the time the current poverty measure was adopted, such programs as food stamps and public housing provided benefits to relatively few families. Since then, they have made important contributions to reducing material hardship in the United States, and it makes no sense for their contributions to be ignored in the official poverty measure. We refer here to nonmedical in-kind benefits; the next section considers medical care benefits and out-of-pocket medical care costs. A major issue concerns the best method to assign an appropriate value to nonmedical in-kind benefits, given that recipients may not value them as highly as the equivalent amount of cash. The Census Bureau in its work over the past decade to develop experimental estimates of poverty based on an adjusted income measure has wrestled with the issue of valuation. We review the approaches that the Census Bureau has adopted at various times and suggest areas for research.[15]

Another issue is which types of benefits to include. The Census Bureau's work to date has covered food stamps, public and subsidized housing, and regular and subsidized school lunches. Benefits from the Low-Income Home Energy Assistance Program (LIHEAP), the Special Supplemental Nutrition Program for Women, Infants, and Children (WIC), and the School Breakfast Program, which are covered in SIPP but not in the March CPS, also seem prime candidates to include. For many other types of in-kind benefits (e.g., Meals on Wheels and other food programs for the elderly and free or subsidized meals or housing from employers), there are limited or no available data and no experience with valuation. A recommendation by the Panel to Evaluate the Survey of Income and Program Participation (Citro and Kalton, 1993:79-80,83) that SIPP use one or more of its topical modules to examine the range of in-kind programs and identify those that may be sufficiently widespread to warrant regular measurement may be the place to start.

The value of employer-provided in-kind benefits that are necessary for

---

[15] Smeeding (1982) initiated the work at the Census Bureau to value in-kind benefits.

work (e.g., child care, parking, training subsidies, or free uniforms or tools) should not be included because the definition of disposable income excludes out-of-pocket costs for child care and other work-related expenses, net of any employer subsidy.[16] Also, employer contributions for pensions should not be included. The National Income and Product Accounts (NIPA) include such contributions as income and, conversely, exclude actual pension income. However, the contrasting approach that has traditionally been followed for poverty measurement, namely, counting pension income as received and excluding pension contributions, makes much more sense for a measure of current economic poverty. Other kinds of employer benefits, such as contributions for life or accident insurance, are more problematic. To the extent they free up resources for consumption, they should be counted as income. However, there are measurement problems. Also, such benefits are difficult to value because of the likelihood that recipients would place a lower value on the benefit than its cost to employers. (This problem affects other in-kind benefits as well, but perhaps not to the same extent; see below.)

Census Bureau Valuation Procedures

The Census Bureau's procedures for assigning values for food stamps, school lunches, and public housing rely on the market value approach, in which the full private market value of the benefit (minus contributions by the recipient) is assigned as income.[17] For food stamps, the procedure is very simple, counting as income the full face (market) value of food stamp benefits that are reported for the year by respondents to the March CPS. For "regular price" school lunches, the procedure for determining the subsidy value uses information from the U.S. Department of Agriculture (USDA) on subsidies per meal for lunches that are provided at the "full established price." (Because of USDA assistance to the states, the full price represents less than the total cost of the meal.) The annualized subsidy value is added to family income for children ages 5-18 whose families reported in the March CPS that they "usually" ate hot lunches at school during the year and did not receive these meals free or at a reduced price. For those children who are reported to have received free or reduced-price school lunches, an additional subsidy value is assigned, also using information from the Department of Agriculture. Unlike food stamps, which function virtually like money, the approach of counting school

---

[16] The alternative approach of adjusting the thresholds would involve adding child care and other work expenses to the thresholds for working families, and then adding the value of employer subsidies to income (see Renwick and Bergmann, 1993, for an example). The net effect would be about the same as under our approach but actually more data-intensive to implement (data would be needed to estimate the threshold amounts and the subsidies).

[17] See Chapter 5 for a description of the effects on poverty rates of adding values to disposable income for these programs with the current valuation methods.

lunch subsidies as income at the full subsidy value is not without problems (see Bureau of the Census, 1993a:ix). Thus, participating families have no choice about the type or quantity of food and may well value the benefit at less than the full subsidy value.

The procedure for valuing rent subsidies for people living in public or subsidized housing is complex (see Bureau of the Census, 1993a:B-1) because the March CPS ascertains residence in such housing but not the rents paid by residents or the rent subsidies. To estimate the subsidy values to add to the CPS income amounts, the Census Bureau uses the results of an analysis from the 1985 American Housing Survey (AHS), updated each year to reflect changes in the Consumer Price Index for housing. In the AHS analysis, the Census Bureau compared the actual gross rent (including utilities) paid by families in subsidized housing to the estimated market rent these families would have been expected to pay if their units had not been subsidized. The comparisons were carried out separately for families in three income groups: under $6,000, $6,000-$9,000, and $10,000 and over. The market rent estimates for each set of comparisons were developed by using the coefficients from a model that related gross rent for two-bedroom nonsubsidized units by region from the AHS to number of bathrooms, number of appliances, number of housing flaws, and presence of satisfactory neighborhood services. The relative subsidies estimated for two-bedroom units were assumed to apply to smaller and larger units.

For 1981-1985, the Census Bureau developed values for in-kind benefits using two other approaches in addition to market value: the recipient value approach and an approach called "poverty budget shares" (see Bureau of the Census, 1986). The recipient value approach attempts to measure the value of a benefit to the recipient, which may be lower than the market value. However, in many cases it is difficult to measure recipient value. The poverty budget shares approach links the value of in-kind benefits to the current poverty measure by placing a limit on the value of specific benefits that is equal to the amount spent on the item by unsubsidized families and individuals with incomes near the poverty level. (The limit is equal to the lesser of the market value or the poverty budget share value.) The assumption is that recipients cannot use "extra" amounts of an in-kind benefit to meet their basic needs for other items.

Comparisons of estimates of nonmedical in-kind benefit values using the three methods indicate that the recipient value approach and, to a lesser extent, the poverty budget shares approach had less effect in lowering poverty rates than the market value approach. Thus, in 1985, the market value approach to adding values for food stamps, school lunches, and subsidized housing to money income reduced the poverty rate by 1.5 percentage points (from 14 to 12.5%)—an 11 percent reduction in the rate (Bureau of the Census, 1986:Table C). The recipient value approach reduced the rate by 1.2

percentage points (to 12.8%), while the poverty budget shares approach reduced the rate by 1.4 percentage points (to 12.6%). These results reflect the more conservative assignment of values to in-kind benefits of the recipient value approach and, to a lesser extent, the poverty budget shares method, compared with the market value approach.

Assessment of Valuation Approaches

The Census Bureau adopted the current market value approach for valuing in-kind benefits and dropped the other two approaches on the basis of recommendations at its 1985 Conference on the Measurement of Noncash Benefits.[18] At this conference, Chiswick (1985) noted that the validity of the market value approach depends on two assumptions: (1) that a household would pay the same market price (on average) as that used in estimating the market value, and (2) that the household would, in the absence of the noncash transfer, have consumed at least that much of the good or service in question. With the exception of food stamps (which are virtually the same as cash), Chiswick argued that the recipient value approach is conceptually superior to the market value approach. The reason is precisely that the assumptions underlying the latter may not hold and, hence, the value that the recipient places on a good or service may be far below the market value.

Some participants at the conference argued against the view that the recipient value approach is the superior concept (see, e.g., Browning, 1985). Also, all of the participants agreed that there is as yet no reliable way of estimating recipient value. Indeed, Chiswick made the point that the Census Bureau's recipient value estimation procedure was instead a "matched estimate" technique, which stratified families, on the basis of their survey responses, into cells defined by income and demographic characteristics and by whether they were subsidized or not. Under this procedure, the cash equivalent value of the subsidy was taken to be the difference between the expenditures on the good or service by unsubsidized and subsidized families within each group. A flaw in this approach was that it ignored the selection bias for participation in assistance programs.

No one at the conference supported the poverty budget shares method, which Chiswick (1985) described as a "bounded market value" approach. The upper limit on the market value assigned to a family for an in-kind benefit was usually the amount spent on the good or service by nonparticipants who were near the poverty level, under the assumption that values in excess of that amount could not always substitute for other needs. Flaws in this approach, as Chiswick noted, were that it treated any benefits above the threshold level as

---

[18] An exception was medical care benefits, for which the Census Bureau adopted a "fungible value" approach; see next section.

having no value to the recipients and that it assumed the same demand for subsidized goods and services among program participants as among near-poverty nonparticipants.

Needed Research and Development

We agree with the Census Bureau's use of market values for food stamps and other nonmedical in-kind benefits, primarily on the ground of operational feasibility. The major problem area concerns public housing, for which it is most likely that recipients would not value the benefit as much as an equivalent amount of cash and for which there are difficulties in accurately ascertaining the market value or the recipient value.

The Census Bureau has changed its procedure for estimating rental subsidies several times over the decade to strive for greater accuracy. Yet there is evidence that problems remain. Thus, the Census Bureau's aggregate estimates of housing subsidies are considerably below the subsidy amounts reported as outlays by the U.S. Department of Housing and Urban Development (HUD). For example, Steffick (1993) cites 1990 total outlays of $13 billion but the Census Bureau estimates $9 billion in total subsidies for that year. The distribution of subsidy amounts among families may also be problematic. As an example, although housing costs vary considerably by geographic area, the Census Bureau's estimates distinguish only the four major regions (see Steffick, 1993, on this point). Finally, the Census Bureau is still using data from the 1985 American Housing Survey, which are now quite old. At a minimum, the Census Bureau should reestimate its model with later AHS data. Ideally, more research should be conducted on methods for valuing housing subsidies.

We note that SIPP affords the opportunity to improve the valuation of nonmedical in-kind benefits. SIPP includes more benefits (specifically, LIHEAP, WIC, and School Breakfast) than does the March CPS and provides more accurate reporting because of more frequent interviews. SIPP also ascertains housing costs (rent and utilities) for people in subsidized as well as unsubsidized housing and so provides a much better basis for imputing rental subsidies than does the March CPS, which lacks housing cost data. The Census Bureau is currently developing an in-kind benefit valuation program for SIPP, and we urge that this work move forward.

Medical Care Needs and Resources

The issue of how best to treat medical care needs and resources in the poverty measure has bedeviled analysts since the mid-1970s, when rapid growth in the Medicare and Medicaid programs (and in private health insurance) led to a concern that the official measure was overstating the extent of poverty among beneficiaries because it did not value their medical insurance benefits. Yet after almost two decades of experimentation, there is still no agreement on the best approach to use. (See Moon, 1993, for a review of past approaches and suggested alternatives.)

Two problems make it very difficult to arrive at a solution that both achieves the necessary consistency between the threshold concept and the resource definition and is feasible to implement. The first problem is that medical care benefits are not very fungible—they may free up resources to some extent, but they by no means have the fungibility of, say, food stamps. There are two reasons that food stamps are essentially interchangeable with money: (1) virtually all households spend at least some money for food, so the receipt of food stamps frees up money income for consumption of other goods and services; (2) the maximum food stamp allowance is low enough that it is unlikely households would receive more benefits than the amount they would otherwise choose to spend on food. Neither of these conditions holds for medical care benefits: not all families have medical care needs during a year, and, although medical care benefits for low-cost services (e.g., a prescription drug or a doctor visit) may free up money income for other consumption, the "extra" benefits received from insurance (or free care) to cover expensive services (e.g., surgery) are not likely to free up money income to the same degree. Hence, approaches that add the value of medical insurance benefits to income without also increasing the thresholds have the perverse effect that sick people look better off than healthy people even though their extra "income" cannot be used to support consumption. In the more common practice of assigning average benefits for groups (i.e., valuing medical benefits at the assumed insurance premium amount), the result is similar—to make sicker groups, such as the elderly or disabled, look better off than healthier groups.

However, any attempt to develop thresholds that appropriately recognize needs for medical care runs into the second problem: that such needs are highly variable across the population, much more variable than needs for such items as food and housing. Everyone has a need to eat and be sheltered throughout the year, but some people may need no medical care at all while others may need very expensive treatments. One would have to develop a large number of thresholds to reflect different levels of medical care need, thereby complicating the poverty measure. Moreover, the predictor variables used to develop the thresholds (e.g., age, or self-reported health status) may not properly reflect an individual's medical care needs during any one year: some people in a generally sicker group may not be sick that year and vice versa for people in a generally healthier group. The result would be that it would be very easy to make an erroneous poverty classification.

A related issue is that, until very recently, hardly any research on this topic considered the question of out-of-pocket medical care costs. Even groups with good medical insurance coverage, such as the elderly, pay some of their medical expenses directly, and the dollar amounts for such expenses as health insurance premiums, deductibles, copayments, and payments for uncovered services can be high. Yet little thought has been given to how to adjust the poverty thresholds or the family resource definition to appropriately account for these costs.

Proposed Approach: Recommendation

We propose an approach that separates the measurement of economic poverty from the measurement of medical care needs and the adequacy of resources to meet those needs. Hence, the concept we propose for the poverty thresholds includes such budget categories as food and housing but not medical care. For consistency, we propose that medical insurance benefits *not* be added to income and that out-of-pocket medical care expenses (including health insurance premiums) be *subtracted* from income.

Although the proposed measure excludes medical care from both the poverty thresholds and family resources, it does not ignore the effects of the health care financing system or of people's health status on economic poverty. If people incur higher out-of-pocket medical care expenses (e.g., because they are sicker or have inadequate or no insurance coverage), their disposable income for comparison to the poverty threshold will be lower, and vice versa. The proposed measure will also be sensitive to any changes in the health care financing system that increase families' disposable income and thereby reduce economic poverty (e.g., more widespread insurance coverage with limits on out-of-pocket expenses), as well as to changes that decrease disposable income and thereby increase economic poverty (e.g., tax increases to pay for health insurance). In contrast, the current poverty measure cannot be sensitive to changes in health care financing, whether these changes increase or reduce families' disposable income.

Although the proposed measure is far better than the current measure in accounting for health care costs and resources, it does not directly assess the extent to which everyone has access to a package of health insurance benefits that protects them against the risk of being unable to afford needed medical attention. Hence, it is very important that research continue on developing indicators of the adequacy of health insurance coverage. We urge that these indicators be cross-tabulated with but kept separate from the economic poverty measure: that measure cannot directly include all aspects of well-being, and it is particularly difficult to try to include medical care in it.

RECOMMENDATION 4.3. **Appropriate agencies should work to develop one or more "medical care risk" indexes that measure the economic risk to families and individuals of having no or inadequate health insurance coverage. However, such indexes should be kept separate from the measure of economic poverty.**

Alternative Approaches

Several participants in the Census Bureau's 1985 Conference on Measurement of Noncash Benefits, including Ellwood and Summers (1985), Ward (1985) and Smolensky (1985), took positions that agree with our recommendation to exclude medical care needs and resources from the poverty measure. But other participants, including Blinder (1985) and O'Neill (1985), argued just as strongly for including medical care benefits (averaged for groups) in income and adjusting the thresholds if needed. (O'Neill thought that the thresholds would not have to be adjusted very much.) Aaron (1985) agreed that it would be difficult to include medical care in the poverty measure, but he was uncomfortable with excluding it entirely. Citing a suggestion by Burtless, Aaron proposed a two-index method of defining poverty as a possible way out of the dilemma: count people as poor if they do not have enough income to meet their nonmedical needs, or if they lack adequate health insurance (or sufficient remaining income to purchase such insurance), or both.

Clearly, considerable controversy surrounds this issue. Hence, we review in some detail the pros and cons of alternative approaches to treating medical care needs and resources in the measurement of poverty—beginning with the current measure—and why we chose our recommended approach.

Current Poverty Measure When they were developed in the early 1960s, the official poverty thresholds implicitly included (through the multiplier) an allowance for some out-of-pocket medical care expenses. Estimates are that such expenses accounted for 4 percent of median income in 1963 (Moon, 1993:3); 7 percent of total expenditures in the 1960-1961 CEX (Jacobs and Shipp, 1990:Table 1); and 5 percent of personal consumption expenditures in the 1960-1961 NIPA (Council of Economic Advisers, 1992:Table B-12). The official thresholds included *no* allowance for medical expenses that could be covered by insurance.

On the income side, the current measure assigns no value to health insurance benefits and makes no adjustments for above-average or below-average out-of-pocket expenditures. Hence, families with above-average expenditures may be erroneously counted as not poor, and families with below-average expenditures may be erroneously counted as poor. The biases are not likely to be offsetting but rather to err in the direction of underestimating poverty, because above-average out-of-pocket medical care expenses can be very high indeed. In the 1987 National Medical Expenditure Survey (NMES), about 60 percent of families had annual out-of-pocket expenses (excluding premiums) that were less than 2 percent of their annual income, but 10 percent had expenses that exceeded 10 percent of their income; see Table 4-1. Over 20 percent of the elderly had expenses that exceeded 10 percent of their income, as did 19 percent of families with annual income below $20,000.

TABLE 4-1 Annual Family Out-of-Pocket Expenses for Personal Medical Care Services as a Percent of Family Income, Percentage Distribution, 1987

Family Characteristics (% of all Families)	Families by Expenses as a Percent of Income[a]							
	No Expenses	0.01–0.99%	1.0–1.9%	2.0–2.9%	3.0–4.9%	5.0–9.9%	10.0–19.9%	20.0% or More
Total[b]	11.0	30.5	17.4	9.7	11.0	10.2	5.6	4.4
Family Income								
Under $20,000 (42%)	17.7	18.3	11.9	8.0	10.9	14.0	10.1	9.0
$20,000–$39,999 (30%)	7.1	32.2	19.8	12.1	13.7	9.9	3.6	1.6
$40,000 or more (27%)	3.6	48.0	23.6	9.9	8.5	5.0	1.0	0.4
Age and Insurance Status								
Under 65								
Any private insurance (64%)	7.1	37.2	20.6	10.3	10.9	8.2	3.4	2.1
Public insurance only (7%)	40.4	24.9	7.5	5.6	4.9	6.2	5.7	4.9
Uninsured (9%)	23.1	21.1	13.2	9.0	8.6	11.5	6.6	6.8
65 or older								
Medicare only (2%)	13.7	12.5	7.3	10.7	11.5	15.0	15.9	13.1
Medicare and public (2%)	33.3	20.0	13.1	6.5	8.2	7.4	3.8	7.7
Medicare and private (16%)	4.2	14.9	13.3	9.4	16.0	18.7	12.7	10.6

SOURCE: Taylor and Banthin (1994:Table 8); data from the 1987 National Medical Expenditure Survey; percentages do not always add to 100 because of rounding.

[a]Expenses include out-of-pocket expenses for inpatient hospital and physician services; ambulatory physician and nonphysician services, including vision care and telephone calls with a charge; prescribed medicines; home health care services; dental services; and medical equipment purchases and rentals for all family members. Expenses exclude health insurance premiums.

[b]Estimated total population is 100,225,000 families, excluding 0.4 percent with zero reported income.

Adding Health Insurance Benefits to Income Work by the Census Bureau and others on valuing health insurance benefits was stimulated by the expansion of health insurance coverage in the public and private sectors. The work began on the assumption that health care benefits could be added to income just like other in-kind benefits (e.g., food stamps), without adjusting the poverty thresholds. Analysts quickly moved from trying to add to income the actual benefits received by a particular individual because this approach had the perverse effect of making sicker people look richer than healthier people. However, as Moon (1993) points out, the preferred strategy of adding average insurance values for groups is hardly better, because it has the effect of making sicker groups (e.g., the elderly or disabled) look richer than healthier groups.

Over the years, the Census Bureau has tried several approaches to valuing Medicare and Medicaid benefits, including a market value approach, a recipient value approach, the poverty budget shares approach, and the current method, called the "fungible value" approach. (See Chiswick, 1985, for a critique of the first three approaches.) The agency has also assigned values to employer-provided health insurance. In all of this work, the Census Bureau has compared estimates of income including values for health insurance benefits to the official thresholds without adjustments.

In brief, the fungible value approach for valuing Medicare and Medicaid benefits starts with the market insurance value but includes only the portion that is determined to be fungible in the sense that it frees up resources that could have been spent on medical care (see Bureau of the Census, 1993a:B-1–B-3). The determination of the fungible portion of Medicare or Medicaid is made by comparing a family's income to a poverty threshold consisting only of food (based on the USDA Thrifty Food Plan) and housing (based on fair market rents determined by HUD). Then for each family, the value of the mean Medicare or Medicaid benefits (or both) for families in the same risk class is added to income to the extent that the family has any income that exceeds the new, lower threshold.[19]

The effects of adding Medicare and Medicaid benefits to income without adjusting the thresholds are dramatic; see Table 4-2.[20] In 1986 (the last year for which estimates are available to compare across valuation methods), the fungible value approach reduced the poverty rate by 1.1 percentage points (or 8%) for the total population and by 2.5 percentage points (20%) for the

---

[19] The risk classes for Medicare are people age 65 and over and the blind and disabled by state. The risk classes for Medicaid are people age 65 and over, the blind and disabled, nondisabled people age 21-64, and nondisabled people under age 21, by state. As an example of the calculation, if a family's risk class had average Medicare benefits of $2,500 per year and $1,000 of income that exceeded its food and housing needs, then only $1,000 of the Medicare benefits would be added to income.

[20] These and other estimates derived from the Census Bureau's experimental poverty series should be viewed as approximate. In most instances, one cannot determine from the published tables the purely marginal effects of a particular change because the tables generally show the *cumulative* effects of more than one change. For example, one definition might add food stamps and the next might also add Medicare. An estimate of the effects of Medicare obtained by comparing poverty rates between the two definitions will thus be affected by interactions between the effects of food stamps and Medicare.

TABLE 4-2 Poverty Rates with and without Insurance Values for Public and Private Medical Care Benefits Under Different Valuation Approaches, Selected Age Groups, 1986, in Percent

Population Group and Medical Care Benefit	Fungible Value[a]	Market Value[b]	Recipient Value[b]
Total Population			
Official definition	13.6	13.6	13.6
Including Medicare only	13.1	N.A.	N.A.
Including Medicaid only	13.1	N.A.	N.A.
Including Medicare and Medicaid	12.5	10.3	12.3
Also including employer-provided insurance	12.0		
People under Age 18			
Official definition	20.5	20.5	20.5
Including Medicare only	20.3	N.A.	N.A.
Including Medicaid only	19.4	N.A.	N.A.
Including Medicare and Medicaid	19.2	16.1	19.0
Also including employer-provided insurance	18.4		
People Aged 25–44			
Official definition	10.2	10.2	10.2
Including Medicare only	10.0	N.A.	N.A.
Including Medicaid only	9.8	N.A.	N.A.
Including Medicare and Medicaid	9.6	8.4	9.6
Also including employer-provided insurance	9.1		
People Aged 65 and Over			
Official definition	12.4	12.4	12.4
Including Medicare only	10.0	N.A.	N.A.
Including Medicaid only	12.3	N.A.	N.A.
Including Medicare and Medicaid	9.9	4.1	8.2
Also including employer-provided insurance	9.8		

NOTE: The Census Bureau uses a single market value approach to estimate the value of employer-provided health insurance benefits; the effects are shown in the fungible value column because the latter is the current preferred approach for valuing public health insurance benefits.

N.A., not available.

[a]Calculated from Bureau of the Census (1988b:Tables F, H).
[b]Calculated from Bureau of the Census (1988a:Tables C, 1).

elderly. The reductions in the poverty rate under the recipient value approach were somewhat larger: 1.3 percentage points (10%) for all people and 4.2 percentage points (34%) for the elderly. The reductions in the poverty rate under the market value approach were quite large: 3.3 percentage points (24%) for the total and 8.3 percentage points (67%) for the elderly.[21]

Adding in the value of employer-provided health insurance further reduces poverty (see Table 4-2), although not to a marked extent.[22] In 1986, the effects were greatest for working-age people 25-44 (reducing their poverty rate by 0.5 percentage point, or 5%) and least for those aged 65 and over (reducing their rate by only 0.1 percentage point, or 1%).

Moon (1993:6-7) terms the current Census Bureau fungible value method for valuing government medical insurance benefits an improvement over previous approaches but still flawed:

> By allowing the value of benefits to fully fill in the gap between food and housing costs and the poverty line, the formula effectively assumes that all resources beyond food and housing would be devoted to medical expenses up to the poverty line. This is an improvement over counting the full value of medical benefits as part of resources, but it still has the essential problem of treating as fungible benefits that can be used for only one purpose. For the elderly, it effectively establishes a new—and lower—poverty threshold equivalent to the food and housing minimum budgets.

If the expansion of health insurance benefits that began in the 1960s had served to offset the out-of-pocket expenses component of the poverty thresholds, then it might have been appropriate to add insurance values to resources in some way without adjusting the thresholds. However, what happened is that demand for medical care increased dramatically: per capita medical care spending more than doubled over the 1970-1990 period, rising from $1,166 to $2,566 (in 1990 dollars). Individuals' out-of-pocket *share* declined, but the real-dollar average of out-of-pocket expenditures increased by 25 percent—from $478 in 1963 to $597 in 1990, both figures representing about 4 percent of per capita median income (Moon, 1993:23). In other words, health insurance paid for increased use of medical services, but it did not reduce average out-of-pocket expenses. One reason is that many forms of insurance require individuals to pay part of their expenses, so that the higher demand for medical

---

[21] The poverty budget shares approach reduced the poverty rate in 1985 (the last year in which this approach was used) by 1 percentage point (7%) for the total population and by 3.1 percentage points (25%) for the elderly, similar to the effect of the fungible value approach (Bureau of the Census, 1986:Tables C, D).

[22] The Census Bureau estimates employer contributions through a model developed from a statistical match of the March CPS and the 1977 National Medical Care Expenditure Survey. The Census Bureau hopes soon to update its model by using data from the 1987 NMES—see Bureau of the Census (1993a:B-3–B-4).

care induced by the availability of insurance coverage carried with it some-what higher out-of-pocket spending.[23]

One can debate the extent to which the poverty thresholds should be raised to allow for the increase in the standard and costs of medical care that has occurred since the 1960s, just as one can debate the extent to which the thresholds should be raised to allow for increases in the overall standard of living. Some spending for medical care services is discretionary (see below), but to add the value of health insurance benefits to income (in whole or in part) but not to add any amount to the poverty thresholds—to allow either for medical care needs that would be covered by insurance or for higher out-of-pocket expenses—is to ignore completely the increased costs of medical care and to assume the fungibility of medical care benefits. This approach is perverse, particularly for people with high health care needs (who may also have above-average out-of-pocket costs). As we recommend above (Recommendation 4.1), poverty estimates of this type are not appropriate.

A Comprehensive Single Index The treatment of medical care needs and resources in the poverty measure must be consistent for both the thresholds and the family resource definition. It must also be complete by taking account of total medical care needs, whether covered by insurance or paid for out of pocket. One option described by Moon (1993) that meets these criteria is to develop a comprehensive single index of poverty that includes both nonmedical and medical needs and resources. Under this approach, the thresholds would have an allowance for medical care spending covered by insurance and an allowance for out-of-pocket expenditures. Correspondingly, the value of each family's insurance coverage would be added to income up to the level of the budget allowance (i.e., there would be no value added for additional insurance coverage). Also, the amount of a family's out-of-pocket expenses that exceeded the average budget allowance would be subtracted from income; if a family had below-average out-of-pocket expenses, the difference would be *added* to income). Because of the great variability in medical care needs, Moon suggested separate thresholds by health care risk category on the basis of such characteristics as family size and health status, which could be proxied by age or measured directly.[24]

---

[23] A study by the Office of Technology Assessment (1992) cautions that a causal relationship between health insurance coverage and increased use of medical care services is not established. However, the literature finds strong evidence of such a relationship (see, e.g., Hafner-Eaton, 1993; Hahn, 1994; Newhouse and The Insurance Experiment Group, 1993; Spillman, 1992; see also the review in Office of Technology Assessment, 1994). These findings support the expectation from economic theory that consumption of medical care, like other goods and services, is sensitive to relative prices (which are lowered by insurance coverage).

[24] Wide variations in total medical care expenditures (covered by insurance and out of pocket) are evident in the 1987 NMES (see Lefkowitz and Monheit, 1991). Thus, people aged 65 and over with Medicare and some private insurance who were in fair or poor health had

This option is consistent and complete, but it has many practical difficulties. On the threshold side, the problem is the necessity to develop a large number of different thresholds, which greatly complicates the poverty measure and distorts comparisons of the ability of different types of families to meet their basic (nonmedical) needs in terms of income-to-poverty ratios (welfare ratios). For each of the various thresholds, it must be decided how large or small to make the allowance for medical care needs.

On the resource side, there are problems with both the out-of-pocket and the insurance components. Some out-of-pocket expenditures are discretionary (e.g., elective cosmetic surgery) or incurred for services that are not strictly needed to treat a physical health problem (e.g., extra laboratory tests or ineffective drugs). To subtract such expenses from income could make people look poor when, in fact, the medical expenses were optional. Unfortunately, there are no data available with which to determine the proportion of out-of-pocket medical care expenses that could be termed discretionary or unnecessary, whether on an average basis or for people in particular health care risk categories (e.g., there are no data to determine the proportion of spending on cosmetic surgery that is in fact elective and not needed for physical health reasons). It seems unlikely that people would choose to pay for discretionary medical care expenses that moved them below the poverty line, but it could happen in some instances.[25]

With regard to the insurance component, there is the problem that people who lack insurance or have inadequate insurance but who either are not sick during the year or who receive uncompensated care could look poor when they are not. This result could come about because such people would have no or an insufficient insurance value added to their income to offset their insurance "needs" on the budget side. It is true that people lacking adequate insurance are more at risk than other people, but depending on their actual health experience during the year, they may not actually be poorer than other people.[26]

A Two-Index Poverty Measure   To try to overcome some of the complexities of combining nonmedical and medical care needs and resources in a single poverty measure, some researchers have suggested a two-index ap-

---

average expenditures of $6,459, compared with $2,575 for those in excellent or good health. For people under age 65 with some private insurance who were in fair or poor health, average expenditures were $3,152, compared with $1,047 for those in good health.

[25] Discretionary and unneeded medical care expenses would likely pose more of a problem for measuring the distribution of disposable income and income-to-poverty ratios across the entire population.

[26] It is one of the healthier age groups—people aged 18-24—who are most apt to report that they lacked health insurance coverage at any time during the year: 29 percent did so in 1992 compared with 15 percent of all people (Bureau of the Census, 1993b:Table 24).

proach. Moon (1993) represents the first attempt to flesh out how such a measure might be implemented. As developed by Moon, a two-index poverty measure would have a nonmedical needs threshold that would be compared with income minus actual out-of-pocket medical care expenditures. It would also have a medical needs threshold that would represent the value of a basic insurance package with no deductible or copayment provisions. This threshold would be compared with the value of a family's insurance package: if the package is insufficient because it requires out-of-pocket payments (e.g., for deductibles or premiums), the family's income (before subtracting actual out-of-pocket payments) would be compared with the nonmedical needs poverty threshold to see if enough additional income is available to cover the required expenses. If a family lacked health insurance coverage, its income would be evaluated to determine if the family could afford to buy a complete insurance package. People would be classified as poor if their family fell below either *one or both* of the nonmedical and medical needs thresholds.

Moon identifies many problems with trying to implement the medical component of a two-index measure. On the threshold side, it would be necessary to specify and price out a basic insurance package, something that would involve considerable judgment. Indeed, Moon suggests that a preferable procedure might be to use estimates of medical care expenditures for people covered by insurance, from such sources as the NMES, perhaps adding a factor to account for insurers' administrative costs. Another problem on the threshold side is that it would not suffice to have a single insurance package (or estimate of expenditures) as the standard: rather, multiple standards would be needed for different size families and for people in different health status categories (perhaps proxied by age). Finally, there would be a need to reprice the various insurance packages (or obtain updated expenditure estimates) at frequent intervals to keep pace with changes in the health care system and the implementation of any changes in the system.

On the resource side, there are many operational problems. Thus, it would be necessary to determine for each family:

• part-year versus full-year coverage. For example, families with Medicaid coverage beginning halfway through the year, after having to spend down their income, should not be assigned the same Medicaid value as families covered all year.

• coverage of family members. Some members may have more complete coverage than others.

• benefits provided by private insurance. Compared with the plan that is costed out for the thresholds, some actual plans might be more generous than needed for some services and not generous enough for others (i.e., there is a problem of fungibility among types of medical care benefits). Data would need to be obtained on plan benefits and also on the copayment requirements for the private insurance plan(s) held by families.

• the status of families without insurance. It would be hard to set an income cutoff to use to determine if families without insurance could afford it if they chose, because—unless the health care system is changed—insurance may not be available at any price to some people.

The advantage of a two-index approach is that it provides a clean measure of nonmedical resources assessed against nonmedical needs and then explicitly measures risk with regard to adequacy of insurance coverage (or ability to purchase such coverage and also pay required out-of-pocket expenses). However, the difficulties in defining the basic insurance package, keeping it up to date with changes in the health care system, and obtaining the necessary information each year on families' actual insurance coverage appear to be overwhelming.

Also, there is a fundamental asymmetry in the concept that underlies a two-index approach. It appropriately treats people with adequate (or more-than-adequate) insurance, in that it compares their insurance coverage with an insurance standard rather than adding insurance benefits to income and assuming that those benefits can be used for nonmedical needs. (This is the big problem in the work to date by the Census Bureau and others on valuing medical care benefits.) It also properly categorizes people with inadequate or no insurance coverage as medically at risk. However, it seems inconsistent to require that the *poverty* count include people who are medically at risk even though they have adequate income to meet their nonmedical needs. Some people who are medically at risk will indeed incur high out-of-pocket medical care expenses that will make them poor on the nonmedical side, but others will be healthy all year (or will have received uncompensated care) and hence will not necessarily be poor on the nonmedical side. To call such people poor because they had a high risk that never materialized seems illogical. Indeed, work by Doyle, Beauregard, and Lamas (1993:Table 1a) with data from the 1987 NMES indicate that a two-index measure could increase the poverty rate by 8 to 9 percentage points (60%) overall and by larger percentages for young adults and workers, even though many of these people had adequate income for their nonmedical needs.[27]

In sum, we conclude that there is a fundamental problem with trying to combine nonmedical and medical care needs and resources in a poverty measure: namely, that the two components are essentially measuring different things. The nonmedical component is assessing on a retrospective basis each family's actual ability to meet its needs during that year for such goods as food

---

[27] Doyle, Beauregard, and Lamas (1993) estimate poverty rates from the 1987 NMES for the following: the current measure; a measure that subtracts average out-of-pocket medical care costs from the thresholds and subtracts both taxes and actual out-of-pocket medical expenses from gross income; a single-index comprehensive measure; and two variations of a two-index measure. See Chapter 5 for an estimate of the effect on poverty rates of the proposed measure.

and housing—needs that are universal and cannot be deferred. The medical component, in contrast, is measuring a *risk* that may not actually materialize. Thus, someone in a high-risk health category may have a good year and need only minimal medical care, but no one can have a year in which he or she does not need to eat. Therefore, including medical care needs and resources in the poverty measure, whether by a single or two-index approach, is to mix apples and oranges: goods (e.g., food), for which needs do not vary greatly within categories (e.g., family size), and medical care, for which actual needs can vary substantially from expected needs or risk.

Separate Measures of Medical Care Risk and Economic Poverty

Given all of the conceptual and operational difficulties with the alternatives, we believe that the proposed approach—namely, to exclude medical care needs from the poverty thresholds and to subtract out-of-pocket medical care expenditures from income—is preferable. However, this approach is not without problems, and we would be remiss not to point them out.

First, there are some practical problems of implementation concerning the quality and sources of data for estimating out-of-pocket medical care expenditures. (These problems are not unique to the recommended approach—they also affect the one-index and two-index approaches described above.) Thus, recall and other errors by survey respondents can diminish data quality (e.g., respondents may report total expenditures rather than the out-of-pocket costs that remain after payments by their insurance plans). With regard to data sources, the March CPS has never asked about medical care costs. SIPP has regularly included a question on out-of-pocket expenses, but it has generally done so only once a panel and only for costs incurred in the month preceding the interview. Clearly, research and development will be needed to obtain data of reasonable quality for use in a poverty measure. It may be that initial implementation should be carried out by means of imputing out-of-pocket medical care expenses from other data sources.[28]

A more serious problem (which also affects other approaches) is that not all out-of-pocket expenses are necessary, and there is no easy way to separate discretionary from needed expenses. We considered capping the amount of

---

[28] The NMES, which about once every 10 years collects very detailed information on medical care treatments and costs from households and from their health care providers and insurers, would be the obvious source for such imputations. Data from the 1987 NMES were used by Doyle, Beauregard, and Lamas (1993) and Weinberg and Lamas (1993) in analyzing the effects of a two-index measure of poverty. NMES may also provide guidance for the measurement of out-of-pocket expenses in SIPP (or the March CPS), although it would clearly not be possible to replicate its in-depth approach. The "bracketing" technique discussed above with reference to reporting of assets could perhaps be used to improve reports of out-of-pocket medical care expenditures in SIPP.

out-of-pocket expenses that would be deducted from income, similar to the proposal to cap the deduction of child care expenses from the earnings of working parents (see below). However, the two situations are not the same. The assumption is that additional child care expenses, above a reasonable allowance to make it possible to work, bring added benefits that the family chooses to pay for, so that, for purposes of poverty measurement, it makes sense to cap the deduction. But it does not make sense to cap the deduction for out-of-pocket medical care expenses when they are incurred to treat an illness or disability.[29] A sick person with high medical care expenditures is not made better off than a healthy person with no or relatively low expenditures; at best, the added expenditures serve only to restore the sick person to a healthy state.

Given that one cannot distinguish between discretionary expenditures (which, ideally, should be disregarded, i.e., not deducted at all) and expenditures that are needed to restore health, we decided not to propose a cap on the deduction for out-of-pocket medical care expenses for the poverty measure. However, this situation could change in the future. For example, if insurance plans that significantly limit families' out-of-pocket liabilities for medical treatment are widely available, then it may well be appropriate to cap the deduction. One could then assume that medical care spending above the limit was discretionary.

Finally, an objection to our proposed approach, voiced by Moon (1993), is that it does not explicitly acknowledge a basic necessity, namely, medical care, that is just as important as food or housing. Similarly, the approach devalues the benefits of having health insurance, except indirectly, in that people who have medical costs that are covered by insurance will be measured as better off than people who have to pay such costs out of pocket.

Moon suggests that one variant of the proposed approach that would acknowledge medical care needs is to have the poverty budget include an allowance for average out-of-pocket expenses. Under this approach, people with above-average expenses would have the difference subtracted from income, and people with below-average expenses would have the difference *added* to income. (Note, however, such a measure would still not acknowledge insurance benefits.) To be completely satisfactory, Moon argues that the poverty thresholds should vary in the allowance they make for out-of-pocket expenses by different family characteristics.

Yet to move in the direction of a poverty measure that accounts for medical care needs and resources leads right back to the complex set of difficulties discussed above for which there appear to be no solutions. Single-index approaches, whether dealing only with out-of-pocket expenses or with

---

[29] Some of these expenses may also be unnecessary, but the consumer (the patient) usually has little control over treatment decisions by providers.

insurance values as well, entail all of the problems with multiple thresholds. Two-index approaches have a similar problem of defining the insurance standard appropriately for different types of families; furthermore, such approaches do not avoid the problem that the medical component is measuring risk, not the ability to satisfy actual needs during a particular year.

Moon (1993:18) suggests that a way out of this morass could be to have a clean nonmedical poverty measure and a *separate* health care risk measure. The two could always be cross-tabulated, but the poverty measure per se would be reserved for the nonmedical component. This suggestion is in fact our proposal. Not only do we recommend a consistent measure of economic poverty, in which disposable income net of out-of-pocket medical care costs is compared with a poverty budget for food, clothing, and shelter, and similar items, but we also support the development of one or more indexes of medical care risk.

The necessity to monitor people's risks of incurring medical care costs that exceed their ability to pay is clear. Current indicators that simply record the presence of any type of health insurance coverage are too simplistic (see, e.g., Bureau of the Census, 1993b:Table 24). What is needed are measures of the adequacy of coverage and the ability to pay for required out-of-pocket costs. It will be difficult to develop good measures, but the effort appears well worth the costs. We repeat, however, that measures of medical care risk should be developed separately from the economic poverty measure. To do otherwise is to overwhelm the poverty measure with operational and conceptual difficulties.

Taxes

Both the concept that underlies the official poverty thresholds and the concept that we propose represent budgets for consumption after taxes; however, the current definition of family resources is before taxes. For consistent measurement, there is little disagreement that income and payroll taxes need to be taken into account: such tax payments represent a mandatory cost of obtaining income and hence are not available for consumption. It seems particularly important to take account of taxes because of frequent changes in tax laws that may leave gross incomes unchanged but affect net incomes to a significant degree.

The Census Bureau has considerable experience with estimating Social Security payroll tax and federal and state income tax liabilities (see below). Improvements in the methodology are certainly possible and should be pursued; also, for completeness, estimates should be developed for local income taxes, where applicable. However, there is no need to wait for further research to implement the tax adjustments that the Census Bureau has already developed.

We do not propose that adjustments be made to income for other kinds of taxes, such as sales, excise, or property taxes. These taxes are an integral part of consumption, and the CEX expenditure data that we recommend be used to develop the reference family poverty threshold include them (e.g., clothing expenditures in the CEX include the applicable sales taxes). It is true that such taxes vary from locality to locality, so that the average amounts included in the thresholds may not be completely appropriate for specific areas (even with the housing cost adjustments by region and size of place). Yet it is clearly not feasible to develop the large number of thresholds that would be needed to take account of different levels of property and other consumption taxes across areas. It might be possible for people with above-average values of consumption taxes to subtract the diffference from income (and vice versa for people with below-average values). However, the costs of obtaining the necessary data would be high and the measurement problems would be great.

Census Bureau Tax Estimation Procedures

For more than a decade, the Census Bureau has published experimental poverty estimates that deduct payroll and federal and state income taxes from annual income as measured in the March CPS (see, e.g., Bureau of the Census, 1993a). The current procedure for imputing Social Security payroll taxes is straightforward. CPS-reported wage and salary earnings are multiplied by the Social Security payroll tax for the employee portion up to the specified limit; CPS-reported net self-employment earnings are multiplied by the (higher) payroll tax rate for the self-employed up to the specified limit; and certain employees (based on unpublished statistics from the Social Security Administration) are assigned noncovered status (e.g., federal government employees and proportions of workers in certain occupation groups).

For imputing federal income taxes, including the refundable Earned Income Tax Credit, the current Census Bureau procedure involves a complex series of operations. The Bureau first assigns members of CPS households to tax filing units, using a set of rules to try to approximate Internal Revenue Service (IRS) filing provisions. Next, the Bureau calculates adjusted gross income by summing reported amounts for wages and salaries, net farm and nonfarm self-employment income, net rental and property income, dividends, interest, income from estates and trusts, private and government pensions, unemployment compensation, and alimony; plus a portion of Social Security income and imputed amounts for net realized capital gains; minus imputed contributions to Individual Retirement Accounts (IRAs). Statistics of Income (SOI) data from the IRS are used for the capital gains and IRA imputations; the May 1983 CPS pension supplement is also used to estimate probabilities for IRA contributions. No attempt is made to adjust for other exclusions from income, such as moving expenses or alimony paid.

Second, the Census Bureau determines which tax filing units itemize deductions and the amount of their deductions. A statistical match of data from the March CPS and the AHS is used to determine mortgage and property tax amounts for homeowners in the CPS; probabilities of itemizing are applied to assign itemizing status;[30] and amounts of itemized deductions are computed using a matrix derived from SOI data.

Third, the Census Bureau computes the standard deduction according to the number of exemptions and calculates tax liabilities using the appropriate tax schedule for the simulated return type. Finally, the Bureau estimates the dependent care tax credit (using data from the June 1982 CPS supplement to estimate probabilities of tax filers paying for child care) and computes the EITC (which can be larger than the tax liability).

For estimating state income taxes for those states with such taxes (44 in 1992), the current Census Bureau procedures involve variants of the federal income tax simulation model. The definitions of tax filing units and adjusted gross income used in the federal model are used in the state models. Not all details of each state's income tax system are simulated, but the important aspects are accounted for. Census Bureau staff have found that their estimates of state income tax liability are biased upwards, probably because they use the federal definition of adjusted gross income and do not incorporate the various adjustments made by a number of states.

Assessment

The simulation of Social Security payroll taxes, as noted above, is quite straightforward. In contrast, there are a number of problems with the simulation of federal and state income taxes (see Nelson and Green, 1986), some of which are particularly important for poverty measurement.

A key problem concerns the determination of dependent members of tax filing units. This classification is essential for computing initial tax liability and for computing the dependent care tax credit and the EITC, both of which are important for the working poor. The March CPS lacks information on whether children in one household are dependents of a taxpayer in another household and, conversely, whether a taxpayer is claiming members of another household as dependents. The March CPS also lacks other information (e.g., child care and homeowner costs) that could improve the accuracy of the tax simulations.

By comparison, SIPP has the advantage of including extensive information relative to federal income taxes. (SIPP also asks about state and local income taxes.) Generally, SIPP panels each year include a tax module that

---

[30] The probabilities of itemizing are derived for homeowners by monthly mortgage categories from the 1979 Income Survey Development Program Research Panel and for renters by adjusted gross income categories.

asks about tax payments for the previous year. (SIPP panels also generally obtain information about dependent care and housing costs.) Questions on tax filing status, number of exemptions, type of form filed (joint, single, etc.), and schedules filed (A, C, etc.) are answered by more than 90 percent of respondents, but questions on adjusted gross income, itemized deductions, tax credits, and net tax liabilities have high nonresponse rates. The primary reason for the nonresponse is that respondents are asked to produce their tax form and use it as the basis for answers to these questions, but only about one-third do so; see Bureau of the Census, no date(a). The Census Bureau has begun work to develop a tax estimation model for SIPP similar to the one used for the March CPS. The SIPP tax information, even with quality problems, should make possible improved estimates of income tax liabilities for families in the survey.

Work-Related Expenses

The current poverty measure takes no explicit account of expenses, such as child care and commuting costs, that are necessary to earn income. As originally developed, the official poverty thresholds implicitly included some allowance for such costs (through the multiplier), but the thresholds have never been adjusted to reflect increases in these costs due to changes in societal work patterns. In particular, many working families face sizable child care expenses that would not have been necessary 30 years ago. Perhaps more important, the fact that the allowance in the official thresholds for work-related expenses is averaged over all families means that the thresholds do not adequately distinguish between the needs of working and nonworking families. To properly assess poverty for both working families and nonworking families, we believe it is incumbent either to develop thresholds that appropriately account for needed work-related expenses or to deduct such expenses from income.[31] Our proposal is to deduct child care and other work-related expenses from income (rather than creating additional thresholds, for the reasons that we presented above).

Child Care

In 1960, an estimated 72 percent of families with children had a parent who could care for the children at home, while the remaining 28 percent had both parents in the work force or were headed by single parents. The situation was just the reverse in 1990, when an estimated 69 percent of families with children had both parents in the work force or were headed by single parents

---

[31] Not discussed here are various arguments for distinguishing between working and nonworking families in terms of the value of time, see Appendix C.

and only 31 percent had a parent at home (estimated from Bureau of the Census, 1992d:Tables 56, 67, 618, 620). While only a fraction of families with both parents (or the only parent in the work force) pay out of pocket for child care, the estimated share of their income that is spent on child care can be significant. Thus, in 1987, one-third of all employed mothers and almost three-fifths of employed mothers with a child under age 5 paid for child care. The average amount they spent accounted for 7 percent of their total family income. Of employed mothers with family income below or near the official poverty line, one-quarter paid for child care, and the average amount they spent accounted for 22 percent of their total family income (O'Connell and Bachu, 1990:Table 7).

In order to more appropriately characterize the poverty status of working versus nonworking families, we propose to deduct weekly out-of-pocket child care costs from the income of families with both parents or the only resident parent in the work force, for each week worked in the year. We further propose to limit the deduction to the earnings of the parent with the lower earnings or to the value of a cap that is adjusted annually for inflation, whichever is lower (see below).

To make this adjustment to income in the March CPS requires imputing child care expenses because the survey does not ask about expenditures, whether for child care or other items. However, information is available on the numbers and ages of children and on the work status of parents with which to make a reasonable imputation. In contrast, SIPP has regularly asked about child care costs, either as part of a detailed child care module or as a single question in one of the other modules. Indeed, we used SIPP data to impute child care costs to the March CPS to analyze the effects on poverty rates of implementing the proposed measure (see Chapter 5).

On the question of how high to set the cap for child care expenses, one possibility is to set it at a percentage of median expenditures, following the procedure that we recommend to derive the food, clothing, and shelter component of the poverty thresholds. Data from the 1990 SIPP indicate that median weekly child care expenditures for working families with such expenses were $44 for families with one child and $51 for families with two or more children.[32] However, amounts that are below these medians may be too low to serve as a *cap*, particularly for larger families, for several reasons. For example, they do not make allowances for such factors as the age of the children, and child care expenditures for children under 5 are considerably higher than for school-age children (see O'Connell and Bachu, 1990:Table 7). Indeed, the relatively low median expense by families with two or more children relative to families with one child is undoubtedly because more families in the former group have older children.

---

[32] Based on tabulations prepared for the panel; dollar amounts are for 1992.

An alternative would be to use the caps specified for the federal income tax dependent care tax credit.[33]   Currently, the IRS limits eligible dependent care expenses to $2,400 a year for one dependent, or $46 per week, and $4,800 a year for two or more dependents, or $92 per week. By comparison, the AFDC program currently allows a maximum deduction of $175 per month ($40 per week) for work-related child care expenses for each child aged 2 years or older and a maximum deduction of $200 per month ($46 per week) for each younger child, giving a maximum deduction for families with two children of $86 per week. The Food Stamp Program has the same limits, and also allows deductions for day care expenses incurred for adult dependents and expenses incurred so that the caretaker can attend school.

Whatever cap is set, the guiding principle that we recommend is that it should represent a reasonable level of expenses necessary to hold a job, excluding additional expenses that parents may elect in order to provide enrichment for their children. In other words, we propose treating child care costs solely from the viewpoint of calculating a measure of disposable income that recognizes that some portion of the earnings of working families is not available for consumption.

We are very much aware that there are many other aspects of child care beyond out-of-pocket costs that are important to examine in order to measure well-being of children (and their parents) in a broader sense. The quality of the care is one key aspect. Families with high child care costs may be less well off in terms of resources available for consumption, but they may have a higher level of overall well-being if their expenditures are for a high-quality program that enhances the development of their children and correspondingly increases the mental comfort of the parents. Indeed, families with high child care costs may be better off on some dimensions than families with no such costs, if the latter situation results from leaving the children at home unattended (rather than because child care is donated by a grandmother or other loving relative or because the family receives a subsidy). As with the treatment of medical care expenditures, we believe that it is important to develop measures of the adequacy of child care, but we underline the necessity of keeping such measures separate from the economic poverty measure.

Other Work-Related Expenses

Most workers incur commuting and other costs (e.g., union dues, licenses, permits, tools, uniforms) to hold a job and, consequently, have less than the full amount of their earnings available for consumption. Hence, we propose to subtract a flat weekly amount for other work-related expenses (updated annually for inflation) from the earnings of each adult for each week worked

---

[33] Watts (1993) recommends this approach, and we adopted it for our analysis in Chapter 5.

in the year. The amount deducted should not exceed the person's earnings. For working families with children, the earnings of the parent with the smaller amount of earnings should limit the combined deduction for child care expenses and that parent's own other work-related expenses.

The reason to deduct a flat amount, rather than actual expenses, is because of the tradeoff that people often make between housing and commuting costs—by choosing a more expensive home closer to work or a less expensive one farther away. The adjustment to the poverty thresholds for geographic area differences in housing costs will be the same for all families in an area (see Chapter 3). For example, within a large metropolitan area that, on average, has higher housing costs relative to smaller areas in a region, the families of people who commute from outlying suburbs with cheaper housing costs will have the same housing cost adjustment as the families of people who commute short distances from more expensive, closer-in neighborhoods. For consistency, then, each worker needs to have the same work expense deduction.

Tabulations that we obtained from Wave 3 of the 1987 SIPP panel provide a basis for designating a flat weekly amount of work-related expenses.[34] They indicate that 84 percent of workers drove to work; 10 percent had parking or public transportation expenses; and 30 percent had other work expenses (e.g., for uniforms). Summing the three categories (driving, other transportation costs, and all other work expenses), 91 percent of all workers had some type of work expense. For workers with low to moderate family incomes (specifically, with per capita family income below the third decile), 74 percent drove to work; 10 percent had parking or public transportation expenses; and 25 percent had other work expenses. In all, 85 percent of these workers incurred some type of work-related expense.

In 1992 dollars, the mean weekly amount for combined work-related expenses for all workers (including those with no expenses) was $29 ($1,450 for a 50-week work year); the median weekly amount was $17 ($850 for a 50-week work year).[35] We believe it would be reasonable to develop an amount for the work expenses deduction as a percentage of the median. For our empirical analysis in Chapter 5, we deducted about $14.40 per week ($720 for a 50-week work year), which represents 85 percent of the median.

Child Support Payments

Since the current poverty measure was developed, the number of parents who live apart from their children has grown, and a large fraction of them incur

---

[34] The 1984-1987 SIPP panels included a work expense module. It would be useful to repeat such a module periodically, to determine if there is a need to realign the amount of the work expense deduction in real terms.

[35] Combined work-related expenses were calculated for the first job reported by each worker in Wave 3 of the 1987 SIPP panel by summing the reported weekly amount for parking and

child support obligations. A recent estimate (Sorenson, 1993), using data from the 1990 SIPP panel, was that 14-18 percent of men aged 18-54 were noncustodial fathers. The range (rather than one number) comes from two factors—nonresponse to the question on parenthood and an apparent under-count of black noncustodial fathers relative to black custodial mothers. About 44 percent of noncustodial fathers paid child support, and, on average, the payments accounted for about 9 percent of their families' incomes (calculated from Sorenson, 1993:Table 3).[36]

The current poverty measure counts child support payments as income to the recipient families, but it does not subtract such payments from the income of the payers. Yet child support payments, which are not discretionary in the sense that gifts of money to another household would be, cannot be used to support consumption by members of a payer's current family. For consis-tency, we propose to subtract child support payments from the income of the paying family (and to continue to count them as income to the recipient family).

The March CPS does not ask about child support payments to another household, and no information is available with which to make a reasonable imputation. The addition of one two-part question—whether the respondent pays child support and, if yes, how much—would remedy this deficiency. SIPP, in contrast, has regularly asked about child support payments, and we used SIPP data to estimate the effect on the poverty rate of subtracting child support payments from the payer's income (see Chapter 5).

Home Ownership Services

Economists have long argued that estimates of families' economic resources, to be comparable for renters and homeowners, need to take account of the flow of services that owners obtain from their homes. Thus, analysts who estimate resources by using a consumption definition almost always add the rental equivalence value (or "imputed rent") for homeowners to their other expen-ditures. The value added is net of owners' actual outlays for mortgage princi-pal and interest, property taxes, and maintenance costs (i.e., nothing is added if owners already have mortgage, tax, and maintenance expenses that equal or exceed the estimated rental equivalence value). The intent is to measure housing consumption in a comparable manner for renters and owners by estimating what an owner would have had to pay in rent (not including

---

public transportation, the reported annual amount divided by 12 for all other expenses (e.g., uniforms), and the reported weekly miles driven to work times the 1987 IRS mileage allowance of 22.5 cents per mile. Mean and median values for all workers were then updated for price changes to 1992.

[36] Presumably, some noncustodial mothers also pay child support, but Sorenson's analysis was restricted to men.

utilities). If the rental equivalence value is not added to homeowners' consumption, then people who own their homes outright or who have housing costs below the rental value of their homes would appear to consume less than renters or homeowners with higher costs.[37]

The same logic applies to resource estimates that are based on an income definition, namely, that people with low or no mortgage payments or other homeownership costs should have a rental equivalence value added to their income to recognize the fact that they do not face the same housing costs as renters or other homeowners. The concept of imputed rent is hardly intuitive or palatable to many people, yet, theoretically, the case is unarguable: owners with low housing costs have more of their income available for consumption of other items (e.g., food) and, hence, not to include imputed rent is to underestimate their income relative to their poverty threshold. The imputed rent value would be net of mortgage and other costs that do not exceed the amount of imputed rent: that is, we do not suggest that homeowners who assume mortgage payments that exceed the rental value of their home obtain a deduction from income. An alternative would be to develop separate thresholds for owners with low or no housing costs and other owners and renters.

Data from the 1991 American Housing Survey indicate that 39 percent of low-income households own their homes, compared with 68 percent of other households.[38] Among low-income households headed by someone aged 65 or older, 61 percent own their homes, compared with 81 percent of other households headed by someone aged 65 or older (Grall, 1994:Tables 4,5). The question is what proportion of low-income homeowners would likely have significant amounts of imputed net rent added to their income. A high proportion of low-income homeowners—66 percent—do not have a mortgage. However, a large proportion of low-income homeowners who do not have mortgages (62%) nonetheless have housing costs (for property taxes, insurance, and utilities) that are 30 percent or more of their income (34% have housing costs that are 50% or more of their income). An even higher proportion of low-income homeowners who have a mortgage (89%) have housing costs that are 30 percent or more of their income (65% have housing costs that are 50% or more of their income) (Grall, 1994:Tables 5,11,12). Overall, perhaps one-fourth of low-income homeowners could have significant

---

[37] Similarly, consumption-based resource estimates typically include the estimated service flows from automobiles and consumer durables (and, correspondingly, exclude actual expenditures on these items).

[38] The AHS "low-income" measure is not the same as the current poverty measure: it uses the official poverty thresholds, but it defines the unit of analysis as the whole household, not the family, and it measures income for the 12 months preceding the interview, which is not necessarily a calendar year. There are other differences as well (see Bureau of the Census, 1991).

amounts of imputed net rent added to their income that could possibly raise them above the poverty line (those owning their homes free and clear with other housing costs less than 30% of income). These homeowners represent one-tenth of all low-income households.

Although, for consistency, imputed net rent should be added to home-owners' income for purposes of poverty measurement, the idea is not easy to implement, at least not in the near term. Rental equivalences can be deter-mined by asking owners what they think their houses would bring in rent. The CEX includes such questions, which could be added to SIPP or the March CPS, but the responses are likely to be subject to reporting errors. Another method is to collect data on housing characteristics (a topic not currently covered in SIPP or the March CPS) and, by means of hedonic regression equations, estimate rental equivalences for houses of particular types (e.g., with one, two, or three bathrooms, with or without air conditioning, etc.). This method requires asking a large number of questions of renters, including net rent and characteristics of their housing for input to the regres-sions, and also of owners, including characteristics of their housing for imput-ing rental equivalence from the estimated regression coefficients. With either method, homeowners must be asked about their mortgage payments and property taxes in order to make a net calculation; SIPP obtains this informa-tion but the March CPS does not.

Finally, some analysts argue (see, e.g., Ruggles, 1990) that it may not always be appropriate to base imputed rent on the characteristics of one's current home. Thus, many elderly people who have paid off their mortgages or have low payments continue to live in homes that are larger than their current needs. It would seem inappropriate to impute a full rental value for a larger-than-needed home, although it is not clear what type of downward adjustment to the value would be appropriate. One approach would be to cap the amount of imputed rent at the level of the housing component of the poverty thresholds to recognize that the imputed rent offsets housing costs but does not represent additional money that is actually available for other con-sumption.

Given the practical difficulties, we do not propose that the income calcu-lated for a family for purposes of poverty measurement now include imputed rent. However, we urge that high priority be given to research to develop data and methods that could make possible a reasonably accurate calculation of imputed net rent. The next regular review of the poverty measure should give serious consideration to revising the income definition to include imputed net rental values in homeowners' income.

Effects of the Proposed Poverty Measure

5

$\mathbf{T}$his chapter presents our analysis of the difference it would make to poverty statistics to adopt the proposed measure in place of the current measure. This analysis has several objectives: to demonstrate the feasibility of implementing the proposed measure; to determine the reasons for important differences in the numbers and kinds of poor people between the proposed measure and the current measure; and to identify problems and areas for further research.

We first describe the data sources and procedures that we used. Next, we present the results we obtained for income year 1992, for which we conducted the most extensive analysis. Two aspects that we explore in detail are the effects of using different equivalence scales for the poverty thresholds and the accuracy of our imputations for out-of-pocket medical care costs and their implications for poverty rates. We then briefly review the data, procedures, and results for the more limited analysis that we were able to conduct for earlier years. Finally, we consider the likely effects on poverty rates of using the Survey of Income and Program Participation (SIPP) instead of the March income supplement to the Current Population Survey (CPS).

In conducting this analysis, we had to wrestle with a number of data problems. Hence, in this chapter we also discuss those problems and make recommendations for improvements in data sources that are needed for more accurate measurement of people's poverty status. The discussion covers data sources for deriving and updating the thresholds, as well as data sources for estimating family resources.

DATA AND PROCEDURES

An extract of the March 1993 CPS provided to the panel by the Census Bureau served as the primary database for our analysis for income year 1992. SIPP is an alternate data source and, indeed, we recommend that SIPP become the basis for official poverty statistics in place of the March CPS (see below).[1] We did use SIPP data to impute some of the elements for deriving disposable income that are not part of the March CPS. Because we have estimates of aggregate poverty rates from the March CPS and SIPP, using the current gross money income definition of family resources, we are reasonably confident of the type of results that we would have obtained had we used SIPP (see below).

Poverty Measure Alternatives

For income year 1992, we conducted two analyses that compared the current measure with the official thresholds and the official definition of family resources (namely, gross money income) to the proposed measure.

The first analysis was designed to illustrate the effects of the current and proposed measures on the kinds of people who are poor, holding constant the official 1992 poverty rate for the total population. For this exercise, we determined the two-adult/two-child family threshold that, together with the proposed threshold adjustments (with a 0.75 scale economy factor) and the proposed family resource definition, resulted in the same 1992 poverty rate as the official rate of 14.5 percent.[2] The official reference family threshold for 1992 was $14,228; the threshold that gave the same result with the proposed measure is $13,175.[3]

The second analysis was designed to illustrate the effects—for the whole

---

[1] We did not use SIPP in our analysis because the Census Bureau had not completed work to develop procedures for simulating income taxes and valuing in-kind benefits with SIPP (this work will be completed in the near future); we did not have the time or resources to undertake such work ourselves. By using the March CPS, we could take advantage of the Bureau's long-standing procedures for estimating taxes and valuing in-kind benefits with that data source.

[2] The 1992 poverty rates that we tabulated from the March 1993 CPS for the current measure are consistent with rates published in Bureau of the Census (1993c). Subsequently, the Census Bureau revised the rates due to the introduction of new population weighting controls derived from the 1990 census results that incorporate an adjustment for the census undercount (see Bureau of the Census, 1995). Thus, the revised official 1992 poverty rate for the total population is 14.8 percent instead of 14.5 percent as previously reported and as we tabulated.

[3] The value of $13,175 has no intrinsic meaning as a reference family poverty threshold. It is an artifact of the analysis, including not only the effects of the other threshold adjustments and definition of resources as disposable money and near-money income, but also the effects of the underlying data, including imputations. In other words, it is simply the result of implementing all other proposed changes and calculating what level of the reference family threshold is necessary to achieve the specified rate of 14.5 percent.

population and various groups—of raising the poverty threshold in real terms as well as implementing the proposed threshold adjustments and family resource definition. For this exercise, we used a two-adult/two-child family threshold of $14,800, representing the midpoint of our suggested range for that threshold of $13,700 to $15,900 (see Chapter 2). We implemented two versions of the proposed measure with the $14,800 reference family threshold: one with a scale economy factor of 0.75 and one with a scale economy factor of 0.65.

Threshold Adjustments

Table 5-1 shows the poverty thresholds for 1992 by family size and number of children for the current measure. Table 5-2 shows the thresholds for three versions of the proposed measure: using a $13,175 reference family threshold to keep the overall poverty rate at 14.5 percent; using a $14,800 reference family threshold and a scale economy factor of 0.75; and using a $14,800 threshold and a scale economy factor of 0.65. Unlike the official thresholds, the proposed thresholds do not distinguish one- and two-person families by whether the head is over or under age 65. We adjusted the thresholds in Table 5-2 for estimated differences in the cost of housing by size of metropolitan area within nine regions of the country; see Table 5-3.

Imputation Procedures for Proposed Resource Definition

For the two analyses, we also implemented the proposed definition of family resources as disposable money and near-money income, adding values for in-kind benefits (food stamps, school lunches, and public housing) to gross money income, and subtracting the following from income: out-of-pocket medical care expenditures (including health insurance premiums), federal and state income and Social Security payroll taxes, child care expenses, and other work-related expenses. Imputations to the March 1993 CPS were the basis for each of these adjustments. The only element of the proposed resource definition that we did not implement was the subtraction of child support payments to another household, because the March CPS does not provide a basis for a reasonable imputation; however, we have an estimate of the likely effect of subtracting child support payments on the aggregate poverty rate from SIPP (see below).

This section describes our imputation procedures (in some cases, the Census Bureau's procedures for which we simply adopted the results) for each component used in the derivation of disposable money and near-money income (see Betson, 1995, for a detailed description). Generally, the goal of our procedures was to use the best and most recent data source and to develop a

TABLE 5-1   Official Poverty Thresholds in 1992, by Family Size and Type

Number in Family (Age of Head)	Number of Related Children Under 18 Years								
	None	One	Two	Three	Four	Five	Six	Seven	Eight or More
One[a]									
<65	$7,299								
65+	6,729								
Two									
<65	9,395	9,670							
65+	8,480	9,634							
Three	10,974	11,293	11,304						
Four	14,471	14,708	14,228	14,277					
Five	17,451	17,705	17,163	16,743	16,487				
Six	20,072	20,152	19,737	19,339	18,747	18,396			
Seven	23,096	23,240	22,743	22,396	21,751	20,998	20,171		
Eight	25,831	26,059	25,590	25,179	24,596	23,855	23,085	22,889	
Nine or More	31,073	31,223	30,808	30,459	29,887	29,099	28,387	28,211	27,124

SOURCE: Bureau of the Census (1993c:Table A).

NOTE: Weighted average thresholds for families of two or more people (which are those commonly cited) are as follows: $9,137 for all two-person families ($9,443 for such families with the householder under age 65, $8,487 for such families with the householder age 65 and over); $11,186 for three-person families; $14,335 for four-person families; $16,592 for five-person families; $19,137 for six-person families; $21,594 for seven-person families; $24,053 for eight-person families; and $28,745 for families of nine or more people (Bureau of the Census, 1993c:Tables A-3, 23). Weighted average thresholds for each family size are the average of the thresholds for the specific categories (e.g., families of size two with no children or one child), weighted by the proportion that each category represents of all families of that size.

[a]A one-person "family" is an unrelated individual, that is, someone living alone or with others not related to him or her.

procedure that preserved as much of the variance and as many of the relation-ships among key variables as possible. (The preservation of variance and key relationships is particularly important for an indicator such as the poverty measure, which relates to one tail of the income distribution.) However, we were limited in available time and resources.[4]

---

[4] Readers interested in replicating our results or in conducting additional analyses may obtain a data file (from the Committee on National Statistics) that contains the March 1993 CPS extract file with our imputed variables and poverty status indicators for the current measure and the proposed measure.

TABLE 5-2 Poverty Thresholds in 1992 Under Proposed Measure, by Family Size and Type

Number in Family	Number of Related Children Under 18 Years								
	None	One	Two	Three	Four	Five	Six	Seven	Eight
$13,175 Reference Family Threshold: 0.75 Scale Economy Factor									
One[a]	$5,262								
Two	8,850	7,834							
Three	11,995	11,083	10,147						
Four	14,883	14,038	13,175	12,293					
Five	17,594	16,796	15,985	15,161	14,322				
Six	20,172	19,411	18,640	17,857	17,063	16,258			
Seven	22,645	21,912	21,173	20,424	19,665	18,898	18,119		
Eight	25,030	24,323	23,608	22,887	22,158	21,420	20,674	19,919	
Nine	27,342	26,655	25,963	25,264	24,559	23,848	23,128	22,402	21,667
$14,800 Reference Family Threshold: 0.75 Scale Economy Factor									
One[a]	$5,911								
Two	9,941	8,800							
Three	13,474	12,450	11,398						
Four	16,719	15,769	14,800	13,809					
Five	19,764	18,868	17,957	17,031	16,088				
Six	22,660	21,805	20,939	20,060	19,168	18,263			
Seven	25,438	24,615	23,784	22,943	22,091	21,229	20,354		
Eight	28,117	27,323	26,520	25,710	24,891	24,062	23,224	22,376	
Nine	30,714	29,943	29,165	28,380	27,588	26,789	25,981	25,165	24,339
$14,800 Reference Family Threshold: 0.65 Scale Economy Factor									
One[a]	$6,680								
Two	10,483	9,432							
Three	13,644	12,741	11,802						
Four	16,449	15,636	14,800	13,938					
Five	19,017	18,267	17,500	16,715	15,910				
Six	21,409	20,707	19,992	19,263	18,519	17,758			
Seven	23,665	23,001	22,326	21,640	20,943	20,232	19,508		
Eight	25,811	25,178	24,536	23,885	23,224	22,552	21,870	21,177	
Nine	27,865	27,258	26,643	26,021	25,390	24,751	24,103	23,445	22,777

NOTE: The thresholds are adjusted by geographic area; see Table 5-3 and text.

[a]A one-person "family" is an unrelated individual, that is, someone living alone or with others not related to him or her.

In-Kind Benefit Values and Taxes

We used the 1992 values that the Census Bureau provided on the March 1993 CPS extract file for in-kind benefits (food stamps, school lunches, and public and subsidized housing) and for federal and state income and Social Security payroll taxes. (See Chapter 4 for a description of the Census Bureau's current in-kind benefit valuation procedures, which use the market value approach,

TABLE 5-3   Housing Cost Adjustments for Proposed Poverty Thresholds

Area and Population Size	Index Value
Northeast	
New England (Connecticut, Maine, Massachusetts, New Hampshire, Rhode Island, Vermont)	
Nonmetropolitan areas and metropolitan areas under 250,000	1.128
Metropolitan areas of 250,000–500,000	1.128
Metropolitan areas of 500,000–1,000,000	1.148
Metropolitan areas of 1,000,000–2,500,000	1.141
Metropolitan areas of 2,500,000 or more	1.209
Middle Atlantic (New Jersey, New York, Pennsylvania)	
Nonmetropolitan areas and metropolitan areas under 250,000	0.908
Metropolitan areas of 250,000–500,000	0.997
Metropolitan areas of 500,000–1,000,000	1.020
Metropolitan areas of 1,000,000–2,500,000	0.975
Metropolitan areas of 2,500,000 or more	1.187
Midwest	
East North Central (Illinois, Indiana, Michigan, Ohio, Wisconsin)	
Nonmetropolitan areas and metropolitan areas under 250,000	0.896
Metropolitan areas of 250,000–500,000	0.959
Metropolitan areas of 500,000–1,000,000	0.987
Metropolitan areas of 1,000,000–2,500,000	0.995
Metropolitan areas of 2,500,000 or more	1.059
West North Central (Iowa, Kansas, Minnesota, Missouri, Nebraska, North Dakota, South Dakota)	
Nonmetropolitan areas and metropolitan areas under 250,000	0.861
Metropolitan areas of 250,000–500,000	0.962
Metropolitan areas of 500,000–1,000,000	0.981
Metropolitan areas of 1,000,000–2,500,000	1.028
Metropolitan areas of 2,500,000 or more	N.A.
South	
South Atlantic (Delaware, District of Columbia, Florida, Georgia, Maryland, North Carolina, South Carolina, Virginia, West Virginia)	
Nonmetropolitan areas and metropolitan areas under 250,000	0.899
Metropolitan areas of 250,000–500,000	0.961
Metropolitan areas of 500,000–1,000,000	1.007
Metropolitan areas of 1,000,000–2,500,000	1.043
Metropolitan areas of 2,500,000 or more	1.119
East South Central (Alabama, Kentucky, Mississippi, Tennessee)	
Nonmetropolitan areas and metropolitan areas under 250,000	0.827
Metropolitan areas of 250,000–500,000	0.935

TABLE 5-3   *Continued*

Area and Population Size	Index Value
East South Central—*continued*	
Metropolitan areas of 500,000-1,000,000	0.947
Metropolitan areas of 1,000,000-2,500,000	N.A.
Metropolitan areas of 2,500,000 or more	N.A.
West South Central (Arkansas, Louisiana, Oklahoma, Texas)	
Nonmetropolitan areas and metropolitan areas under 250,000	0.858
Metropolitan areas of 250,000-500,000	0.911
Metropolitan areas of 500,000-1,000,000	0.942
Metropolitan areas of 1,000,000-2,500,000	0.962
Metropolitan areas of 2,500,000 or more	1.005
West	
Mountain (Arizona, Colorado, Idaho, Montana, Nevada, New Mexico, Utah, Wyoming)	
Nonmetropolitan areas and metropolitan areas under 250,000	0.888
Metropolitan areas of 250,000–500,000	0.976
Metropolitan areas of 500,000-1,000,000	1.039
Metropolitan areas of 1,000,000–2,500,000	1.003
Metropolitan areas of 2,500,000 or more	N.A.
Pacific (Alaska, California, Hawaii, Oregon, Washington)	
Nonmetropolitan areas and metropolitan areas under 250,000	0.969
Metropolitan areas of 250,000–500,000	1.018
Metropolitan areas of 500,000-1,000,000	1.028
Metropolitan areas of 1,000,000–2,500,000	1.104
Metropolitan areas of 2,500,000 or more	1.217

NOTES: Housing cost indexes calculated from 1990 census data on gross rent for apartments with specified characteristics, adjusted to reflect the share of housing in the proposed poverty budget; see Chapter 3. Nonmetropolitan areas are combined with metropolitan areas of less than 250,000 population because of restrictions on geographic area coding in the CPS and SIPP.

N.A., not applicable.

and for a description of the Census Bureau's tax simulator. Because of the Census Bureau's procedures to protect confidentiality on the public-use March CPS files, care must be taken in subtracting taxes for high-income people so as not to inadvertently move them below the poverty line. Also, the portion of taxes due to realized capital gains should not be subtracted because such gains are not part of the proposed resources definition.)

Out-of-Pocket Medical Care Expenditures

The March CPS does not contain any information on medical care expenses (out-of-pocket or otherwise), although it does provide some relevant information that is helpful for imputation purposes, such as age and health insurance coverage. We imputed out-of-pocket expenses by using tabulations provided by the Agency for Health Care Policy and Research (AHCPR) from the 1987 National Medical Expenditure Survey (NMES), aged to represent the 1992 population.[5] AHCPR prepared separate multivariate tabulations for families (and unrelated individuals) for which the head was under age 65 or age 65 and older. The tabulation for families headed by someone younger than 65 cross-classified the age of head and type of health insurance coverage (private, public, or no insurance) by family size, family annual income-to-poverty ratio, and race of head. The tabulation for families headed by someone age 65 or older included the same variables, except that the categories for type of insurance coverage were different (Medicare and private, Medicare and public, all other).[6]

Because of the small sample size of the NMES, we had to combine many of the cells in these two very large multivariate tabulations to have a minimum of 100 observations in each cell. The tabulation that we used for families headed by someone younger than age 65 cross-classified health insurance status (covered, not covered) by family size (one, two-three, four or more people), by race of head (black, other), and by annual income-to-poverty ratio (less than 1.50, greater than or equal to 1.50). The tabulation that we used for families headed by someone aged 65 or older cross-classified the age of head (under 75, 75 and older) by income-to-poverty ratio (under 1.50, greater than or equal to 1.50) and by family size (one, two or more people). For each category in these two tabulations, we had the weighted counts of families with no out-of-pocket medical care expenditures and with non-zero expenditures within each of 10 expenditure ranges. Out-of-pocket expenditures included health insurance premiums, copayments, deductibles, and all other health care expenditures paid directly by the family. The lower bounds for the 10 expenditure ranges were $1, $500, $1,000, $1,500, $2,000, $2,500, $5,000, $7,500, and $12,500.

The imputation of out-of-pocket expenditures to the March 1993 CPS was a multistep procedure. The first step was to determine whether the individual CPS record would be imputed to have any out-of-pocket expenditures. For families who reported receiving Medicaid, we assumed that they would have no out-of-pocket medical expenditures.[7] For non-Medicaid families, we randomly assigned a fraction of these families to have some out-

---

[5] A multiple regression would have been preferable for imputation purposes (because it would then have been possible to introduce more variation), but it could not be obtained within the time and resources available.

[6] Although type of health insurance coverage is captured in these tabulations, differences in generosity of coverage within type (e.g., differences among state Medicaid programs) are not.

[7] This assumption is an approximation, as the generosity of Medicaid programs varies across states, and some families with Medicaid coverage do incur out-of-pocket medical expenditures. See Taylor and Banthin (1994:Table 2) for estimates from the 1987 NMES of out-of-pocket expenses by type of insurance coverage.

of-pocket medical expenditures on the basis of their characteristics and the computed probabilities from the NMES tabulations. If the family was assigned to have out-of-pocket medical expenditures, we devised an imputation procedure so that these families were assigned a level of expenditures consistent with the distribution of expenditures tabulated with their characteristics from the NMES. The object of this two-step procedure was to impute a set of medical expenditures that would reflect the entire distribution of expenditures and not to impute to all families the average level of expenditures consistent with their characteristics (see Betson, 1995).

Child Care Expenses

The March CPS does not contain any information on child care expenses, although it does have information on the number and age of children and employment status and weeks worked for the parents, which is needed for imputation purposes. We imputed child care expenses by using four regression equations from the 1990 SIPP panel. Two logit regressions estimated, respectively, the probability that a single parent who worked and a two-parent family in which both parents worked would pay for child care. Then, two ordinary-least-squares regressions estimated, for those single-parent and two-parent working families who paid for care, the total weekly amount. The single-parent working family equations included as independent variables the race of the head, the number of children of various ages, the region of residence, and the log of total family income. The two-parent working family equations included the same variables plus the proportion of family earnings accounted for by the earnings of the mother. (A number of model specifications were tested before deciding on these regression models.)

For weekly child care amounts, the probability that a family would have paid for child care was computed using the estimated logit equations. On the basis of this probability, the family was randomly assigned either to have or to have not paid for child care. If the family was imputed to have paid for child care, the second estimated equation and the family's characteristics were used to predict an average amount of child care for the family. A random "shock," whose standard deviation was derived from the standard error of the estimated equation, was then added to this average amount.

This weekly amount was then multiplied by the number of weeks worked by the head of single-parent families or by the secondary worker of two-earner families. A cap was imposed so that the annual amount imputed could not exceed the earnings of the parent with the lower earnings or the value of the ceiling on eligible expenses for the dependent care tax credit of $2,400 per year for one child and $4,800 for two or more children.

Other Work-Related Expenses

The March CPS does not contain any information on work-related expenses, although it does report the employment status and weeks worked of each adult. We imputed work expenses to each worker aged 18 and over. For each week worked, we assigned a work expense value of $14.42, representing an annual amount of $750 for a 52-week work-year (or $720 for a 50-week work-year—see Chapter 4). The amount assigned was not allowed to exceed the worker's annual earnings. Also, for any parent for whom child care expenses were imputed (the parent in each family with the lower annual earnings), the combined child care and other work expense deduction was not allowed to exceed the parent's annual earnings.

The value of the work expense deduction was derived on the basis of analyzing work expense data from Wave 3 of the 1987 SIPP. We computed median weekly work expenses for the first job reported for all workers aged 18 and over (including those reporting zero values). The estimated median weekly value in 1992 dollars was $17 (see Chapter 4 for details of the calculation). The amount that we deducted from earnings for each week worked ($14.42) is 85 percent of the median value.

Distribution of Imputed Values

On average, we imputed $2,872 in deductions for out-of-pocket medical care expenses, child care expenses, and other work-related expenses, or 8.5 percent of gross money income for the average unit (families and unrelated individuals). As would be expected, the dollar amount imputed increased linearly with gross money income and decreased on a percentage basis. As shown in Table 5-4, the imputed deduction for the sum of these three expense categories is $669 for the family at the 10th percentile of the distribution (10.7% of gross money income); $3,007 for the family at the 50th percentile (median) (11.1% of gross money income); and $4,898 for the family at the 95th percentile (5.2% of gross money income). Higher amounts, both in dollars and as a percentage of gross money income, were imputed for these expenses for the reference family of two adults and two children (see Table 5-4); this results from the high proportion of workers among this family type.

RESULTS

Effects with a Constant Poverty Rate

In our first analysis, we implemented the current measure with the official 1992 threshold of $14,228 for a two-adult/two-child family and the proposed measure with a threshold of $13,175 for this family type and a scale economy factor of 0.75. By design, the proposed measure under this scenario produces about the same 1992 poverty rate (14.54%) and number of poor people (36.9 million) as the current measure (14.52% and 36.9 million). However, they are not all the same people.

TABLE 5-4 Distribution of Gross Money Income, with Amounts Deducted for Out-of-Pocket Medical Care Expenditures, Child Care Expenses, and Other Work-Related Expenses, 1992, in Dollars

Percentile of Gross Money Income	All Families[a]			Two-Adult/Two-Child Families		
	Gross Money Income	Deductions[b]		Gross Money Income	Deductions[b]	
		Dollar Amount	Percent		Dollar Amount	Percent
10th	6,282	669	10.7	15,798	2,648	16.8
20th	10,768	1,429	13.3	24,364	4,142	17.0
30th	15,544	2,042	13.1	31,005	4,629	14.9
40th	20,971	2,518	12.0	37,275	5,656	15.2
50th (median)	27,088	3,007	11.1	43,387	5,894	13.6
60th	34,210	3,516	10.3	49,816	5,669	11.4
70th	42,916	3,956	9.2	56,993	6,108	10.7
80th	54,538	4,416	8.1	66,633	6,926	10.4
90th	74,240	4,651	6.3	86,667	6,641	7.7
95th	93,818	4,898	5.2	99,451	6,946	7.0
Average	33,857	2,872	8.5	46,583	5,243	11.3

[a]Includes unrelated individuals.

[b]Average of imputed out-of-pocket medical care expenses (including health insurance premiums), child care expenses, and work-related expenses for families with gross money income 2.5 percentiles below to 2.5 percentiles above each percentile value (e.g., deductions for families at the 10th percentile are averaged over families with gross money income between the 7.5 and 12.5 percentiles).

The proposed measure moves 7.4 million people out of poverty, and it moves about 7.4 million people into poverty. (A total of 29.5 million people, 80% of the poverty population, are poor under both measures.) Most of the movement occurs near the poverty line. Thus, 87 percent of the 7.4 million people who are no longer categorized as poor move from the category of income between 50 and 100 percent of the poverty line to the category of income between 100 and 150 percent of the poverty line. Similarly, 79 percent of the 7.4 million people who are newly categorized as poor move from the category of income between 100 and 150 percent of the poverty line to the category of income between 50 and 100 percent of the poverty line; see Table 5-5.

Table 5-6 shows the effect of the proposed poverty measure on the composition of the poor population. By age, somewhat more poor people are adults aged 18-64 and somewhat fewer poor people are adults aged 65 and older under the proposed measure in comparison with the current measure, while the proportion of children under age 18 among the poverty population is about the same under both measures. By race, somewhat more poor people

TABLE 5-5 Change in Poverty Status and Income-to-Poverty Ratio
Under the Current and Proposed Poverty Measures, with Total Poverty
Rate Held Constant at 14.5 Percent, 1992

Poverty Status and Income-to-Poverty Ratio	Number of People (millions)	Percent Distribution Within Category
People Moved out of Poverty	7.35	100.0
Current measure: income <50% of threshold		
Proposed measure		
Income 100–150% of threshold	0.45	6.1
Income 150–200% of threshold	0.00	0.0
Income 200% or more of threshold	0.00	0.0
Current measure: income 50–100% of threshold		
Proposed measure		
Income 100–150% of threshold	6.42	87.3
Income 150–200% of threshold	0.47	6.4
Income 200% or more of threshold	0.01	0.1
People Moved into Poverty	7.37	100.0
Current measure: income 100–150% of threshold		
Proposed measure		
Income <50% of threshold	0.02	0.3
Income 50–100% of threshold	5.81	78.8
Current measure: income 150–200% of threshold		
Proposed measure		
Income <50% of threshold	0.00	0.0
Income 50–100% of threshold	1.47	19.9
Current measure: income 200% or more of threshold		
Proposed measure		
Income <50% of threshold	0.00	0.0
Income 50–100% of threshold	0.07	0.9
People Poor Under Both Measures	29.54	100.0
Current measure: income <50% of threshold		
Proposed measure		
Income <50% of threshold	8.47	28.7
Income 50–100% of threshold	6.10	20.6
Current measure: income 50–100% of threshold		
Proposed measure		
Income <50% of threshold	1.50	5.1
Income 50–100% of threshold	13.47	45.6
People Not Poor Under Both Measures	209.71	100.0
Current measure: income 100–150% of threshold		
Proposed measure		
Income 100–150% of threshold	14.79	7.1
Income 150–200% of threshold	3.48	1.7
Income 200% or more of threshold	0.25	0.1

TABLE 5-5 *Continued*

Poverty Status and Income-to-Poverty Ratio	Number of People (millions)	Percent Distribution Within Category
People Not Poor Under Both Measures—continued		
Current measure: income 150–200% of threshold		
Proposed measure		
Income 100–150% of threshold	11.75	5.6
Income 150–200% of threshold	9.41	4.5
Income 200% or more of threshold	2.37	1.1
Current measure: income 200% or more of threshold		
Proposed measure		
Income 100–150% of threshold	5.44	2.6
Income 150–200% of threshold	20.88	10.0
Income 200% or more of threshold	141.34	67.4

NOTE: The reference family (two-adult/two-child) threshold for the current measure is $14,228; for the proposed measure keeping the overall poverty rate constant, it is $13,175. The total U.S. population is 253.97 million.

are white and somewhat fewer poor people are black under the proposed measure. By ethnicity, somewhat more poor people are Hispanic under the proposed measure. The proposed measure also markedly reduces the proportion of poor people who are categorized as one-person families (either living alone or with others not related to them); this effect is largely due to the scale economy factor (see below).

The most significant effect of the proposed measure is on the proportions of poor people in families that receive welfare and in families with one or more workers. For families that receive Aid to Families with Dependent Children (AFDC) or Supplemental Security Income (SSI), their share of the poverty population decreases from 40 to 30 percent. For families with workers, their share of the poverty population increases from 51 to 59 percent. The proposed measure also noticeably affects the proportion of poor people in families that lack health insurance; their share increases from 30 to 36 percent. Finally, the proposed measure alters the regional composition of the poverty population. The share of poor people who reside in the Northeast and West increases under the proposed measure, while the share of poor people who reside in the South and, to a lesser extent, the Midwest decreases.[8]

Another way to consider the differences in the current and proposed measures is to look at the poverty rates for various groups. While the overall poverty rate of 14.5 percent is the same under both the current and the proposed measures, the rates for some groups differ appreciably; see Table 5-7. Of

---

[8] See Table 5-3 for the states in each region.

TABLE 5-6 Composition of the Total and Poverty Populations Under the Current and Proposed Measures, with Total Poverty Rate Held Constant at 14.5 Percent, 1992

Population Group	Percent of Total Population	Percent of Poor Population	
		Current Measure[a]	Proposed Measure[b]
Age			
Children under 18	26.3	39.6	39.2
Adults 18–64	61.5	49.6	51.8
Adults 65 and older	12.2	10.8	9.0
Race			
White	83.6	66.8	69.3
Black	12.5	28.6	25.7
Other	3.9	4.6	5.1
Ethnicity			
Hispanic	8.9	18.1	20.9
Non-Hispanic	91.1	81.9	79.1
Family Size			
One person	14.5	21.7	15.7
Two persons	23.2	15.8	17.1
Three or four persons	42.3	33.5	37.4
Five or more persons	20.1	29.0	29.8
Welfare Status of Family			
Receiving AFDC or SSI	9.9	40.4	29.9
Not receiving AFDC or SSI	90.1	59.6	70.1
Work Status of Family			
One or more workers	81.1	50.8	58.9
No workers	18.9	49.2	41.1
Health Insurance Status of Family			
No health insurance	13.7	30.1	35.7
Some health insurance	86.3	69.9	64.3
Region of Residence			
Northeast	20.0	16.9	18.9
Midwest	24.0	21.7	20.2
South	34.4	40.0	36.4
West	21.6	21.4	24.5

[a]A threshold of $14,228 for two-adult/two-child families.
[b]A threshold of $13,175 for two-adult/two-child families, with a 0.75 scale economy factor; see text for discussion.

course, there are significant differences in poverty rates among groups under the current measure: for example, the rate for children (22%) is 50 percent higher than the overall rate of 14.5 percent; the rate for people in families receiving AFDC or SSI (59%) is 310 percent higher than the overall rate; and the rate for people in working families (9%) is 37 percent lower than the overall rate (see first column of Table 5-7). Hence, it is important to find an

TABLE 5-7 Poverty Rates by Population Group Under the Current and Proposed Measures, with Total Poverty Rate Held Constant at 14.5 Percent, 1992

Population Group	Poverty Rate (%)		Percentage Point Change	
	Current Measure[a]	Proposed Measure[b]	Actual	Standardized[c]
Age				
Children under 18	21.87	21.66	-0.21	-0.14
Adults 18–64	11.70	12.23	0.53	0.66
Adults 65 and older	12.90	10.80	-2.10	-2.36
Race				
White	11.60	12.04	0.44	0.55
Black	33.15	29.76	-3.39	-1.48
Other	17.39	19.06	1.67	1.39
Ethnicity				
Hispanic	29.43	34.03	4.60	2.27
Non–Hispanic	13.06	12.62	-0.44	-0.49
Family Size				
One person	21.75	15.77	-5.98	-3.99
Two persons	9.91	10.74	0.83	1.22
Three or four persons	11.50	12.84	1.34	1.69
Five or more persons	20.98	21.60	0.62	0.43
Welfare Status of Family				
Receiving AFDC or SSI	59.39	44.04	-15.35	-3.75
Not receiving AFDC or SSI	9.60	11.30	1.70	2.57
Work Status of Family				
One or more workers	9.09	10.55	1.46	2.33
No workers	37.91	31.70	-6.21	-2.38
Health Insurance Status of Family				
No health insurance	31.95	37.87	5.92	2.69
Some health insurance	11.76	10.83	-0.93	-1.15
Region of Residence				
Northeast	12.29	13.81	1.52	1.80
Midwest	13.10	12.21	-0.89	-0.99
South	16.89	15.36	-1.53	-1.32
West	14.39	16.48	2.09	2.11

NOTE: The poverty rates are for individuals: They are determined on the basis of comparing the income of their family (or one's own income if an unrelated individual) to the appropriate threshold.

[a]A threshold of $14,228 for two-adult/two-child families.

[b]A threshold of $13,175 for two-adult/two-child families, with a 0.75 scale economy factor; see text for discussion.

[c]See text for derivation.

appropriate metric for comparing poverty rates between the two measures. One such metric is to present results in terms of percentage changes in the poverty rate for each group; however, it is awkward to speak of percentage changes in a percentage. A method that is equivalent but more readily interpretable is to present results in terms of percentage point changes in the poverty rate in which these changes are standardized for each group to be comparable to the total population (see last column of Table 5-7).[9]

In standardized terms, the proposed measure increases the poverty rate by more than 1 percentage point for the following groups: people in two-person families, 1.2; people of other races (not white or black), 1.4; people in three- or four-person families, 1.7; Northeasterners, 1.8; Westerners, 2.1; Hispanics, 2.3; people in working families, 2.3; people in families not receiving AFDC or SSI, 2.6; and people in families without health insurance, 2.7. In contrast, the proposed measure decreases the poverty rate by more than 1 percentage point (in standardized terms) for the following groups: people in families with some health insurance, −1.2; Southerners, −1.3; blacks, −1.5; adults aged 65 or older, −2.4; people in families without workers, −2.4; people in families receiving AFDC or SSI, −3.8; and one-person families, −4.0.

Effects with a New Threshold

For our second analysis, we implemented the current measure with the official 1992 threshold of $14,228 for a two-adult/two-child family and the proposed measure with a threshold of $14,800 for this family type and two different scale economy factors—0.75 (alternative 1) and 0.65 (alternative 2). The value of $14,800 is the midpoint of our suggested range ($13,700–$15,900) for the starting reference family threshold. The purpose of this analysis was to determine the effect on the overall poverty rate, as well as the effect on groups, of raising the poverty threshold in real terms in addition to implementing the recommended adjustments to the threshold and family resource definition.

The Overall Rate

Under the proposed measure with a $14,800 reference family threshold and a 0.75 scale economy factor for 1992, 46.0 million people are poor, and the poverty rate is 18.1 percent, compared with the official count of 36.9 million and the official rate of 14.5 percent. With the same threshold and a 0.65 scale economy factor, the 1992 poverty rate is 19.0 percent.

---

[9] The procedure is to determine the ratio of the current poverty rate for the total population to the rate for the group and apply that ratio to the percentage point change for the group. This procedure standardizes the percentage point changes by treating each group as if it had the same poverty rate as all people.

The net effect of implementing the proposed measure with a higher threshold is to increase the number of poor, but not all of the movement is in the same direction. Under alternative 1 (0.75 scale economy factor), 4.2 million people are moved out of poverty and 13.3 million people are moved into poverty (32.7 million people are poor under both measures). As in the analysis with a constant poverty rate, most of the movement occurs near the poverty line. Thus, 93 percent of the 4.2 million people who are no longer categorized as poor move from the category of income between 50 and 100 percent of the poverty line to the category of income between 100 and 150 percent of the poverty line. Conversely, 72 percent of the 13.3 million people who are newly categorized as poor move from the category of income between 100 and 150 percent of the poverty line to the category of income between 50 and 100 percent of the poverty line.

Below, we show in broad terms the effects of the proposed changes to the thresholds and to the family resource definition on the increase in the overall poverty rate, which is 3.6 percentage points for alternative 1 and 4.5 percentage points for alternative 2 (see "Marginal Effects" for a more detailed decomposition):

Type of Change	Alternative 1	Alternative 2
All changes	+3.6	+4.5
$14,800 threshold	+0.7	+0.7
0.75 scale economy factor	−0.7	N.A.
0.65 scale economy factor	N.A.	-0-
Housing cost index	+0.1	+0.1
Proposed resource definition	+2.0	+2.0
Net interaction effect	+1.5	+1.7

The use of a higher reference family threshold accounts for only 0.7 percentage point of the increase in the poverty rate. The use of a 0.75 scale economy factor (alternative 1) offsets the effect of a higher reference family threshold: it decreases the poverty rate by 0.7 percentage point. In contrast, the use of a 0.65 scale economy factor (alternative 2) has no effect, which is why the overall increase in the rate is higher for alternative 2 than for alternative 1. (See the discussion below as to why the two scale economy factors have these different outcomes.) Adjusting the threshold for geographic area differences in the cost of housing has little effect on the overall poverty rate for the nation as a whole.

In contrast, the changes to the family resource definition account for a large part of the increase in the poverty rate, 2.0 percentage points.[10] There is

---

[10] This amount is the sum of the effect of each specific change—e.g., adding the value of in-kind benefits to income or subtracting child care costs from income—considered alone.

also an interaction effect, calculated as the total effect minus the sum of the marginal effects of all the components, which can increase or decrease the rate. An example of a positive interaction effect is that of a working family that is not poor when its taxes, child care expenses, and other work-related expenses are considered in isolation, but that becomes poor when its expenses on all of these items are considered together. This interaction effect accounts for 1.5 percentage points of the increase for alternative 1 and 1.7 percentage points of the increase for alternative 2.

Groups

Implementing the proposed measure with a higher threshold increases the poverty rate for most population groups. The pattern of effects is similar to that seen in the previous analysis that held the overall poverty rate constant; see Table 5-8. In standardized terms, alternative 1 increases the poverty rate by 5.0 or more percentage points (compared with the overall increase of 3.6 percentage points) for several groups: people in two-person families, 5.2; Northeasterners, 5.7; Hispanics, 5.7; Westerners, 5.7; people in families lacking health insurance, 5.9; people in families of three or four persons, 6.3; and—the largest increase—people in working families, 7.3. It increases the poverty rate by less than 2.2 percentage points for a few groups: Southerners, 2.1; elderly people, 1.9; blacks, 1.1. It actually *decreases* the rate by more than 1 percentage point for two groups: people in welfare families, −1.5; and one-person families, −1.8. (The increases in the poverty rate for other groups are within 1 percentage point of the overall increase.)

Perhaps the most striking effect of the proposed measure is on the distribution of the poor population between working and welfare families. People in working families make up 51 percent of the poor under the current measure; under alternative 1, they make up 61 percent of the poor. This increase represents a net shift of 9.4 million working family members who are not classified as poor under the current measure who are so classified under the proposed measure. People in welfare families make up 40 percent of the poor under the current measure; under alternative 1, they make up 29 percent of the poor. This decrease represents a net shift of 1.5 million welfare family members who are no longer classified as poor under the proposed measure. Despite these shifts, however, the poverty rate for welfare families remains considerably higher than the rate for working families.

In comparing the effects of the two equivalence scales in the proposed measure, the use of a 0.65 scale economy factor (alternative 2) increases the poverty rate for most groups by 0.5-1.0 percentage point more than the use of a 0.75 scale economy factor (alternative 1). There are a few striking exceptions to this general pattern, shown in Table 5-8. For the elderly, alternative 2 increases their poverty rate by an additional 3.9 percentage points over

TABLE 5-8   Poverty Rates by Population Group Under the Current and Proposed Measures, 1992

| Population Group | Poverty Rate (%) | | | Percentage Point Change—Standardized[a] with Proposed Measure | |
| | Current Measure | Proposed Measure | | | |
		Alternative 1	Alternative 2	Alternative 1	Alternative 2
Total population	14.52	18.12	19.02	+3.60	+4.50
Age					
Children under 18	21.87	26.44	26.35	3.03	2.97
Adults 65 and over	12.90	14.56	18.00	1.89	5.74
Race and Ethnicity					
White	11.60	15.26	16.14	4.58	5.68
Black	33.15	35.62	36.76	1.08	1.58
Hispanic[b]	29.43	40.98	40.88	5.70	5.65
Family Size					
One person	21.75	19.09	23.83	−1.78	1.39
Two persons	9.91	13.45	15.10	5.18	7.60
Three or four persons	11.50	16.52	16.81	6.34	6.70
Five or more persons	20.98	26.19	24.74	3.61	2.60
Welfare or Work Status					
Receiving AFDC or SSI	59.39	53.40	55.12	−1.46	−1.04
One or more workers	9.09	13.66	14.11	7.30	8.02
Without Health Insurance	31.95	44.87	46.03	5.87	6.40
Region of Residence					
Northeast	12.29	17.09	18.19	5.67	6.97
Midwest	13.10	15.43	16.27	2.58	3.51
South	16.89	19.37	20.29	2.13	2.92
West	14.39	20.06	20.83	5.72	6.50

NOTE: Both alternatives use a two-adult/two-child poverty threshold of $14,800; for alternative 1 the scale economy factor is 0.75; for alternative 2 it is 0.65. The poverty rates are for individuals: They are determined on the basis of comparing the income of their family (or one's own income if an unrelated individual) to the appropriate threshold.

[a]See text for derivation of standardized percentage point changes.

[b]Hispanics may be of any race.

alternative 1. In other words, the equivalence scale has more of an effect on the elderly than on other groups. This finding also holds for one-person families and members of two-person families, for which, in comparison with other groups, alternative 2 makes more of a difference in their poverty rates than does alternative 1. Indeed, the results for these groups are not unrelated, as a very high proportion of the elderly are in one- and two-person families.[11]

---

[11] In 1992, 31 percent of the elderly lived alone (compared with 12 percent of all people age 15 and older); another 54 percent lived with a spouse (Bureau of the Census, 1993d:Table 71). Note that the category of one-person "families" or unrelated individuals includes those living with other unrelated individuals in a larger household, as well as those living alone.

Finally, in contrast to the pattern for all other groups, measure 2 *decreases* poverty for five-person and larger families by 1 percentage point compared with measure 1. (See below for further discussion of equivalence scale effects.)

Marginal Effects

This section considers the effects of the individual components of the proposed poverty measure, including the various adjustments to both the thresholds and the family resource definition. We show why, for example, the proposed poverty measure increases the poverty rate for people in working families and decreases the rate for people in welfare families. Table 5-9 shows the marginal effect on the rate for specific groups of making each of the following changes in isolation: the adjustment to the thresholds for geographic area differences in the cost of housing, the use of a 0.75 scale economy factor, the use of a 0.65 scale economy factor, adding the value of in-kind benefits to income, subtracting out-of-pocket medical care expenses from income, subtracting income and payroll taxes from income, subtracting child care expenses from income, and subtracting other work-related expenses from income. Not shown is the marginal effect of a particular reference family threshold or the net interaction effect.[12]

The adjustment to the thresholds for area differences in the cost of housing increases the overall poverty rate by a negligible amount (see Table 5-9, first column). This result is expected because the housing cost adjustment is an index with values higher and lower than 1, which should approximately balance out overall. By region, the housing cost index has marked effects, increasing the poverty rate in the Northeast by 2 percentage points and in the West by 1.7 percentage points (all figures are standardized). In contrast, the housing cost index decreases the poverty rate in the South by 1.1 percentage points and in the Midwest by 0.8 percentage point. The housing cost index has negligible effects on the poverty rate for other groups, with the exception of Hispanics, who reside disproportionately in East and West coast cities with higher-than-average housing costs; the index increases their poverty rate by 1.1 percentage points.

The use of an equivalence scale with a scale economy factor of 0.75 reduces the overall poverty rate by 0.7 percentage point. In contrast, the use of a scale economy factor of 0.65 has almost no effect on the poverty rate. The

---

[12] For the total population, as noted above, the marginal effect of a $14,800 reference family threshold (compared with the current threshold of $14,228) is to increase the overall poverty rate by 0.7 percentage point; the net interaction effect increases the rate by 1.5 and 1.7 percentage points for alternatives 1 and 2, respectively. In the analysis that keeps the overall poverty rate constant, the marginal effect of a $13,175 reference family threshold (compared with the current threshold of $14,228) is to decrease the rate by 1.2 percentage points; the interaction effect decreases the rate by 0.2 percentage point.

effects of the two scale economy factors are similar for most groups, with the exceptions noted above and discussed below.

The addition to gross income of values for in-kind benefits has a marked effect on reducing the overall poverty rate—1.7 percentage points. The reduction in the poverty rate from adding the value of in-kind benefits is particularly large for several groups: the elderly, −2.2; Northeasterners, −2.3; and people in welfare families, −2.5. The reduction in the poverty rate from this change to the resource definition is least for people in families without health insurance, −1.1 percentage points.

The subtraction from gross income of out-of-pocket medical care expenses (including health insurance premiums) has a large effect on increasing the overall poverty rate—2.1 percentage points. The increase in the poverty rate from this component is particularly large for several groups: people in families without health insurance, 2.9; people in families with workers, 3.0; people in two-person families, 3.2; and elderly people, 3.5. The increase in the poverty rate from this component is less striking for blacks, 1.0; and people in welfare families, 0.5.

The subtraction of taxes increases the overall poverty rate by 0.5 percentage point. (The EITC does not fully offset payroll and state income taxes.) The subtraction of child care expenses has a smaller effect (0.3 percentage point), which is expected because this deduction applies only to working families with children in which both parents (or one if there is just one) work and the family pays for child care. The subtraction of other work-related expenses increases the overall rate by 0.8 percentage point. Summing the marginal effects of these three components, the result is an increase in the overall poverty rate of 1.6 percentage points. The increase in the poverty rate from subtracting these three components from income is much less for the elderly, 0.2 percentage point; there is also a smaller-than-average effect for blacks, 1.0 percentage point, and for people in welfare families, 0.4 percentage point. For people in working families, there is a larger-than-average effect: subtracting these three components from income increases their poverty rate by 2.9 percentage points.

We do not have a directly comparable estimate of the effect of child support payments on poverty rates. Tabulations prepared for us from the 1990 SIPP panel, which compare aggregate poverty rates under the current measure and under a measure in which child support payments are subtracted from income, indicate that the effect might be to increase the overall poverty rate by about 0.3-0.5 percentage point, similar to the effect of child care expenses.

Looking across all of the components provides insight as to why the proposed measure disproportionately affects the poverty rates under alternatives 1 and 2 for some groups relative to the overall increase of 3.6 to 4.5 percentage points. For example, the poverty rate for welfare family members *decreases* by 1 percentage point (on a standardized basis), although it remains

TABLE 5-9 Effect of Individual Components of the Proposed Measure on Percentage Point Changes in the Official Poverty Rates, 1992

Population Group	Marginal Percentage Point Change in the Poverty Rate[a]			
	Housing Cost Index	Scale Economy Factor 0.75	Scale Economy Factor 0.65	In-Kind Benefits
Total Population	0.09	−0.73	−0.02	−1.65
Age				
Children under 18	0.11	−0.33	−0.33	−1.79
Adults 65 and over	−0.03	−2.07	1.26	−2.15
Race and Ethnicity				
White	0.01	−0.89	−0.03	−1.61
Black	0.07	−0.49	−0.06	−1.84
Hispanic[b]	1.12	−0.15	−0.19	−1.68
Family Size				
One person	0.02	−3.99	−1.58	−1.47
Two persons	0.01	0.40	1.95	−1.42
Three or four persons	0.15	0.44	0.80	−1.92
Five or more persons	0.09	−0.28	−0.86	−1.60
Welfare or Work Status				
Receiving AFDC or SSI	0.21	−0.40	−0.02	−2.50
One or more workers	0.03	−0.78	−0.34	−1.66
Without Health Insurance	0.04	−0.60	−0.25	−1.06
Region of Residence				
Northeast	1.98	−0.95	0.04	−2.26
Midwest	−0.81	−0.95	−0.11	−1.66
South	−1.10	−0.56	0.16	−1.46
West	1.73	−0.69	−0.33	−1.52

NOTE: The poverty rates are for individuals: They are determined on the basis of comparing the income of their family (or one's own income if an unrelated individual) to the appropriate threshold.

very high. This occurs because welfare families benefit proportionately more than others from in-kind programs, including health insurance (as reflected in lower out-of-pocket medical care expenses) and are proportionately less adversely affected by taxes and work expenses. Conversely, the rate for working family members increases by a full 7-8 percentage points (on a standardized basis). Such families are proportionately more affected than others by subtracting out-of-pocket medical care costs, taxes, child care, and other work-related expenses.

The poverty rate for members of families without health insurance increases by 6 percentage points (on a standardized basis), mainly because there is a proportionately smaller effect for these families of adding values for in-kind benefits and a proportionately larger effect of subtracting out-of-pocket medi-

Out-of-Pocket Medical Costs	Taxes	Child Care Costs	Other Work Expenses
2.09	0.47	0.28	0.81
1.62	0.25	0.40	0.74
3.52	0.11	0.00	0.08
2.54	0.55	0.29	0.93
1.04	0.24	0.27	0.45
1.94	0.41	0.22	0.71
1.56	0.93	0.00	0.69
3.15	0.29	0.31	0.82
2.37	0.10	0.49	1.07
1.58	0.65	0.25	0.59
0.47	0.02	0.16	0.24
3.00	0.78	0.56	1.58
2.91	0.70	0.33	1.14
2.09	0.45	0.22	0.64
2.39	0.54	0.40	1.01
2.07	0.47	0.25	0.79
1.81	0.38	0.26	0.76

[a]The effect of changing only the single component on the official 1992 poverty rate for the group (see Table 5-8). The effect is expressed in standardized percentage points; see text for derivation.

[b]Hispanics may be of any race.

cal care costs. Conversely, the poverty rate for blacks increases by less than 2 percentage points (on a standardized basis) because proportionately more blacks are in welfare families and proportionately fewer are in working families. Finally, the poverty rate for children increases by 3 percentage points—or close to the overall increase—because poor children are members of both welfare families and working families.

Equivalence Scale Effects

Use of the panel's proposed equivalence scale has significant implications for poverty rates for certain groups relative to the equivalence scale that underlies the current measure. Also, the choice of a scale economy factor—0.75 or

TABLE 5-10   Effect of Alternative Scale Economy Factors in the Proposed Measure on Poverty Rates, by Family Size, 1992

Family Size	Official Poverty Rate (%)	Percentage Point Change Due to Scale Economy Factor[a]		Percent of Population in Each Category	
		0.75	0.65	Total	Children
One person[b]	21.75	−3.99	−1.58	14.5	0.2
Two persons	9.91	+0.40	+1.95	23.2	5.7
Three persons	12.03	+0.91	+1.63	19.5	19.7
Four persons	11.05	0.00	0.00	22.8	35.5
Five persons	16.56	−0.34	−0.55	11.9	22.2
Six persons	22.24	−0.24	−0.99	4.8	9.6
Seven or more persons	35.07	−0.18	−1.26	3.3	7.1
Total	14.52	−0.73	−0.02	100.0	100.0

NOTE: The poverty rates are for individuals: They are determined on the basis of comparing the income of their family (or one's own income if an unrelated individual) to the appropriate threshold.

[a]The percentage point changes are standardized: they represent the percentage point changes for each family size category times the ratio of the overall poverty rate to the rate for that category. Both scale economy factors were applied to a threshold of $14,228 for the reference two-adult/two-child family.

[b]Includes people living alone or with others not related to them.

0.65—makes a difference for some groups. To explore these effects more fully, we analyzed poverty rates for people in specific family sizes, from one-person families (i.e., unrelated individuals) to families of seven or more persons; see Table 5-10. Specifically, we compared the official rates to rates developed with the same threshold for a two-adult/two-child family ($14,228), but with different thresholds for other family types calculated from the proposed equivalence scale formula with a scale economy factor of 0.75 or 0.65.[13] The only factor that we change in these comparisons is the equivalence scale: that is, we do not change the reference family threshold (up or down) or the resource definition or adjust the thresholds for differences in cost of housing.

Because the threshold for the reference family does not change, the current poverty rate of 11 percent for people in four-person families should not change across the three measures, and, in fact, it does not. The rates for people in other family types do change, in varying ways.

The scale economy factor of 0.75 affects the poverty rates for people in

---

[13] The formula is as follows: scale value = $(A + 0.70K)^{0.75 \text{ (or 0.65)}}$, where A is the number of adults in the family and K is the number of children under age 18. To develop the thresholds, the scale value for each family type is converted to a ratio to the scale value for the reference two-adult/two-child family and applied to the threshold for that reference family.

smaller and larger families, but, with one exception, the effects are small. The exception is the category of one-person families, for which the 0.75 factor reduces their poverty rate by almost 4 percentage points (on a standardized basis) compared with the official rate. One can see why this occurs by looking at Figure 3-5 (in Chapter 3): the equivalence scale value for one-person families with the 0.75 factor is lower than the current scale value, while the scale values for other family types are very similar. The difference in the scale values for one-person families stems from the fact that the current measure assumes that unrelated individuals need almost 80 percent as much as two-adult families, but the proposed equivalence scale with the 0.75 scale economy factor assumes that unrelated individuals need only about 60 percent as much as two-adult families. (Expressed another way, the current measure assumes that two-adult families need only 29% more than one-adult families, while the proposed scale with the 0.75 factor assumes that they need 68% more. These relationships are not quite the same when the second person in a family is a child; see Chapter 3.)

The scale economy factor of 0.65 affects poverty rates to a moderate extent for people in almost all family size categories, although the net effect for the total population balances out to almost zero. The 0.65 factor reduces poverty for unrelated individuals (although not as much as the 0.75 factor) and also for people in families of five, six, and seven or more persons. In contrast, it increases poverty for people in two-person and three-person families. The reason for these results is that the 0.65 factor assumes greater economies of scale than either the measure with the 0.75 factor or (in most instances) the current measure. Hence, the 0.65 factor generally produces higher scale values than the other two measures for two- and three-person families and lower scale values for families of five or more persons. (The scale value for unrelated individuals with the 0.65 factor is between the other two values for this group; see Figure 3-5.)

In sum, the scale with the 0.75 factor has little effect on poverty for most family size categories but a large (negative) effect on unrelated individuals; the scale with the 0.65 factor has moderate effects on every category. Neither scale affects poverty among children to any degree because almost 80 percent of children are in families of 3-5 persons, for which the effects tend to balance out. In contrast, because 85 percent of the elderly are in families of one or two persons (with 54% in the latter category), the scale with the 0.75 factor lowers the poverty rate for the elderly by a significant amount, while the scale with the 0.65 factor has the opposite effect (see Table 5-9).

Accuracy of Medical Care Expense Imputations

The imputation of out-of-pocket medical care expenses is the component with the biggest single effect on the overall poverty rate under the proposed measure, increasing the rate by 2.1 percentage points in standardized terms. Clearly, a question is the adequacy of the imputation procedures.

One way to assess their adequacy is to inspect the results for reasonableness. Thus, the results we obtained meet such obvious tests as that the amounts imputed, in total and by characteristics, match the dollar totals obtained from the NMES data. Also, the imputed amounts make sense in relation to families' income levels: for families with gross money incomes around the median, we imputed an average of about $2,150 for out-of-pocket medical care expenses; for families with incomes around the 10th percentile, we imputed an average of only $450 for such expenses. (Table 5-4 shows the combined amount of deductions for out-of-pocket medical care, child care, and other work-related expenses that were imputed to families at different points in the income distribution.)

Some recent research studies provide information to evaluate alternative imputation procedures for out-of-pocket medical care expenditures, including ours. Weinberg and Lamas (1993) estimated poverty rates for 1989 under several measures, including some that took account of out-of-pocket medical care costs that they imputed to the March 1990 CPS by using 1987 NMES data. Specifically, they imputed mean 1987 expenditures, updated to 1989 with the Consumer Price Index (CPI) for medical care, to people under age 65 categorized by age group (under 5, 6-17, 18-44, 45-64) and health insurance coverage (any private insurance, public insurance only, uninsured) and to people aged 65 and older categorized by health insurance coverage (Medicare only, Medicare and other public coverage, Medicare and private coverage, uninsured). Because they also made some other changes to the poverty definition, it is not possible to estimate precisely the marginal effect on poverty rates of subtracting their imputed values for out-of-pocket medical care costs. Roughly, it appears that the effect would be to increase the 1989 poverty rate of 12.8 percent by 5.4 percentage points (Weinberg and Lamas, 1993:Table A-2); this increase is 6.1 percentage points standardized to the 1992 poverty rate of 14.5 percent.

Doyle, Beauregard, and Lamas (1993) used the 1987 NMES itself, projected forward to income year 1991 and calibrated to the March 1992 CPS, to estimate poverty rates with the current definition and measures that excluded out-of-pocket medical care costs. (They also estimated poverty rates with variations of a two-index approach.) For one measure, they calculated out-of-pocket expenses in the same manner as Weinberg and Lamas (1993) (i.e., by using subgroup means); for another measure, they used the actual out-of-pocket expenditures reported in the NMES for each family unit. With subgroup means, they estimated that the subtraction of out-of-pocket medical care costs would increase the 1991 poverty rate of 14.2 percent by 1.9 percentage points; with the use of actual NMES expenditure data, they estimated that the increase would be 1.1 percentage points (Doyle, Beauregard, and Lamas, 1993:Table 2a).[14]

Hence, there are four estimates, including the panel's, of the effect on poverty of subtracting out-of-pocket medical care costs (including health insurance premiums) from income (standardized to 1992):

• 6.1 percentage points, with group means imputed to the March 1990 CPS (Weinberg and Lamas, 1993);

• 2.1 percentage points, with the more elaborate imputation procedure that we carried out on the March 1993 CPS;

• 1.9 percentage points, with group means imputed to a 1987 NMES file calibrated to the March 1992 CPS (Doyle, Beauregard, and Lamas, 1993); and

• 1.1 percentage points, with actual expenditure data from a 1987 NMES file calibrated to the March 1992 CPS (Doyle, Beauregard, and Lamas, 1993).

Clearly, the effect on the poverty rate of subtracting out-of-pocket medical care costs from income is less with the use of actual data than with imputed data. Also, a more elaborate imputation (e.g., that conducted by the panel) produces less of an effect than a simpler imputation. These findings are as expected because the distribution of out-of-pocket medical care costs is highly skewed: many people have relatively low costs, while some people have high costs that raise the average, even within subgroups. Hence, an imputation procedure (particularly a simple one) is likely to overstate the expenses of enough people so as to overstate the increase in the poverty rate. Finally, there is an unexplained difference attributable to the use of a different survey file: namely, estimates of the effect on the poverty rate of subtracting out-of-pocket medical care costs with the NMES are lower than those with the March CPS, even when the same procedure of imputed subgroup means is used.[15]

Overall, it is not possible to draw a definitive conclusion about our approach because of the differences in the data and procedures used to calculate each of the estimates. However, it appears that our estimate is roughly consistent with all the available work, although it may somewhat overstate the

---

[14] Again, these are rough estimates because Doyle, Beauregard, and Lamas also made other changes to the poverty measure, specifically, excluding taxes from income and reducing the official poverty thresholds by 3.6 percent to account for average out-of-pocket medical care expenses for the total population. A tabulation run for the panel, which provides a better estimate of the marginal effect, estimated an increase in the poverty rate of 0.8 percentage point with the approach of using actual expenditure data from the NMES. (This tabulation kept taxes in the income definition and lowered the official thresholds.)

[15] One factor that may contribute to the difference is that Doyle, Beauregard, and Lamas (1993) updated the 1987 NMES expenditure data by changes in the national health accounts rather than by the change in the medical care component of the CPI.

effect on the poverty rate of subtracting out-of-pocket medical care costs from income. For the elderly, our measure may somewhat *understate* the effect on the poverty rate. Thus, Doyle, Beauregard, and Lamas (1993:Table 2a) estimate that subtracting out-of-pocket medical care expenses would raise the poverty rate for the elderly by 6.8 percentage points, compared with our estimate of 3.5 percentage points; see Table 5-9 (both increases are standardized to the poverty rate for the total population).

The treatment of out-of-pocket medical care costs is clearly a topic for which further work is needed. As a first priority, improved imputation procedures should be developed for both the March CPS and SIPP. Data from the next round of the NMES (scheduled for 1996) should prove very helpful in this regard. Work should also be done to explore ways of obtaining reasonable estimates of actual expenses in SIPP, acknowledging that SIPP (let alone the March CPS) cannot obtain the kind of detailed information on medical care costs that is the focus of the NMES. A mixed strategy may prove optimal: asking some broad questions on expenses in SIPP and using the more detailed NMES information to adjust the responses appropriately.[16] In any case, we stress the importance of accounting for out-of-pocket medical care costs in the poverty measure. Even the lower bound for the estimated increase in the poverty rate represents a significant effect. Moreover, by taking account of such expenses, the poverty measure will be able to contribute to tracking the effects of changes in the health care financing system on families' resources for consumption.

Prior Income Years

Data and Procedures

It is clear from the analysis that implementation of the proposed poverty measure will have important effects on the overall poverty rate in total and for various population groups. What is less clear is the effect on time trends. We attempted to conduct the same kinds of analyses reviewed above for 1992 with the March 1990, 1984, and 1980 CPS files. For the current measure, we used the official thresholds for 1992, 1989, 1983, and 1979. For the proposed measure, we used a $14,800 reference family threshold for 1992 and thresholds for the earlier years that reflect changes in spending on food, clothing, and shelter by two-adult/two-child families projected backwards from 1992; Con-

---

[16] The method of "bracketing" responses, that is, asking respondents who answer "don't know" whether the amount is above or below certain levels (e.g., $100, $500, $1,000, $5,000, $10,000) may improve the completeness of reporting of out-of-pocket medical care expenses in SIPP. The bracketing method has been used successfully for asset reporting in the Health and Retirement Survey (see Chapter 4) and will be used in the next round of that survey for out-of-pocket medical care expenses.

sumer Expenditure Survey (CEX) expenditure data were used to calculate the thresholds for the proposed measure (see Chapter 2, especially Table 2-7).

In the calculation of disposable income, we used the values for taxes and in-kind benefits that were developed by the Census Bureau and supplied with the extract file for each year. For child care and other work-related expenses, we adjusted the amounts that we used for our imputations for income year 1992 backwards to the earlier years by the change in the overall CPI. These adjustments do not seem unreasonable, although they do not capture price changes specific to these particular expenses, nor do they reflect other relevant changes that may have occurred over the period (e.g., in the proportion of working families that pay for child care). In the case of out-of-pocket medical care expenditures, we concluded that a simple price adjustment, even using the medical care component of the CPI, could be very problematic, particularly given the large effect of this component. With regard to cost-of-housing differences, the March CPS files for earlier years provide less geographic identification so that it would be difficult to implement a sufficiently detailed index. Hence, we computed poverty rates for 1979, 1983, 1989, and also 1992 that made all of the proposed changes with the exception of the subtraction of out-of-pocket medical care expenditures from income and the adjustment of the thresholds for housing cost differences. Child support payments are also not accounted for because of the absence of data in the March CPS with which to make a reasonable imputation.

Results

With either a 0.75 or a 0.65 scale economy factor (alternative 1 or 2), the proposed measure produces poverty rates that differ somewhat from the rates under the current measure for 1992 and preceding years; see Table 5-11.[17] The differences are more pronounced when one compares percentage point changes in the poverty rate for different periods:[18]

	Percentage Point Increase		
	Current	Proposed Measure	
Time Period	Measure	Alternative 1	Alternative 2
1979–1983	+3.5	+3.9	+3.8
1983–1989	−2.4	−2.0	−1.9
1989–1992	+1.7	+1.3	+1.5
1979–1992 (overall)	+2.8	+3.3	+3.4

[17] Because we do not subtract out-of-pocket medical care costs, the differences for 1992 are smaller than shown above; presumably, the differences for earlier years are also smaller than would be the case if out-of-pocket medical expenses were deducted from income.

[18] The percentage point changes under the proposed measure are standardized to the official rate in the first year of each time period.

TABLE 5-11   Poverty Rates Under the Current and Proposed Measures: 1992, 1989, 1983, 1979

Measure	1992	1989	1983	1979
Poverty Rate (%)				
Current measure	14.52	12.82	15.24	11.70
Proposed measure[a]				
0.75 scale economy factor	14.59	13.21	15.16	11.36
0.65 scale economy factor	15.25	13.69	15.64	11.80
Percentage Point Change under Proposed Measure[b] (standardized to 1992)				
0.75 scale economy factor	+0.07	+0.44	−0.08	−0.42
0.65 scale economy factor	+0.73	+0.99	+0.38	+0.12
Marginal Change Due to				
0.75 scale economy factor	−0.73	−0.69	−0.55	−0.62
0.65 scale economy factor	−0.02	−0.16	−0.10	0.06
Addition of in-kind benefits	−1.65	−1.76	−1.38	−2.21
Subtraction of taxes	0.47	0.76	1.03	0.60
Subtraction of child care costs	0.28	0.33	0.24	0.24
Subtraction of other work expenses	0.81	0.82	0.68	0.74

NOTES: The reference (two-adult/two-child) family thresholds are as follows:

	1992	1989	1983	1979
Current measure	$14,228	$12,575	$10,097	$7,355
Proposed measure	14,800	12,986	10,038	7,565

The poverty rates are for individuals: They are determined on the basis of comparing the income of their family (or one's own income if an unrelated individual) to the appropriate threshold.

[a]Excludes adjustments for out-of-pocket medical care costs and geographic area differences in the cost of housing.

[b]Standardized percentage point changes represent the percentage point changes for a time period times the ratio of the official poverty rate in 1992 to the official rate for the period. Marginal percentage point changes are also standardized to 1992.

Over the entire period from 1979 to 1992, the proposed measure shows a somewhat higher increase in the poverty rate than the current measure. One reason for the difference is that such in-kind benefits as food stamps were more widely available in the 1970s than in the 1980s. The proposed measure reflects this change; the current measure does not.[19] Both the proposed and the current measures show an increase in the poverty rate from the economic recession in the early 1980s, a decline in the poverty rate from the economic

---

[19] As shown in Table 5-11, adding the value of in-kind benefits to income reduces the poverty rate by a larger amount in 1979 than in later years.

recovery of the mid- and late 1980s, and another increase in the rate from the recession in the early 1990s. However, the proposed measure shows a larger increase in the poverty rate from 1979 to 1983 because of such factors as the curtailment of in-kind benefits in the early 1980s and somewhat higher taxes on the working poor, which are captured in the proposed measure but not the current measure. The recent expansion of the Earned Income Tax Credit (EITC) is also captured in the proposed measure, which shows a smaller increase in the poverty rate from 1989 to 1992 than the current measure.

Our analysis of time trends is limited by our inability to develop reasonable imputations for many components of disposable income. We believe that it would be possible, with further work, to produce a more definitive analysis of changes in the poverty rate over time under the current measure and the proposed measure. For example, data from the predecessors to NMES in 1977 and 1980 could be used to develop imputations for out-of-pocket medical care expenses; data from the 1984 SIPP panel could be used to develop imputation regressions for child care expenses for earlier years; and data from the 1980 census could be used to develop geographic cost-of-housing indexes for earlier years. We support such work in order to develop a time series for comparison and to facilitate the transition to a new measure.

Historically, it is likely that the major differences between the current measure and the proposed measure would be most evident, not in the 1980s, but in the 1970s, when the Food Stamp Program and other antipoverty programs exhibited their largest growth. Because of data limitations, it does not seem feasible to construct estimates with the proposed measure for years before 1979. In the future, the proposed measure should provide a more accurate picture of the effects of important government policy initiatives that affect disposable income.

For example, changes in the health care financing system that affect out-of-pocket medical care costs or changes in tax provisions that affect disposable income would be reflected in the proposed measure; they cannot affect the poverty rate under the current measure. To provide some illustrations of this point, we simulated the effects on the poverty rate of policy changes that are scheduled to occur in a future year or that could conceivably be implemented in the future—making the assumption that the changes were actually implemented in 1992.

For one simulation, we estimated families' net taxes as if the legislated expansion of the EITC, which is scheduled to take full effect in 1996, were in effect in 1992. The result is to reduce the 1992 poverty rate under the proposed measure from 18.1 to 17.2 percent (using a $14,800 reference family threshold and 0.75 scale economy factor).

For another simulation, we estimated families' disposable income as if changes in health care financing (whether instituted publicly or privately) had placed a cap on families' out-of-pocket costs for medical care. Under one scenario, we assumed that such a cap limited families' expenses to a maximum of $3,000 ($1,500 for an unrelated individual); under another scenario, we assumed that the cap limited families' expenses to a maximum of $2,000 ($1,000 for an unrelated individual). We applied these caps to the imputed values of out-of-pocket medical care expenses in our data file for 1992. The result is to reduce the 1992 poverty rate under the proposed measure from 18.1 percent to 17.2 percent for the higher cap and from 18.1 percent to 16.6 percent for the lower cap.

Poverty Rates Using SIPP

For the reasons described above, our analysis was conducted entirely with extracts from the March CPS. However, we recommend (see below) that SIPP become the source of the nation's official poverty statistics, beginning when the survey is redesigned in 1996. A question is what effects the use of SIPP, compared with the March CPS, will have on poverty rates. Table 5-12 presents a time series of poverty estimates for the total population based on the official thresholds and gross income data from the March CPS, SIPP, and the CEX, as well as estimates of poverty based on the official thresholds and a consumption or expenditure definition of family resources from the CEX.

In looking at the income-based estimates, the poverty rates from SIPP for 1984-1991 are consistently lower than the rates from the March CPS: the difference ranges from 2.6 to 3.6 percentage points. This pattern suggests if we had analyzed our measure with SIPP, the result for 1992, using a $14,800 reference family threshold, would have been poverty rates of 14.9 to 15.8 percent (depending on the scale economy factor) instead of the rates of 18.1 to 19.0 percent that we obtained with the March CPS. In other words, the increase in the rate—compared with the official rate of 14.5 percent—would have been 0.4 to 1.3 percentage points instead of 3.6 to 4.5 percentage points.

In turn, the March CPS rates for the years 1980-1991 are lower than the rates from the CEX, particularly in the years after 1983. These results suggest that surveys with a focus on measuring income in fact capture more income (at least at the lower end of the income distribution) and, hence, produce lower poverty rates. Indeed, the rates from SIPP, which is the survey with the greatest focus on income, are close to the CEX rates that use a consumption or expenditure-based definition of resources.[20]

---

[20] Preliminary unpublished estimates of CEX consumption-based and expenditure-based poverty rates by Christopher Jencks (private communication) are lower than those shown above. Income-based poverty rate estimates from the CEX, March CPS, and SIPP would be lower by about 1 percentage point if food stamps were added to income. Food expenditures that are paid for by food stamps are included in the consumption- and expenditure-based measures.

TABLE 5-12 Poverty Rates Calculated from the Consumer Expenditure Survey, Current Population Survey, and Survey of Income and Program Participation, 1980–1991

| | Percent Poor of the Total Population | | | | |
| | Income Definition | | | Consumption/Expenditure Definition | |
Year	CEX[a]	March CPS[b]	SIPP[c]	CEX Consumption[d]	CEX Expenditures[e]
1980	13.7	13.0	N.A.	8.2	10.1
1981	14.3	14.0	N.A.	N.A	8.8
1982	15.8	15.0	N.A	N.A.	11.3
1983	16.1	15.2	N.A.	N.A.	10.2
1984	17.6	14.4	11.5	9.9	10.2
1985	17.6	14.0	10.7	N.A.	10.1
1986	18.9	13.6	10.3	N.A.	9.4
1987	15.0	13.4	10.8	N.A	9.7
1988	15.8	13.0	10.0	9.3	9.5
1989	15.2	12.8	N.A.	N.A.	9.7
1990	N.A.	13.5	10.1	N.A.	N.A.
1991	N.A.	14.2	10.6	N.A.	N.A.

[a]Estimates from Slesnick (1991b:Table 7).
[b]Estimates from Bureau of the Census (1992c:Table 2).
[c]Estimates from unpublished tabulations, Bureau of the Census. The 1985 estimate is an average of the rates estimated from the 1984-1985 panels.
[d]Estimates from Cutler and Katz (1991:Table 13). The estimates are crudely adjusted for use of the personal consumption deflator to update the thresholds instead of the CPI; a strictly comparable CPI-based poverty rate estimate for 1988 in Cutler and Katz (1992:Table 3) is 10.3 percent. Consumption is defined as all out-of-pocket expenditures minus spending on insurance, pensions, and Social Security plus net imputed rent for homes and vehicles.
[e]Estimates from Slesnick (1991b:Table 7).

There are several reasons that SIPP poverty rates are lower than the rates from the March CPS: SIPP obtains more complete reporting of transfer income (e.g., Social Security, SSI, and unemployment compensation); SIPP obtains higher reported numbers of recipients for most income types, and, with more income sources reported, there is a greater likelihood that respondents' total income will be above the poverty line; SIPP asks self-employed people about their income or cash "draw" from their businesses, rather about their net profit or loss; and SIPP obtains a better match of family composition with income data, which has been shown to reduce the poverty rate (see Bureau of the Census, 1993c:xxii; Coder and Scoon-Rodgers, 1994; see also Appendix B). Recent Census Bureau research (Lamas, Tin, and Eargle, 1994) also suggests that a small fraction of the difference between the SIPP and March CPS poverty rates is due to higher attrition of low-income people from SIPP for which the weighting adjustments do not completely compensate.

However, allowing for the attrition effect would still produce a 2-3 percentage point difference in the poverty rates estimated by the two surveys.

With regard to poverty rates for various groups, Census Bureau tabulations for 1987 and 1988 indicate that differences between SIPP and the March CPS are similar for most groups under the current measure, with the CPS rate always higher. For example, for 1987, the March CPS rate was 124 percent of the SIPP rate for the total population, 124 percent for men, 125 percent for women, 128 percent for people aged 18 to 64, 123 percent for Hispanics, and 132 percent for whites. For blacks, the March CPS rate was only 107 percent of the SIPP rate, and for children it was 115 percent. For the elderly, the CPS rate was 140 percent of the SIPP rate. The patterns were similar for 1988 (Short and Shea, 1991:Table D-3). These results suggest that differences between the March CPS and SIPP would be similar under the proposed measure for most groups, with the March CPS rate exceeding the SIPP rate in every case. In the next section, we consider explicitly the role of SIPP in poverty measurement and the overall need for improved data.

DATA SOURCES

Critically important for the measurement of poverty is the availability of appropriate, high-quality, and timely data—both for developing and updating the poverty thresholds and for estimating the resources available to families and individuals. We experienced first-hand the problems of inadequate data on family resources in analyzing the effects of implementing the proposed poverty measure in place of the current measure. Similarly, in attempting to understand the behavior of the proposed method for updating the poverty thresholds (see Chapter 2), we faced inadequate time-series data on consumer expenditures.

We note specific data problems and possible solutions in many places throughout our report. In this section we pull together in broad terms our proposals for improvements to support appropriate and accurate poverty measurement now and into the future. We first consider needed improvements for estimating families' resources in terms of disposable money and near-money income. On the resource side of the ledger, the data requirements are particularly pressing because of demands for fast release of the latest poverty statistics and the need for large sample sizes to support reliable comparisons across population groups, geographic areas, and time periods. A fundamental issue for resource estimation is which of the two major income surveys in the United States—the March CPS or SIPP—should provide the basis for official poverty statistics with the proposed definition.

We then look briefly at issues of estimating disposable income for surveys that are focused on other topics (e.g., health or housing) but need background variables on income and poverty for analysis purposes. We take a similar brief look at these issues for the decennial census, which provides small-area income and poverty statistics that are not obtainable in surveys. Finally, we consider needed improvements to data on consumption and expenditures. Deficiencies in the existing series must be remedied, if there is ever to be the possibility of using a consumption-based definition of family resources.

Recommendations

The proposal to define family resources for the poverty measure as disposable money and near-money income requires a wide array of high-quality information on families' demographic characteristics, money income, in-kind benefits, expenses, and assets. The March income supplement to the CPS, which to date has been the source of the nation's official poverty statistics, only partly meets these requirements now and is unlikely to meet them all in the future. Consequently, imputations would be required to fully implement the proposed family resource definition with March CPS data. In general, despite reporting problems with surveys, it is much preferable to have actual rather than imputed data. Imputation procedures are unlikely to reproduce fully the relationships and variations that exist in the population, and they may well introduce errors. There is an alternate source that we believe can provide the needed data, namely, the relatively new SIPP.

From our comparative review of the current and likely future capabilities of the two surveys (see below), we conclude that SIPP should become the primary source of official income, poverty, and related statistics, beginning when a redesign of the survey takes effect in 1996. The SIPP design, questionnaire, and methodological research program should give priority to implementation of the poverty measure.

To facilitate the transition to a new poverty measure with a new data source, the Census Bureau should produce concurrent series of poverty statistics from both SIPP and the March CPS. Also, many analysts will want to continue to develop poverty estimates from the March CPS so the Census Bureau should regularly issue public-use files from both the March CPS and SIPP that are suitable for this purpose.

RECOMMENDATION 5.1. **The Survey of Income and Program Participation should become the basis of official U.S. income and poverty statistics in place of the March income supplement to the Current Population Survey. Decisions about the SIPP design and questionnaire should take account of the data requirements for producing reliable time series of poverty statistics using the proposed definition of family resources (money and near-money income minus certain expenditures). Priority should be accorded to methodological research for SIPP that is relevant for improved poverty measurement.**

A particularly important problem to address is population undercoverage, particularly of low-income minority groups.

RECOMMENDATION 5.2.   To facilitate the transition to SIPP, the Census Bureau should produce concurrent time series of poverty rates
from both SIPP and the March CPS by using the proposed revised
threshold concept and updating procedure and the proposed definition of family resources as disposable income.   The concurrent
series should be developed starting with 1984, when SIPP was first
introduced.

RECOMMENDATION 5.3.   The Census Bureau should routinely issue
public-use files from both SIPP and the March CPS that include the
Bureau's best estimate of disposable income and its components
(taxes, in-kind benefits, child care expenses, etc.) so that researchers
can obtain poverty rates consistent with the new threshold concept
from either survey.

Data Sources for Income

The March CPS

The March CPS has several important advantages: large sample size (over
60,000 households); timeliness (reports and data files are typically available
within 6 months of data collection); and the fact that analysts both inside and
outside the Census Bureau are comfortable with the data.   However, the
March CPS has many limitations for measuring poverty with the proposed
resource definition.[21]

The March CPS collects information for each adult household member
on previous year's money income from a large number of sources and also asks
about participation in the major in-kind benefit programs. However, its
coverage of in-kind programs is not complete. Moreover, it does not ask
about expenses that we propose to deduct from income, such as out-of-pocket
medical care expenditures, child care costs, other work-related expenses, and
child support payments. The March CPS also does not ask questions that
would facilitate accurate estimation of income taxes, such as number of dependents (including those outside the household), whether the household item-
izes deductions, etc. The March CPS does not ascertain characteristics of
rented housing needed to value public subsidies or characteristics of owned
housing needed to impute equivalent rents. Finally, it does not ask about
assets or lump sum receipts, which may be needed for supplementary short-
term poverty measures, if not for the official annual measure.

---

[21] For a detailed description of the March CPS, see Appendix B.

Indeed, the March CPS cannot be used to construct poverty measures for shorter (or longer) periods than a year. Moreover, the annual data it provides present a number of technical difficulties. In particular, family composition as defined in March may not reflect the composition during the income reference year, which can result in an erroneous assignment of poverty status. With regard to data quality, many income questions in the March CPS have high nonresponse rates: overall, 20 percent of estimated total income from the CPS represents imputed rather than reported values. There are other kinds of reporting errors as well.

The problems with the March CPS are tractable in principle (e.g., more questions could be added or steps taken to improve quality). In practice, however, it would be difficult to effect further improvements because the March CPS is a supplement to the monthly labor force survey that is the basis of the nation's monthly unemployment statistics. The primary focus of the Bureau of Labor Statistics (BLS), which sponsors the monthly CPS, and the Census Bureau, which collects it, is to maintain and enhance the quality of the monthly labor force data. All of the supplements, including the March income supplement, are of secondary priority. One consequence is that fairly high nonresponse rates to the income supplement are tolerated so as not to reduce the likelihood that households will cooperate with the next month's employment questions. Also, the recent major redesign of the CPS, involving a new sample, revised questionnaire, and revised data collection and processing systems, focused on the main labor force component and not the supplements. The income supplement will benefit from some of the changes, such as the introduction of computer-assisted interviewing, but no special effort was made to revisit the questionnaire or other features of the income supplement itself.

The Alternative of SIPP

Recognizing the inherent limitations of the March CPS as long ago as the early-1970s, a federal interagency committee sponsored by the U.S. Office of Management and Budget proposed that a new income survey be fielded to improve the scope and quality of the information available on income and the effects of government assistance programs. This proposal ultimately led to the creation of SIPP, which began in 1983 (see Committee on National Statistics, 1989:Ch. 4). Currently, SIPP is designed as a longitudinal survey that follows the adult members of samples or "panels" of about 20,000 households. A new panel is introduced every February and followed over a period of 32 months, with interviews at 4-month intervals. The survey is scheduled for a major redesign beginning in 1996.[22]

---

[22] See Appendix B for a detailed description of SIPP.

SIPP has already made important contributions to knowledge about the dynamics of income receipt and program participation, health insurance coverage, asset holdings, and other topics related to material and other dimensions of well-being. SIPP has also made important strides toward obtaining higher quality income data than in the March CPS (e.g., nonresponse rates for many income sources are significantly lower), although there are still problems to overcome. With specific regard to poverty measurement, SIPP asks (or has asked) questions to obtain virtually all of the information needed to implement the proposed family resource definition. On the negative side, SIPP experienced significant start-up problems, including delays in release of data products and budget cuts that necessitated reductions in sample size and number of interviews.

A panel of the Committee on National Statistics (CNSTAT) recently completed a thorough review and evaluation of SIPP, recommending changes to begin with the 1996 panel (Citro and Kalton, 1993). These changes, taken together, promise to significantly improve the usefulness of the survey for both longitudinal and cross-sectional analyses of income, program participation, and related topics. They include:

• extending the length of each panel (i.e., each new sample of households whose members are followed over time) from 32 to 48 months;

• following children as well as adult members of the households originally included in each panel, even if they move to other households;

• introducing new panels every 2 years, so as to reduce the complexity of the survey (compared with the current design of introducing a new panel every year) and still maintain the ability to produce yearly time series for income, poverty, program participation, and other statistics;

• enlarging the sample size of each panel so that about 55,000 households are available for cross-sectional estimates by combining two panels, compared with 38,000 under the current SIPP design (for fully funded panels) and 62,000 in the March CPS;[23] and

• making maximum use of the planned introduction of computer-assisted interviewing and database management system technology to improve data quality and timeliness.

The CNSTAT Panel to Evaluate SIPP concluded that these changes would make it possible for SIPP to produce timely income statistics of high reliability. Noting the limited ability to make further improvements to the March CPS, the SIPP panel recommended that, over time, SIPP replace the March CPS for purposes of producing income, poverty, and related statistics.[24]

---

[23] The CNSTAT SIPP panel believed that further expansion of sample size would be possible once planned improvements in data collection and processing are put into place.

[24] The CPS would, of course, continue to include income items for use in labor force analyses.

We are in full agreement with the recommendation that SIPP become the basis for the nation's official poverty and related statistics. The March CPS does not collect all of the information needed for poverty measurement, has problems with the quality of the information that it collects, and does not have much room for further improvement. In contrast, SIPP collects most of the needed information, has achieved quality improvements, and, because of its focus on income, has ample opportunity for further improvements in both the scope and the quality of income-related data. The best time to put this recommendation into effect would be in 1996, when other changes to the survey are made.

Orienting SIPP to Poverty Measurement

A decision to use SIPP to produce the official poverty data means that all aspects of the survey should be reviewed to determine their suitability for providing the most accurate statistics possible under the proposed measure. A key aspect for review is the proposed redesign of the survey. Although the Census Bureau has accepted many of the recommendations of the CNSTAT Panel to Evaluate SIPP, it has decided against the recommendation for a design that would have two panels of about 27,000 households each in the field each year, with new panels introduced every 2 years. Instead, the Census Bureau has proposed a design that would have one large panel of 50,000 households in the field each year, with new panels introduced every 4 years.

The Census Bureau's design has the advantage of maximum sample size in a single panel for purposes of longitudinal analysis. For cross-sectional analysis, the two designs are equivalent: the two panels in the field each year under the CNSTAT SIPP panel's design can readily be combined to produce the same sample size as the single, larger panel of the Census Bureau's design.

Longitudinal estimates are important, but we believe that the time series of annual poverty rates and other statistics is paramount and that the design must support the production of reliable annual estimates. In this regard, the Census Bureau's proposed design provides no overlap between panels. Hence, every 4 years, it will be hard to determine if changes in the poverty rate are real or due to the introduction of a new panel in place of an old panel that may have uncorrected attrition bias or other problems.[25]

Since most attrition of sample cases from SIPP occurs by the end of the first year of a panel, there may be problems of attrition bias with the CNSTAT SIPP panel's design as well as the Census Bureau's, as the former does not

---

[25] Attrition bias can occur when attrition rates differ between groups: for example, higher rates of attrition for low-income people could produce a downward bias in the poverty rates. Adjustments to the survey weights are usually made to compensate for attrition bias, but the adjustments may not be adequate.

refresh the sample for cross-sectional estimates more frequently than every 2 years. Research on attrition and the most appropriate corrective actions is obviously needed, whichever design is used, and the Census Bureau has stated its commitment to such research for SIPP. However, it is still the case that attrition bias or other problems with a panel that may affect the poverty estimates cannot be fully assessed with a nonoverlapping design.

Indeed, a nonoverlapping design also limits the possibility of using SIPP for longitudinal analysis of important policy changes, such as changes in the welfare or health care systems. Ideally for such analysis, one wants information for a sufficient length of time before a change in order to accurately character-ize people's behavior under the old policy regime. One then wants informa-tion for as long as possible after the policy change to assess the effects on behavior. However, if policy changes take effect near the beginning or end of a 4-year panel under the Census Bureau's design, information either before or after the change will be limited, reducing the ability to adequately evaluate the effects. In contrast, under the design of the CNSTAT Panel to Evaluate SIPP, there will likely always be a panel in the field that is suitable for analysis of before-and-after effects, albeit with a smaller sample size.

In addition to considering the best survey design for purposes of poverty measurement, the SIPP questionnaire should be reviewed to determine what changes may be required. Thus, some questions may need to be added at least occasionally (e.g., work expenses) or asked more frequently (e.g., child care expenses or child support payments), while others may need to be modified. In some cases, such as the estimation of tax liabilities, it may make sense to collect a limited set of variables that will enhance the Census Bureau's simula-tion model rather than to try to collect detailed information directly.[26]

Finally, from the perspective of improved poverty measurement, we urge that high priority be given to several areas of methodological research for SIPP. First, questionnaire research should be pursued to develop ways to improve the quality of reporting of wage and salary income in SIPP, which falls short of independent estimates (very likely because many people report net rather than gross pay). Second, research should be conducted to improve the weighting process so that the weights adequately account for the higher rates of attrition evidenced by low-income population groups (see Appendix B on both these points).

Third, and very important, research should be conducted to improve population coverage in SIPP. A problem that affects all household surveys, including SIPP and the March CPS, is that not all people who are associated with sample households are in fact listed as household residents. Particularly subject to undercoverage are low-income minority groups. For example, it is

---

[26] See Citro and Kalton (1993:Chap. 3) for suggestions of content changes to SIPP that generally comport with the proposed resource definition for the poverty measure.

estimated that as many as 20 percent of black men are missed in the March CPS and SIPP, relative to the population counted in the decennial census. Undercoverage rates are even higher for young black men (Citro and Kalton, 1993:Table 3-12; see also Appendix B). The Census Bureau has initiated a program of coverage research to better understand coverage problems and develop effective countermeasures (Shapiro and Bettin, 1992), and we urge that this work go forward. We note, however, that household surveys, by their nature, overlook some population groups, including the homeless and people in institutions. The decennial population census (see below) includes these groups, although coverage is far from complete.

Transition

We are reasonably confident that use of SIPP data will show the same effects of the proposed poverty measure as shown in the March CPS, with the exception of lower overall rates. However, its use as the official source of poverty statistics represents another change in addition to the significant changes that we propose in the measure itself. To aid in making the transition and to help evaluate the SIPP-based estimates, it would be helpful for the Census Bureau to produce, for some period, concurrent time series of poverty rates from the March CPS and SIPP by using the proposed revised thresholds (updated each year with new CEX data) and the proposed disposable income resource definition. Admittedly, the construction of disposable income with the March CPS is complicated by the necessity for extensive imputations: in addition to imputation procedures for taxes and nonmedical in-kind benefits that already exist, the Census Bureau would need to develop imputation procedures for out-of-pocket medical expenditures, child care expenses, and child support payments.[27] However, we believe that such procedures can be developed, using data from such sources as SIPP and NMES, and that it would be very useful for researchers and policy analysts to have concurrent series. Any imputations that are performed, whether on the March CPS or SIPP, should be evaluated as to their quality and the sensitivity of the resulting poverty rates to the form of the imputation.

The concurrent series should be developed going forward from 1996 when the new SIPP design is implemented, and also going backward to 1984 when SIPP was first introduced. In the case of the latter estimates, some imputations will be required for SIPP as well as for the March CPS; also, small sample size for many SIPP panels will be a problem. Nevertheless, the

---

[27] For child support payments, adequate imputations will require the addition of a question to the March CPS that asks whether families provide support to children outside their household (ideally, the question would ask the amount as well, obviating the need for an imputation procedure).

"backcasting" exercise should provide results that are helpful to analysts in historically assessing poverty trends under the proposed measure.

Finally, for the foreseeable future, the Census Bureau should routinely issue public-use files from both the March CPS and SIPP that include the Bureau's best estimate of disposable income and its components (taxes, in-kind benefits, child care expenses, etc.). Although many researchers will make the transition to using SIPP for analysis purposes, it is likely that others will continue to use the March CPS for some kinds of poverty analysis, particularly analyses related to labor force behavior (which is the focus of the regular CPS). Hence, it is important that researchers have ready access in the March CPS data files to income variables constructed under the new resource definition as well as variables for the new thresholds: to use the new thresholds with income variables that represent the old resource definition would result in inappropriate estimates of poverty.

Research Recommendations

Income Data in Other Surveys

Many federally sponsored surveys in addition to the March CPS and SIPP (e.g., the American Housing Survey, Consumer Expenditure Survey, National Health Interview Survey, National Medical Expenditure Survey) collect income data. Because the focus of these surveys is on some other topic, they cannot typically afford the questionnaire space to collect detailed income information, although they need to obtain some income measures as background variables for analysis purposes. Often, income-to-poverty ratios are desired because such measures adjust for differences in family size and composition. Our recommendation to measure poverty on the basis of families' disposable money and near-money income may present a problem for surveys with limited room for questions not directly germane to their primary focus.

We encourage work by agencies to determine the best set of questions to include in surveys that require income and poverty measures as background variables. Given limited questionnaire space, we believe that it is more important to include questions that will permit estimating disposable income (e.g., questions on net pay, child care costs, and food stamp benefits) than it is to include questions to distinguish among a large number of components of gross money income (e.g., types of cash transfers or property income).[28]

We also encourage research by agencies on adjustments that may be needed for the greater extent of income underreporting that is likely to occur

---

[28] In 1990, the Interagency Forum on Aging-Related Statistics issued a set of guidelines for income questions to include in surveys of the elderly. That effort might serve as a model for work to develop guidelines for survey questions to support measurement of disposable income.

because a survey cannot ask about as many income components as are included in SIPP or the March CPS. Research with the March CPS, SIPP (and its predecessor, the Income Survey Development Program) has demonstrated that probing for more different sources of income elicits higher levels of reporting compared with asking broad categories (see Appendix B).

Finally, and most important, we urge research by agencies on methods to develop poverty estimates for surveys with limited income information that are comparable to the estimates that would result from having complete information with which to calculate disposable money and near-money income. Comparisons of poverty rates from SIPP based on a full implementation of the disposable income concept with rates based on a partial implementation (e.g., based on money income only, or money income, taxes, and nonmedical in-kind benefits only) could form the basis for developing appropriate adjustment factors for other surveys. Alternatively, agencies might come up with some rough-and-ready imputation procedures to use for estimating disposable income from limited survey information (e.g., a table for imputing out-of-pocket medical care expenditures based on type of health insurance and the number and age of family members).

> **RECOMMENDATION 5.4. Appropriate agencies should conduct research on methods to develop poverty estimates from household surveys with limited income information that are comparable to the estimates that would be obtained from a fully implemented disposable income definition of family resources.**

Income Data in the Decennial Census

Another source of income information is the decennial census, which provides data every 10 years for small geographic areas for which reliable estimates cannot be obtained in household surveys. The census also includes population groups, such as the institutionalized and the homeless, that are typically excluded from household surveys (although census estimates of the homeless are of doubtful quality). Income and poverty data from the census are used in many kinds of analyses; they also serve such important governmental purposes as allocation of federal funds to states and localities. For example, census estimates of the number of school-age children in poverty are used to allocate federal funds to school districts for programs to aid disadvantaged children.

Questionnaire space in the decennial census is even more limited than in most surveys. Over the decades, the number of income questions has been expanded, but, in the 1990 census, only 8 types of income were ascertained, compared with more than 30 in the March CPS and more than 60 in SIPP. No information was obtained about taxes, in-kind benefits, medical costs, work expenses, child support payments, or assets. Consequently, it is not possible to construct poverty estimates from census data with the proposed disposable income definition of families' resources.

Yet, as we have demonstrated, poverty statistics that are based on gross money income cannot distinguish between groups that differ in important ways (e.g., working versus nonworking families) or capture the effects of important government policy changes. Hence, we believe it is critical for agencies to conduct research on methods to adjust census small-area poverty estimates to more closely approximate the estimates that would obtain with a disposable income resource definition. Again, the basis for such adjustments could be analysis of poverty rates with SIPP: for example, comparing rates estimated with a disposable money and near-money income definition to rates estimated with a gross money income definition for various groups. If key population groups (e.g., the elderly, minorities) were distributed about equally across the country instead of residing disproportionately in some areas, then it might not be necessary to conduct research on methods for adjusting census small-area poverty estimates to approximate a disposable income definition of resources. The reason is that most uses of census poverty statistics are relative in nature: for example, allocating shares of a fixed total amount of federal funding to areas according to their poverty rate relative to the nation as a whole.

Also, while recognizing the constraints on the census questionnaire, we urge serious consideration of adding perhaps one or two simple yes–no questions that would facilitate adjusting the census poverty estimates. For example, questions on whether a family received food stamps or paid for child care in the past year or had health insurance coverage would be very helpful in developing appropriate adjustment factors.[29]

RECOMMENDATION 5.5. **Appropriate agencies should conduct research on methods to construct small-area poverty estimates from the limited information in the decennial census that are comparable with the estimates that would be obtained under a fully implemented disposable income concept. In addition, serious consideration should be given to adding one or two questions to the decennial census to assist in the development of comparable estimates.**

Expenditure Data

Unlike many other developed countries, the United States does not have adequate data with which to develop a poverty measure that uses a consump-

---

[29] At present, planning for the year 2000 census is exploring ways to reduce the content of the census questionnaire and to determine alternative sources of data, such as a continuing large-scale sample survey with most of the census content (see Edmonston and Schultze, 1995). Whether income questions are included in the census or in a census-like questionnaire that is fielded at more frequent intervals, the issue of obtaining information for developing appropriate poverty estimates remains.

tion- or expenditure-based definition of resources; hence, there is virtually no practical alternative to using an income-based definition. Of course, there are many arguments in favor of an income definition, but there are also strong arguments in favor of a consumption or expenditure definition. We believe it is important to consider improvements to the Consumer Expenditure Survey that would permit its use in estimating resources for poverty measurement purposes.[30]

We propose use of the current CEX for deriving and updating the poverty thresholds, for which the data requirements are not as demanding as they are for estimating resources (e.g., sample sizes can be smaller). However, even for this purpose, we believe it is important to consider improvements to the survey. In general, improvements to the CEX would be very useful to support research and policy analysis on consumption and savings behavior and the relationship of consumption, income, and wealth.

The most costly improvement to explore would be an expansion of the sample size. A major expansion, from 5,000 households or consumer units (the number provided for analysis purposes by the Interview Survey component of the CEX) to 50,000-60,000 households (i.e., the sample size of SIPP or the March CPS) would be required for the CEX to serve as the vehicle for estimating resources. A more modest expansion—perhaps doubling the current sample size—would improve the quality of the data for updating the poverty thresholds under the proposed procedure. More generally, such an expansion would make the data more useful for analyzing trends in expenditures and consumption patterns across population groups.

Another area to explore is the development of methods to reduce recall and other reporting errors and to improve the survey's response rate. We surmise that the length and complexity of the questionnaire may be major factors in impairing response. The CEX questionnaire is far more complex than the SIPP questionnaire. The latter has often been criticized for length and complexity, but the burden it poses is less than it would appear for the many people who have relatively few sources of income. In contrast, most people spend money on a wide variety of goods and services and hence must answer most of the detailed questions in the CEX. We understand that the current level of detail may be needed for purposes of respecifying the market basket for the CPI (which is done about once every 10 years); however, a more streamlined questionnaire might be more effective for the purposes of poverty measurement and other analytical uses of expenditure data. One possibility could be to embed a more detailed survey for a subsample of respondents within a larger, more streamlined survey.

Yet another area to explore concerns the overall CEX design, which currently consists of two separate surveys (the Diary Survey and the House-

---

[30] See Appendix B for details about the CEX.

hold Interview Survey) that comprise separate samples and cannot be linked at the individual respondent level. It would be very useful to consider designs that provide more complete reporting of expenditures for individual families in the sample. Also, it would be useful to explore designs that follow family members over time, so that complete expenditure patterns are obtained on an annual basis. Currently, families that move are not followed; instead, interviews are conducted with the new residents.

The kinds of changes to the CEX that could improve its usefulness for poverty measurement and other analysis purposes would not be easy to implement and would likely be expensive (particularly in the case of an increased sample size); however, the potential benefits could be great. A useful first step would be for BLS to conduct or commission a study that evaluates the CEX and assesses the costs and benefits of changes to the survey that could make it more useful for poverty measurement and other purposes. We urge prompt undertaking of such a study. Furthermore, we hope that improvements to the survey that stem from the review can be implemented in time to provide useful input to the next 10-year review of the poverty measure.

> RECOMMENDATION 5.6. **The Bureau of Labor Statistics should undertake a comprehensive review of the Consumer Expenditure Survey to assess the costs and benefits of changes to the survey design, questionnaire, sample size, and other features that could improve the quality and usefulness of the data. The review should consider ways to improve the CEX for the purpose of developing poverty thresholds, for making it possible at a future date to measure poverty on the basis of a consumption or expenditure concept of family resources, and for other analytic purposes related to the measurement of consumption, income, and savings.**

Other Issues in Measuring Poverty

6

The formulation of a poverty measure requires decisions about several issues in addition to the concept and method by which to set and update the thresholds and the appropriate definition of family resources. In this chapter we address three such issues: the time period over which poverty is measured; the unit of analysis on which the measurement occurs (e.g., family or household) and the related issue of the unit of presentation of analysis; and the types of summary measures that are reported to indicate the extent of poverty across time and among population groups. We conclude with a discussion of some of the limitations of any economic measure of poverty.

TIME PERIOD

The current U.S. poverty rate is an annual rate.[1] It uses an annual accounting period in which an annual need standard is compared with an annual measure of resources. Operationally, families are interviewed each March in the Current Population Survey (CPS) and asked about their income for the preceding calendar year. The resulting calculation of the poverty rate is reported to the nation in a *Current Population Report*, P-60 series, each fall for the preceding year.

Recommendation

There are several arguments for retaining the annual accounting period, and overall, we find them persuasive. First, not doing so would interrupt the time series of annual poverty rates extending back to the 1960s. Second, an annual

---

[1] Poverty measures in other countries (which typically do not have official status) are also in most instances annual; the measures in the United Kingdom are exceptional in their use of a subannual (weekly/monthly) need standard and resource definition.

period for measuring income seems natural. People file tax returns that pertain to their income and deductions for a calendar year. Assistance programs that are geared to the tax system (notably, the Earned Income Tax Credit) also use an annual accounting period. Third, there is widespread acceptance of the view that families can smooth consumption and accommodate fluctuations in income over the period of a year. One would not necessarily want to have a poverty measure that counts as poor such people as teachers, who use winter savings to tide them over the summer, or construction workers, who use summer savings to tide them over the winter.

Of course, no one accounting period or measure is right for all purposes, and the use of the poverty measure should affect the choice. One important use is as a general social indicator for evaluating the socioeconomic health of the nation and for measuring progress toward reducing economic insufficiency for the whole population and for particular groups. For this purpose, the length of the measurement period may matter less than whether different time periods result in different trends over time or different poverty rates for key groups, such as the elderly and children. An annual measure is arguably as appropriate as any other for this important purpose.

Another important use of the poverty measure is as a benchmark against which to evaluate the effectiveness of government assistance programs—in terms of whether benefits are provided primarily to people who are poor (on a pretransfer basis) and whether the benefits move recipients out of poverty. For such programs as Supplemental Security Income (SSI), which assists low-income elderly and disabled people who commonly remain in the program for long periods, determining the proportion of program participants who are poor or not poor on an annual basis is quite appropriate.

In contrast, for such programs as food stamps and Aid to Families with Dependent Children (AFDC), which use a short accounting period and may provide benefits to people for periods as short as a few months, an annual calculation is not always appropriate. As an example, consider the case of someone who loses a job and has few other resources, applies for and receives food stamps for, say, a period of 3 months, and then obtains a job that pays good wages for the remainder of the year. Such a person would be classified as a food stamp recipient during the year but with an annual income that might be well above the annual poverty level. Hence, it would look as if the program had provided benefits inappropriately, when, in fact, it had served its goal of helping someone with a short-term need. For analyses of these kinds of programs, one would like to have a shorter term poverty measure, either in place of or as a supplement to an annual measure. Other programs, which are designed to address such root causes of poverty as low levels of education and lack of training, may need to be assessed on a longer term basis than a year. For these programs, one might want a poverty concept applicable to a segment of the life cycle.

Although the evaluation of assistance programs is important, we view this use of the official poverty measure as secondary to its use as a key social indicator. Although there are arguments for shorter and longer accounting periods for indicator purposes, we believe that it makes most sense to continue to calculate the official poverty statistics on an annual basis. To supplement the annual statistics, we support initiatives to develop and publish shorter term measures of poverty that can facilitate evaluation of such programs as AFDC and food stamps. Because of the eligibility rules of these programs—specifically, their requirement that families use up most assets before applying for benefits—it will probably be necessary to include asset values in the family resource definition for poverty measures that use an accounting period of less than a year. Such shorter term measures may also serve as more timely indicators of trends in poverty (although other readily available measures, such as monthly unemployment rates and program caseloads, may serve the same purpose).

We also support work on developing longer term measures of poverty. This is an area that calls for more research and evaluation, given the lack of consensus about desirable measures. We note that by using the Survey of Income and Program Participation (SIPP) as the basis for poverty measurement in place of the March CPS, it becomes possible to develop both annual and subannual poverty measures on a consistent basis, as well as measures that use an accounting period of somewhat longer than a year. For measures with still longer time horizons, it is necessary to turn to a data source like the Panel Study of Income Dynamics (PSID).[2]

RECOMMENDATION 6.1. **The official poverty measure should continue to be derived on an annual basis. Appropriate agencies should develop poverty measures for periods that are shorter and longer than a year with data from SIPP and the Panel Study of Income Dynamics for such purposes as program evaluation. Such measures may require the inclusion of asset values in the family resource definition.**

Short-Term Measures

Short-term poverty, as Ruggles (1990) argues, is a meaningful concept. While it is probably impossible to be poor for only one day, no matter how limited one's resources, and quite possible to get by for a week in the face of limited resources, it is more difficult to delay expenses such as rent over periods as short as 1 or 2 months. Indeed, programs designed to provide short-term economic assistance, such as AFDC and food stamps, typically use a 1-month

---

[2] The PSID, which began in 1968, is a long-running panel survey in which about 9,000 families are interviewed on an annual basis; see Appendix B.

accounting period. The objection to short-term measures is that they may overstate poverty by counting as poor people who can defer expenditures or draw on resources acquired in an earlier period to tide them over a temporary shortfall.

Although the differences are not great, the evidence from analyses of recently available SIPP data shows that the shorter the accounting period, the higher the poverty rate. Thus, rates estimated on a 4-month accounting period are typically between 1 and 2 percentage points higher than rates estimated on an annual accounting period (see, e.g., David and Fitzgerald, 1987; Engel, 1989; Lerman and Yitzhaki, 1989). In analysis of poverty spells that began during the first 15 months of the 1984 SIPP panel, Ruggles (1988a) similarly concluded that annual measures of poverty miss a considerable number of short spells of poverty.[3]

Unfortunately, no evidence is available about the extent to which short-term poverty measures might produce not only different levels but also different trends over time in comparison with an annual measure. There is limited evidence on the differences that might result in poverty rates for several population groups. Williams (1986) reported virtually no difference by family type between annual and average monthly poverty measures calculated from the 1984 SIPP panel. Ruggles' analysis (1988a), however, suggests that under a shorter rather than under a longer accounting period, a smaller proportion of the poor would be people in single-parent female-headed families.

In an analysis of program participation in the 1984 SIPP panel, Williams (1986) found evidence for the idea that a short-term poverty measure would be more suitable than an annual measure for evaluating assistance programs that use a short accounting period. Thus, 90 percent of recipients of AFDC and food stamps were in poverty at least 1 month, even though only 64-70 percent of recipients were in poverty on an annual basis.

If one wanted to develop a short-term poverty measure to supplement the annual measure to use for such purposes as program evaluation, a major issue would be to determine how short a period would be appropriate. The main argument against a monthly accounting period is that it overstates true hard-

---

[3] Annual data from the PSID produce longer estimated spell durations than do monthly data from SIPP. For example, using the PSID, Duncan, Smeeding, and Rodgers (1992) find that 37 percent of poverty spells in the United States are still in progress after 3 years; in contrast, using SIPP, Ruggles (1988a) finds that only 12 to 24 percent (depending on the definition used) are still in progress after just 1 year. Presumably, SIPP is picking up short intrayear poverty spells that are missed in the PSID. Consider the case of someone who is poor for 2 consecutive years on the basis of comparing annual income to an annual poverty threshold, but who, using monthly income and monthly thresholds, is poor for the first 8 months, not poor for the next 4 months, and poor again for the last 12 months. With this pattern of income receipt, Duncan, Smeeding, and Rodgers, using PSID, will identify one spell of poverty lasting 2 years, and Ruggles, using SIPP, will observe two shorter spells.

ship, given that people can shift expenditures through time to at least a limited extent. However, it is not clear how to evaluate the merits of, say, a 2-month, 4-month, or 6-month period.

A related issue concerns the treatment of resources. Assistance programs that use a monthly accounting period also typically include an asset test (with a ceiling on countable assets generally in the range of $1,000-$3,000). Researchers have argued that accounting for asset values in some way would enable the development of a more realistic short-term poverty measure. However, accurate estimation of assets poses greater difficulties than accurate estimation of income, and there are also issues of how to value assets for purposes of poverty measurement (see Chapter 4).

Several researchers have constructed and assessed the effects of measures of poverty that take account of assets. For example, David and Fitzgerald (1987) analyzed the 1984 SIPP, adding the capitalized value of reported interest income from the prior wave (assuming a fixed 6% rate of interest) to the family's current income to estimate a "crisis" measure. They found that this measure of poverty was always lower than the official measure derived on the basis of money income alone, and the difference was somewhat greater the shorter the accounting period:[4]

	Crisis Measure (%)	Official Measure (%)
On a monthly basis	11.0	14.0
On a 4-month basis	11.3	13.2
On an annual basis	10.4	11.3

David and Fitzgerald (1987) found that, on average, 21 percent of people who were counted as income-poor on a monthly basis did not experience a crisis when their interest-generating assets were taken into account; the corresponding figure for people who were income-poor on a 4-month basis was 14 percent. In general, the gross money income resource definition overstated short-term transitions: of those entering or exiting poverty from 1 month to 4 months later, 40 percent never experienced a crisis. Also, David and Fitzgerald (1987) found that such assistance programs as AFDC and SSI are targeted to those in crisis and not to income-poor people with financial assets.

SIPP makes possible the regular derivation and publication of short-term poverty measures, including measures that take account of families' asset hold-

---

[4] Monthly poverty rates are averages over 12 months; 4-month rates are averages over three 4-month periods. David and Fitzgerald (1987) subtracted reported interest income from families' resources to avoid double counting. Note that the "official" annual rate of 11.3 percent they obtained from the 1984 SIPP is several percentage points lower than the official rate from the March CPS. David and Fitzgerald obtained similar results for a measure that also added the capitalized value of stocks and rental property to families' resources. The reason is that 94 percent of those in crisis poverty on the basis of their income and interest-generating assets did not have stocks or rental property.

ings (see Chapter 5 and Appendix B). David and Fitzgerald (1987) suggest that a 4-month accounting period could be optimal, given the SIPP design of interviews at 4-month intervals.

Some publication issues arise with the use of a subannual accounting period for the poverty measure. For example, if the accounting period is 4 months, 4-month poverty rates could be reported every 4 months (with a likely lag of 5-6 months to allow for data processing and analysis). Such rates might serve as more timely indicators of economic distress in the population, although other readily available measures might serve the purpose just as well (e.g., monthly unemployment rates or counts of program participants, both of which are available on a timely basis). To determine how closely short-term poverty rates track the business cycle, it could be useful to develop 4-month (or even monthly) measures from SIPP for 1984-1994. One could then determine the correlations with economic trends and also how closely the rates track other indicators, such as monthly unemployment rates. If the correlations with other indicators are high, then there would be less need to publish short-term poverty rates on a frequent basis.

An alternative to publication every 4 months (or every month in the case of a monthly measure) would be, each year, to publish 4-month rates, averaged over the three such periods in the year (again with a likely lag, as in the March CPS, of 5-6 months). Such an approach would smooth any seasonal variation in the estimates. In addition to average 4-month rates, an option would be to report the proportion of people each year who had at least one 4-month period of poverty (i.e., to report an ever-poor rate).

Long-Term Measures

Duncan (1992) and Duncan, Smeeding, and Rodgers (1992) argue strongly for the calculation of a long-term measure of poverty in addition to short-term and annual poverty measures. The characteristics of people who are chronically or persistently poor differ from those who are temporarily poor. Programs that are designed to tackle root causes of poverty and to invest in human capital and economic potential over the long term need to be evaluated by these longer term measures of poverty. Indeed, there is some preliminary evidence, according to Duncan (1992), that the duration of economic deprivation is an important predictor of such developmental outcome variables as completion of high school or teenage pregnancy.[5] However, there are many

---

[5] Duncan (1992) notes that few developmental studies have been done that use an adequate measure of family income; however, the existing studies find that economic resources affect outcomes independent of other measures of socioeconomic status (e.g., occupation or education of parents) and that longer periods of deprivation have greater adverse effects.

conceptual, methodological, and data-related difficulties in constructing useful and feasible long-term poverty measures.

Based largely on analysis of the PSID, researchers have built up a picture of persistent versus temporary poverty. Lillard and Willis (1978:1004), for example, reported that the probability of a man in poverty in 1967 being in poverty again the following year, on the basis of his earnings, was 34 percent for whites and 61 percent for blacks.

Rodgers and Rodgers (1993) review the subsequent literature. They focus on what they call chronic poverty, in which, in either recurrent spells or long continuous spells, "income is less than needs during a long and continuous period of time" (Rodgers and Rodgers, 1993:29). They develop the notion of chronic poverty on the basis of a measure of permanent income compared with permanent needs. Using the PSID data for the period since the late 1970s, they conclude that about one-third of measured poverty in the United States as of 1987 can be regarded as chronic, and that over the period they studied, "poverty not only increased, it became more chronic and less transitory in nature" (Rodgers and Rodgers, 1993:51). They also conclude that "the poorest group identified consists of people living in families headed by African-American females without high-school diplomas, for whom chronic poverty is about twelve times as intense as in the entire population" (Rodgers and Rodgers, 1993:52).

Ruggles (1990) also reviews a large number of studies of longer term poverty and reports that estimates of the persistently poor vary from 6 to 80 percent of estimates of the single-year poor. The differences are due to differences in the population studied, the definition of poverty used, and the number of years in which one must be poor in order to be classified as persistently poor. Ruggles concludes that a best-guess estimate is that 40-50 percent of those poor in a single year will remain poor for some years to come.

As another example of this literature, Adams and Duncan (1988), in a study of urban poverty, estimated that 13.4 percent of urban people were poor in 1979, 34.6 percent were poor in at least 1 year between 1974 and 1983, and 5.2 percent were "persistently poor"—defined as poor in 8 of 10 years or 80 percent of the years covered.[6] Hence, the persistently poor were about 40 percent of the single-year poor (consistent with Ruggles's estimate) and 15 percent of the ever poor. The single-year poor were more likely than nonpoor people to be black, poorly educated, and living in female single-parent families; the persistently poor were even more likely to have these characteristics.[7]

---

[6] To permit comparison of PSID data with the decennial census, Adams and Duncan (1988) defined "urban" areas to be central counties of metropolitan areas that contained a population of one million or more people. There were 56 such counties (of 3,137 U.S. counties) in 1980.

[7] For another example of long-term poverty analysis and a comparison between metropolitan and nonmetropolitan residents, see Hoppe (1988).

In a paper prepared for the panel, Duncan (1992) notes that there is no agreement in the literature on the optimal form of a measure of long-term poverty. He and Rodgers and Rodgers (1993) distinguish several measures. One measure considers the length or duration of spells of poverty. There are technical issues involved in adjusting for spells that are still in progress at the time of the survey (the censoring problem). Spell analysis is also sensitive to the treatment of missing data. In general, these spell-based measures do not address the phenomenon of multiple spells and hence, as Ashworth, Hill, and Walker (1992) note, are not able to address distributional questions because the unit of analysis is the spell rather than the person or family unit.[8]

A second measure considers the proportion of workers or families whose incomes fall below the poverty threshold in x out of y time periods. These measures are easy to implement but attach no extra weight to consecutive periods of deprivation. A related measure takes the sum of the income over an extended period and compares it to the sum of income needs over that same period, thus focusing on the average of income compared with need. This type of measure puts weight on the extent or intensity of any income inadequacy instead of simply treating poverty as an in-or-out dichotomy in which having a few dollars above poverty in one period may be offset by having many dollars below poverty in another period. However, it also implicitly assumes that a family unit can shift income around as needed within the whole time interval selected.

A third measure considers an income-generating model with an error-component structure. Such a model allows the estimation of the pattern of income over some period of time, based on a multivariate model that controls for observed characteristics that systematically affect income and that characterizes the autoregressive and random components of the error term in that statistical model. These modeling efforts are most useful in studies of the composition of poverty and in policy discussions of the effects of one or another intervention that might affect the unit's characteristics or the effect of those characteristics on the generation of income.

To obtain any type of long-term measure of poverty requires using a data source other than the March CPS. Under the planned redesign of SIPP, it will be possible to obtain measures with a maximum accounting period of 4 years. (The 1993 SIPP panel will also be extended for a total of 10 years, with annual interviews after the first 3 years of 4-month interviews.) The PSID makes it possible to develop measures for accounting periods of virtually any length;

---

[8] In the first 16 months of the 1984 SIPP panel, Ruggles (1988b) found that 32 percent of all people experiencing at least one spell of poverty experienced multiple spells. Ashworth, Hill, and Walker (1992), with data from the PSID, look at poverty over the entire span of childhood, distinguishing such patterns as poor every year, poor only 1 year, poor occasionally, or having recurrent spells of poverty.

however, the small sample size and attrition problems greatly limit disaggregated analysis (see Appendix B).

Longer term poverty measures are almost always proposed as a supplement to annual or shorter term measures. It would seem desirable, for consistency, to have some measures that are derived within a common framework. For example, with SIPP (as redesigned), it would be possible to produce 4-month measures, annual measures, and measures of the proportion of single-year poor who are still poor 1, 2, or 3 years later. Another consistency issue concerns the treatment of assets. If assets are accounted for in short-term measures, the question is whether and how they should be accounted for in long-term measures.

A publication issue with regard to longer term measures concerns the frequency of reporting. It seems unlikely that such measures would show large year-to-year changes; hence, it might be preferable to publish them at intervals of, say, 2 years or longer.

In summary, considerable progress has been made in understanding longer term poverty, but there is not yet a consensus regarding the best measure. We encourage continued research that can further illuminate the nature and composition of long-term poverty and that evaluates the merits and uses of alternative measures.

UNIT OF ANALYSIS AND PRESENTATION

"Unit of analysis" is often used to refer to the unit for which statistics are tabulated and presented. However, in measuring poverty, one must first define the groups of people whose economic resources are to be pooled in determining poverty status. The subsequent decision is whether to present statistics in terms of those same units or to present them for other kinds of units; we use "unit of presentation" to designate this latter decision. One might, for example, have the family as the unit of analysis on which the poverty determination is based and then for the unit of presentation report the number of individuals in poverty.

Unit of Analysis

Throughout this volume we have discussed poverty as a characteristic of a family. We have defined a threshold level of income below which a family is defined to be impoverished, and we have discussed a concept of family income that can be compared with that threshold in making the determination of whether that family is or is not "in poverty." The current official U.S. poverty measure (see Bureau of the Census, 1993c:App. A) takes a family that resides in the same household as the unit of analysis; it includes unrelated individuals (whether living alone or with others), who are defined as single-person families for this purpose.[9]

Recommendations

There are reasons to consider other units of analysis, such as the individual or the household (see discussion below), but we find no compelling evidence at this time to move away from the family concept. Hence, we recommend continuing that practice with one important modification: families should be defined to include cohabiting couples.[10] Such couples typically pool resources, and many of them exhibit considerable stability, so that it seems to make sense to treat them like married-couple families for purposes of poverty measurement.

The topic of resource sharing (or lack of sharing) among family and household members is one that merits further study. We support research on how resources are allocated among the adults and children in a family. We also support research on the extent to which unrelated roommates in a household share resources. The results of such research may suggest a further modification to the unit of analysis for poverty measurement at a future date.

> **RECOMMENDATION 6.2. The official measure of poverty should continue to use families and unrelated individuals as the units of analysis for which thresholds are defined and resources aggregated. The definition of "family" should be broadened for purposes of poverty measurement to include cohabiting couples.**

> **RECOMMENDATION 6.3. Appropriate agencies should conduct research on the extent of resource sharing among roommates and other household and family members to determine if the definition of the unit of analysis for the poverty measure should be modified in the future.**

Discussion

The family is but one of three possible units of analysis that might serve as the basic unit in measuring poverty in the nation. The other two are the household and the individual. We consider important distinctions among these

---

[9] No determination of poverty status is made, however, for unrelated people who are under age 15 because no information on their income is available.

[10] In the CPS, cohabiting couples are defined as two unmarried people of the opposite sex living in the same household who are listed as roommates/unmarried partners. Their households may contain children under age 15 but not other adults. The decennial census question on household relationship separates the response categories of "housemate or roommate" and "unmarried partner." The latter category is taken to represent cohabiting couples.

three and the advantages and disadvantages of each for purposes of measuring poverty.[11]

The Census Bureau defines families and households as follows (Rawlings, 1993:B-2):

> • family: a group of two persons or more related by birth, marriage, or adoption and residing together; all such persons (including related subfamily members) are considered as members of one family.
> • household: all the persons who occupy a housing unit . . . . A household includes the related family members and all the unrelated persons, if any, such as lodgers, foster children, wards or employees who share the housing unit. A person living alone in a housing unit, or a group of unrelated persons sharing a housing unit as partners, is also counted as a household.

For purposes of poverty measurement, as noted earlier, the definition of "family" includes every unrelated person, whether living alone, with roommates or partners, or with but not related to a family. Hence, the use of a household definition would result in a smaller number of larger units: for example, two or more roommates living together would be counted as one household rather than as two or more single-person families. In contrast, the use of an individual or person definition would result in a number of single-person units equal to the total population of the United States living in households (including both family members and unrelated people).[12]

To measure poverty, one establishes a threshold level of income for a unit and then compares the actual income level to that threshold, so logically this could be done for the family, the household, or the individual. The question is which unit, in principle, should be used as the basis for the measurement? The answer is not self-evident, because the three units differ in the extent to which the members jointly pool their income or share their consumption. If all the members of a family or of a household necessarily experienced the same level of income and monetary well-being, then that would be the unit of analysis one should use in measuring poverty. If there were such a unit and if the poverty threshold were set correctly for that unit and the unit's income level was estimated correctly, then the members of that unit would either *all* be in poverty or *all* be out of poverty.

But that condition is surely not met for every family or for every house-

---

[11] There are also variations in the definitions of family and household, which we do not explore. For example, the United Kingdom in the early 1980s switched the unit of analysis for low-income statistics from the family to the household; however, its definition of "family" was the nuclear family, consisting solely of the parent(s) and children under age 18. In contrast, the Census Bureau's definition of family includes all related persons in a household, regardless of age or specific relationship.

[12] There are, of course, other persons in the nation who do not live in households, residing instead in such institutions as jails, hospitals, and group homes or living as homeless persons.

hold. Some family members may be deprived of a full share of the family's
income, and others may consume far more than the average. Similarly,
household members may be in quite different economic circumstances even
though they share the same living quarters and jointly use a bundle of consumer durables. So neither of these units is the perfect solution for measuring
poverty.

Using the individual person as the unit of analysis has considerable appeal,
at least analytically. But what of a dependent family member who has no
independent income and is supported by the income provided by another
family member? It is not evident how to estimate that dependent person's
income level, which makes it difficult to use the individual as the basis of
measurement of poverty.

And what of the expenditure on jointly consumed items such as the
location of the house in a safe neighborhood or the heat and light in the
house? It is also not easily determined how to allocate those expenditures
among the individuals who share in their consumption. These jointly consumed items represent a component of the consumption bundle in which the
several family or household members do in fact have a common level of
resources, if not a common level of utility or satisfaction from them. So even
if there were very complete information available about the income received
by each person in every household or every family, because of the joint use or
consumption of many items, it would not be a simple or straightforward task
to determine who received benefit from that income and therefore who was
and who was not "in poverty."

Since the joint consumption of many durables and some services contrib-
utes to the economies of scale that promote living together in one household
and sharing income, there is a sound rationale for using the larger multiperson
unit, the family or household, instead of the individual, as the basic unit for
defining poverty. But not all the expenditures in a family or household unit
are shared equally among its members. Thus a measurement that assumes that
all members of the unit are either in poverty or out of poverty cannot be
correct in every instance.

We know of no perfect solution to this dilemma. In reality, there is some,
but incomplete, pooling of household or family income and joint consumption, and so a choice must be made in the unit of analysis for measuring
poverty. That choice has long been noted and is often discussed in reports and
essays on the definition of poverty. The extensive and thoughtful review
conducted by the 1976 Poverty Studies Task Force, for example, discussed
this issue (U.S. Department of Health, Education and Welfare, 1976:
Vol.1:34,100). Ruggles (1990:121-124) stressed that the choice should depend on "what one believes about how income is shared among family and
household members." In a more analytic discussion, Atkinson (1989:17-24)
noted the "fragmentary statistics to bear out the anecdotal evidence that there

is significant inequality" among family members and reviewed underlying assumptions that can justify one or another unit as the basis for the unit of analysis in the definition of poverty.

Lazear and Michael (1988) provide an extensive literature review of this issue and offer extensive empirical evidence of differences in the expenditures on behalf of adults and children in U.S. households based on data from the Consumer Expenditure Survey (CEX). These efforts and those in the United Kingdom by Young years ago (1952), by Pahl more recently (1989), an essay by Jenkins (1991), and calculations by Townsend (1979) that illustrate poverty rates among men and women based on their individual incomes, all emphasize the need for further research on intrafamily resource allocation. Although there has been progress in this area in the past decade or two, there is neither sufficient clarity nor consensus to provide a strategy for cracking apart the family unit to measure individual levels of poverty at this time. We believe that further work on this issue could provide the capacity to do so in the future.

Faced with the choice among three possibilities as the appropriate unit of analysis—the family, the household, or the individual—we recommend that the family continue to be used, with one important modification (see below). We have noted the difficulties of using the individual as the unit of analysis. In deciding between the family and the household, our choice is based partly on the precedent that the family has served as the unit of analysis for the measurement of poverty for many years. It is also based partly on our decision to propose an income-based definition of resources instead of an expenditure-based definition, as the pooling of income is, we believe, greater within a family unit than it is among the roommates and various subunits that constitute many households.[13]

Another reason for this choice is the stability of the unit. Although the composition of both households and families frequently changes, since we have used a time frame of one year for the measurement of poverty, the stability of the family unit is probably greater than the stability of multiperson household units over a 12-month period.

There has developed in the past two decades a form of living arrangement that lies analytically somewhere between a family and a household and is now common enough to require a judgment as to how to treat it. It is cohabitation, a form of living together in a marriage-like relationship with an expectation of some longevity but not recorded by a marriage license. By the definitions of the Census Bureau, couples living in cohabitational units are

---

[13] Whichever definition is used for poverty measurement—family or household—poverty statistics would also include unrelated individuals living alone in their own households. The difference is that, with a family definition, unrelated individuals living together in a household are also treated as one-person "families" rather than as a multiperson household.

households but not families. The Census Bureau reports that by 1992 there were 3.3 million "unmarried-couple households," most of whom are cohabiting couples; two-thirds do not include any children under age 15 while one-third do include children. The number of these unmarried-couple households rose from 523,000 in 1970 (estimated by the Census Bureau), a sixfold increase, and the Bureau reports that the ratio of these couples per 100 married couples rose from 1 per 100 in 1970 to 6 per 100 in 1992 (Saluter, 1992:xv and Table K).

We recommend that these couples be treated as families, not as separate one-person units, in the measurement of poverty. The rationale for this extension is that, on average, these cohabitational units last at least 1 year in duration and many, if not a majority, end in a formal marriage, so that the pooling of income and the sharing of expenditures extend well beyond 1 year on average.[14]

We also support research on resource sharing among other kinds of household members, such as roommates, who may pool income for such items as food and housing. In general, we urge continued research on the complex issues of the apportioning of resources among family members within a family and on the nature and extent of resource sharing within family and household units. For accurate measurement of poverty, more research is needed on the extent of unequal allocations within consumer units and the amounts of cross-unit transfers. Also needed are empirical research-based suggestions of algorithms for calculating individual-level consumption.

Research on resource sharing (whether intrafamilial or among unrelated individuals in households) should include an assessment of the likely magnitude of the effects on poverty rates of changing the unit of analysis (e.g., defining roommates as well as cohabiting couples as "families" or completely replacing the family definition with a household definition). In general, moving from a smaller to larger unit of analysis will probably reduce the poverty rate, for two reasons. First, the larger the unit, the lower its poverty threshold relative to its size, thus requiring less income per person for the larger unit to be below the poverty line. (The exception is for measures in which the equivalence scale has a scale economy factor of 1.0, assuming no scale economies with increasing unit size.) Second, the larger the unit of analysis, the more opportunity for "excess" income of one or more family or household members to offset lower income of other members.

These effects were illustrated dramatically when the United Kingdom shifted from the nuclear family to the household as the unit of analysis for its poverty measure: the poverty rate for the total population dropped by 25

---

[14] For analyses of cohabitation in the past decade, see Bumpass and Sweet (1989); Laumann et al. (1994:Ch. 13); Thornton (1988); and Willis and Michael (1994); for the United Kingdom, see Kiernan and Estaugh (1993).

percent. The drop was particularly large for single adult children still living at home, who had been treated as separate units under the old definition but as sharing in the resources of the household under the new definition (Johnson and Webb, 1992). The effect in the United States of moving from a family-based to a household-based measure would not likely be as large because of the more inclusive way in which the family is already defined.

Unit of Presentation

Having selected a unit of analysis, that is, the unit for the measurement of poverty status, a decision is needed on the unit of presentation. Census Bureau reports from the March CPS have typically presented poverty statistics for both families and individuals; SIPP-based reports of poverty transitions have used individuals as the sole unit of presentation.[15]

The recent Committee on National Statistics (CNSTAT) Panel to Evaluate SIPP considered this issue (Citro and Kalton, 1993:172-176). The panel noted that statistics for family (and household) units are useful for such purposes as government and business planning, which often requires information on families or households for targeting purposes. However, for policy analysis and research on such topics as income inequality and the effects of government policies on poverty, the panel concluded that the use of household or family units can be misleading because smaller families or households are counted as equal to larger units.

Ruggles (1990:123) provides a telling example of the effect of using families rather than individuals as the unit of presentation. The annual poverty rate for *families* headed by an elderly person is *higher* than that for other families, while the poverty rate for elderly *people* is *lower* than that for other people. The reason is more elderly people who are poor than those who are not poor live in small family units, while the reverse is true for the nonelderly. Hence, the elderly poor are a higher proportion of *families* in poverty than of *people* in poverty. Clearly, the family-based measure can distort the picture of the types of people who are disproportionately poor.

The CNSTAT SIPP panel observed that another argument for using people as the unit of presentation relates to statistics that are developed on the basis of longitudinal data, such as the monthly demographic and income information in SIPP. The panel recommended that annual poverty rates from

---

[15] Care must be taken in using CPS reports to be sure one understands the unit of presentation in a particular table. Thus, CPS reports include separate tables of poverty statistics for families of two-or-more people and for unrelated individuals (who are treated as one-person families for purposes of poverty measurement). CPS reports (like SIPP reports) also include tables for all people who are members of households. In each case, poverty status is determined on the basis of family characteristics.

SIPP be developed by aggregating the monthly information.[16] Poverty rates calculated in this manner will be more accurate than rates calculated from the March CPS: unlike SIPP, the CPS assumes that the people in each family in March were together for the entire preceding year for which income is measured. When this assumption does not hold (e.g., in the case of a divorced or widowed person who was married for some or all of the preceding year), an erroneous poverty classification may result (see Appendix B).

Although poverty statistics can readily be developed with the SIPP monthly data for people (using the information on their families' characteristics), to develop such statistics for households or families as such poses a conceptual problem. The difficulty is how to define these units longitudinally, given that their composition changes. For example, it may be easy to decide that a married couple that has a baby should be treated as the same family before and after the birth. A more difficult question is how to treat the couple if they later divorce. Is the parent who retains custody of the child the continuation of the original family and the other parent a new one-person household, or does the original family end at the time of the divorce and do two new units begin?

Any longitudinal household or family definition will produce units that exist for only part of the year, and a decision must then be made on whether to count part-period units the same as full-period units. In view of these and other problems, the CNSTAT SIPP panel recommended that the Census Bureau continue the practice of developing person-based longitudinal income, poverty, and program statistics for SIPP reports, with attribution of household, family, and program unit characteristics to people. In the case of annual statistics from the March CPS and SIPP that are designed for comparison purposes, that panel recommended that the tables from both sources should use attribute-based person measures.

We believe that these reasons are convincing for presenting poverty statistics for people. However, users could be misled, and we urge a clarifying note accompanying the presentation. Since by definition all those in a family are either in poverty or not in poverty, the presentation of the "number of people in poverty" might be misunderstood as an independent person-by-person calculation instead of a single calculation for the family unit. A clarifying note with the person counts should minimize that risk.

INDEXES OF POVERTY

By comparing the poverty threshold with the corresponding income estimate for each economic unit, its poverty status is determined. After determining

---

[16] The procedure is to determine each person's monthly family income and monthly poverty threshold corresponding to monthly family composition, aggregate the monthly income and threshold values over the year, and divide to obtain the person's poverty ratio.

the poverty status of all units, there is a question about how to quantify and report that status. The current official U.S. poverty index is a head-count ratio. The head-count ratio measures the proportion of the population with incomes below their poverty thresholds. That head count, expressed as a proportion of the population (e.g., 14.5% for the year 1992), or expressed as a number of people (e.g., 36.9 million people in 1992), is the accustomed way in which poverty is reported in the United States (Bureau of the Census, 1993c:viii).

There are many other ways in which the poverty status of the population might be expressed, and they are typically independent of the concept of poverty, the threshold levels, or the particular definition of income. For example, the Census Bureau currently publishes statistics on the aggregate and mean "poverty gap," or the difference between the income of the poor (or of particular groups) and their poverty thresholds. The Census Bureau also publishes statistics on the proportion of people with family incomes below specified proportions of the poverty thresholds (75%, 50%, etc.)

Recommendation

We recommend continuing the practice of using the head count and head-count ratio, which are familiar and readily understandable, as the basic statistics on poverty. We also recommend supplementing the head-count ratio by other indexes, which provide additional important information—specifically, statistics on the average income of the poor and the distribution of income of the poor. Finally, we recommend publication of the head-count ratio and supplemental statistics for measures in which family resources are defined net of government taxes and transfers. All of these additional statistics need to be carefully interpreted, but they add a needed depth of understanding about the extent of poverty in the United States.

> RECOMMENDATION 6.4. **In addition to the basic poverty counts and ratios for the total population and groups—the number and proportion of poor people—the official poverty series should provide statistics on the average income and distribution of income for the poor. The count and other statistics should also be published for poverty measures in which family resources are defined net of government taxes and transfers, such as a measure that defines income in before-tax terms, a measure that excludes means-tested government benefits from income, and a measure that excludes all government benefits from income. Such measures can help assess the effects of government taxes and transfers on poverty.**

Alternative Indexes

The head-count ratio has several advantages over other possible indexes of poverty. It enables the continuation of the 30-year time series of annual poverty rates. It is easy to calculate and to understand and is intuitively appealing. The public, as well as policy makers, readily grasp what the number and the proportion represent. Some analysts also argue that it is a relatively easy index to use in forecasting the effects of various public policy proposals, and, as such, is a convenient tool for policy analysis.

Our reason for recommending supplements to the head-count ratio is that the amount of information provided by that ratio is limited. Many important changes in the circumstances of the poor are not reflected in it. For example, a transfer made to a poor individual does not change the head-count ratio if the person remains in poverty, even though that person is made better off. Consider a $1,000 transfer to either a family just below poverty or a family far below poverty. In the first case, the transfer may raise that family out of poverty and lower the head-count ratio, thus lowering the poverty index as it is currently measured. In the second case, the same $1,000 transferred to a family far below poverty, and arguably in even greater need, would not lower the head-count ratio if it did not raise the family above the poverty threshold. The head count would still be correct in both cases, but it would not reveal any benefit from the second transfer and would not, therefore, convey a full and accurate picture.

In a seminal paper, Sen (1976) asserted that an ideal poverty index should include three elements: (1) the relative number of poor, indicating the incidence of poverty; (2) the average shortfall of the poor below the poverty threshold, indicating the average deprivation of the poor; and (3) the distribution of income among the poor, indicating relative deprivation among the poor. The head-count ratio only satisfies the first of the three criteria, indicating the incidence of poverty. This index does not reveal the average level of deprivation: it provides the same number if all of those in poverty are $1 below the poverty line or if each of them has only $1 of income. Similarly, the head-count ratio does not indicate the distribution of income among the poor. As a result of these shortcomings, the head-count ratio has potential for misuse. For example, programs to reduce poverty that are targeted on those just below the poverty line will reduce the ratio more than programs of the same budgetary cost aimed at the poorest poor people, those far below the poverty line.

Sen (1976) and Rodgers and Rodgers (1991), among others, have proposed a list of specific properties by which one might evaluate the appropriateness of any proposed poverty index. One such property is monotonicity: that is, the index should decrease for an income increase of a poor person even if that increase does not move the person across the poverty line (as well as, of course, if that increase does move the person across the poverty line). Conversely, the index of poverty should increase for an income decrease of a poor person already below the poverty line. The "poverty gap" has this property, as it is a calculation of the difference between the income of the poor and their poverty thresholds.

A variety of poverty indexes have been proposed that integrate different combinations of the properties suggested for a good index. For example, a number of alternative indexes can be expressed as normalized weighted sums of the poverty gaps of the poor (e.g., indexes of Clark, Hemming, and Ulph, 1981; Foster, Greer, and Thorbecke, 1984; Kakwani, 1980; Rodgers and Rodgers, 1991; Sen, 1976; Takayama, 1979; Thon, 1979—see also Atkinson, 1989; Blakorby and Donaldson, 1980; and the review by Foster, 1984.) These indexes take into account not only the proportion of the population that is poor and the mean income of the poor, but also the distribution of income among the poor.

The statistical advantages of one or another of these indexes as an official poverty statistic, however, must be balanced against possible drawbacks. First, it is imperative that the indexes, like the underlying concept of poverty, have a clear and intuitive interpretation that can be easily understood by those with little or no training in statistics. As Ruggles (1990:29) argues:

> As the indexes become more and more complex it can be difficult even for analysts who are familiar with them to pinpoint the sources of change from period to period or to predict how alternative indexes will react to specific changes in the distribution of income or consumption.

This can be the case even with fairly elementary poverty measures; the situation is greatly exaggerated with more complex measures. In contrast, Kapteyn (1977) argues that as a given measurement is used over time, it gains acceptance and understanding regardless of its complexity. He contends, therefore, that attention should be on the development of the "best" measure rather than the least complex one. Second, as suggested by Atkinson (1989), a poverty index may be satisfactory for certain analytic purposes, even if it does not give unambiguous poverty rankings under all conditions.

Kundu and Smith (1983) review a number of poverty indexes and contend that none of them simultaneously meets all the desirable axiomatic properties by which they judged those indexes. Choices clearly must depend on the nature of the poverty index and its intended use. As an example, Hagenaars (1987) suggests that if the poverty line were an absolute boundary between survival and starvation, then the proportion or the number of poor should take priority over all other considerations.

We are persuaded that the head count and the head-count ratio are of considerable value and should be continued as the primary measures of poverty in the United States. They are intuitive and easy to calculate, even though they fall short of many of the properties considered desirable by those with expertise regarding poverty indexes. To compensate for these shortfalls and to provide a more complete picture of poverty, we are equally persuaded that there should be indicators of both the mean income level and the distribution of income among the poor. These indicators, however, should be kept separate from the head-count ratio, again, for reasons of understandability.

The Census Bureau already produces estimates of the mean poverty gap (or income deficit) each year for both all poor people and various groups, although it is not an official measure of poverty (see, e.g., Bureau of the Census, 1993c). This index measures the average difference between the poverty threshold and the income of the poor. In addition, the Census Bureau produces estimates of the distribution of income among the poor in terms of the proportion falling below specified fractions of the poverty threshold, such as the proportion below 75 percent or 50 percent. (The Census Bureau also publishes the proportion with incomes near poverty, e.g., those below 125% of the poverty threshold.) Together, these statistics provide understandable information on the average deprivation of the poor and the distribution of income among them.

We suggest that the Census Bureau continue to develop such statistics, although we believe that a measure of the *average income* of the poor would be more useful and understandable than the average poverty gap. Also, for statistics on average income (as well as for the poverty gap), it is most important to compute them by groups as well as for all poor people. This is important because different groups have different poverty thresholds, so that a mean income value of, say, $10,000, has different implications for a group with a poverty threshold of, say, $12,000 than for a group with a threshold of, say, $15,000. In this regard, it would be most useful to publish a weighted average poverty threshold, reflecting the composition of the poor population, to accompany statistics on the average income of the poor.[17]

Finally, it is important in the text of reports on poverty to point out limitations of specific indexes. We have noted that the head count and head-count ratio (and changes in them) do not provide any information about the underlying mean and distribution of the income of the poor. Similarly, a measure of mean income does not provide information about the income distribution. Also, it is important to caution about drawing unwarranted conclusions from particular indexes—for example, the poverty gap is not a measure of the amount of money that the government would have to spend to eliminate poverty (see Chapter 8, on behavioral responses to government

---

[17] We note that Orshansky (1965a:14), in her original work on the poverty measure, provided exactly this type of information, namely, average income of the poor for groups and average income of the poor for the total population, compared with an average weighted poverty threshold.

policies). Also, the number of people who are very far below the poverty line may be overestimated because of underreporting of income or the reporting of business losses by self-employed people. Nonetheless, such indicators can enrich understanding of the nature and scope of economic poverty in the United States and how it changes over time.

Indexes with Alternative Resource Definitions

The Census Bureau currently publishes indexes for "experimental" measures of poverty that use alternative definitions of family resources. Thus, Bureau of the Census (1995) provides head counts and head-count ratios for estimates of poverty under 18 resource definitions, the official definition and 17 alternatives. For example, definition (2) subtracts government transfers from income; definition (3) subtracts government transfers and adds realized capital gains; definition (4) is the same as (3) with the addition of employer-provided health insurance benefits; and definition (5) is the same as (4) with the subtraction of Social Security payroll taxes. These and the other experimental measures are designed to illustrate the effects on the poverty rate of defining family resources in different ways—specifically, the effects of excluding various government taxes and including various transfers, as well as the effects of including some kinds of asset holdings (e.g., owned homes) in income.

Measures of this type have a number of problems and must be carefully interpreted. We commented above (in Chapter 4) about the inappropriateness of resource definitions that are inconsistent with the poverty threshold concept (e.g., definitions that add the value of medical care benefits without appropriately adjusting the thresholds). Also, the Census Bureau's practice of specifying definitions in a cumulative fashion is problematic from the perspective of isolating the effect of particular components on the poverty rate. Thus, it is not possible to conclude that the difference between, say, definition (4) and definition (5) is the marginal effect of the added component of subtracting Social Security payroll taxes because of the possible interaction effects of the added component with other changes to the resource definition in the two definitions. (In contrast, in Chapter 5, we present estimates of the marginal effect on poverty rates of each of the proposed changes to the current poverty measure, considered separately, as well as an estimate of the interaction effect.)

Most important, great care must be exercised in attempting to assess the policy implications of differences in poverty rates under alternative resource definitions. People's responses to such government policy changes as the elimination of taxes or benefit programs are likely to result in very different poverty rates than those seen in comparing the current measure with measures that use a different resource definition but in which the real world remains the same. For example, families who currently receive benefits from such government programs as food stamps or Social Security are not likely to have the same private income if these programs did not in fact exist (e.g., they might increase their work hours or delay retirement). Hence, properly speaking, poverty rates calculated under alternative resource definitions assess the implications of an instantaneous change in government programs before there is time for people to adjust their behavior.

Nonetheless, we think it is useful to produce poverty head-count ratios (and other indexes, such as the average income of the poor) under some alternative resource definitions. In particular, we believe it would be useful to publish poverty statistics for measures in which resources are defined net of government taxes and transfers. Several such measures could be useful: one in which resources are defined in before-tax terms, one in which resources are net of taxes but exclude benefits from means-tested government programs (whether cash or in-kind), and one in which resources exclude benefits from all government programs, whether means tested or not. Again, the statistics from such measures must be interpreted with care and caveats about their use provided in the text of reports on poverty: because of behavioral responses, the poverty rate in a world without government taxes or government assistance programs would likely differ from the rate under these measures. Nonetheless, when compared with the proposed poverty measure, such before-tax and transfer measures should be helpful for evaluating the effects of government policies and programs on poverty.

THE LIMITED SCOPE OF
MEASURING ECONOMIC POVERTY

The body of this report focuses on the concept and measurement of economic poverty. We conclude this chapter by noting three limitations in the scope of our efforts: the limited dimension of impoverishment on which we focus; the need for a richer understanding of the meaning and consequences of impoverishment for adults and, especially, for children; and the need for a deeper understanding of the causes of poverty and the potential private and collective actions that might reduce its prevalence and its adverse effects.

First, although the measure of economic poverty is a very powerful social indicator, it speaks only to one dimension of deprivation—economic or material deprivation, fairly narrowly defined. Measures of other types of deprivation—psychological, physical, social—and the overlap with the economic poverty measure are also needed. Many other dimensions of impoverishment can exist, from anxiety and fear about one's personal safety when living in a high-crime neighborhood or with abusive family members to suffering from inadequate medical care and from homelessness to loneliness to helplessness. These, too, need to be conceptualized, measured, and their prevalence recorded across groups and over time. The joint incidence of these other aspects of impoverishment with economic poverty is, one suspects, quite high, but not complete. In describing the extent of impoverishment in the United States, these nonmonetary indices would provide important added information.

Second, in this volume we have not explored, analytically or descriptively, the material circumstances of those who are poor: for example, what household goods they have or how they allocate their resources among categories of consumption. Also, we have not asked about the consequences of economic poverty in terms of other dimensions of impoverishment. We encourage research that asks how economic poverty is linked to families' day-to-day lives—for example, to family violence, homelessness or frequent moves to different households, safety of their neighborhoods, or access to friends, services, and jobs. Similarly, the consequences of economic poverty for access to health care and social services, for an individual's self-esteem, mental and physical health, school achievement, prospects for employment, marriage, and parenting all deserve much more research attention. Also, we have not considered in this volume how the consequences of economic poverty differ by an individual's age or other characteristics. These other, less easily quantified indexes of well-being that may or may not be associated with economic poverty are also deserving of study in order to have a fuller understanding of the lives of the poor and a more complete documentation of the consequences of living in poverty.

Consider, in this regard, the life experiences of children who are poor. Evidence suggests that children living in poor families under the current measure score lower on cognitive, language, and achievement tests and exhibit higher rates of grade failure, of placement in special education, and of dropping out of high school (see Baydar, Brooks-Gunn, and Furstenberg, 1993; Brooks-Gunn, Guo, and Furstenberg, 1993; Fitzgerald, Lester, and Zuckerman, 1995; Haveman, Wolfe, and Spaulding, 1991; Huston, 1991; Huston, McLoyd, and Garcia Coll, 1994; Ramey et al., 1992). Children's physical health indicators, such as low birthweight, failure to thrive, and chronic illnesses, also have been shown to be related to measured poverty (Adler et al., 1994; Brooks-Gunn, 1990; Egbuonu and Starfield, 1982; Eisen et al., 1980; Klerman, 1991; McCormick et al., 1991; Parker, Greer, and Zuckerman, 1988; Stein et al., 1987). Moderate to severe behavior problems in children are also linked statistically to economic poverty (see, e.g., Rutter, 1989).

At the same time, other social and demographic characteristics of families are associated with negative child and adolescent outcomes, including parents' education, age, and occupation and household structure (i.e., two- or one-parent households). Controlling for such characteristics in statistical models of child outcomes generally diminishes but does not eliminate the association between economic poverty and these outcomes. Such findings underscore the importance of considering other dimensions of poor children's lives that contribute to the probability of decrements in all realms of development.

Not only can the adverse effects of economic poverty on children's lives be clearly documented, but children are also disproportionately among the poverty population in the United States. Presently, one in five children in the United States is living in poverty according to the official measure, with the percentage being slightly higher for children aged 6 and under, compared with the rate of those of elementary and high school age (Hernandez, 1993).

The costs of children in poverty are experienced not only by the children themselves, but also by society. Children have great value to their families and communities. As is often said, children are the nation's most important resource; in their well-being lies the reflection of the character of society today as well as its hopes for tomorrow. Children are an important human resource; their success in school and their eventual success in the workplace are essential for a productive society. Being reared in a household with limited economic resources is disproportionately associated with higher rates of crime, violence, underemployment, unemployment, and isolation from the larger community.

Children are dependent on others for their well-being and because of their dependence, they enter or avoid poverty by virtue of their family's economic circumstances. They typically cannot alter their poverty status by themselves, at least until they approach late adolescence, so it is fitting to focus special attention on them in any study of poverty.

Third, and last, this volume does not address the broad and well-researched topics of the causes of economic poverty or issues in the development of policies to reduce its prevalence or its adverse effects. Those topics are well beyond the scope of the panel's work.

7

Use of the Poverty Measure in Government Assistance Programs

The current official U.S. poverty measure has been not only an important statistical indicator; it has also had direct policy uses in government programs that are designed to help low-income families whose resources fall below a standard of need. Many programs have their own need standard for eligibility, but a significant number link their standard to the official poverty thresholds (or a multiple of them). In most cases, the link is actually to the poverty guidelines derived from the thresholds, and, consequently, we use the term guidelines in this chapter.[1]

Another program use of the poverty measure has been for allocation of federal funds to states and localities. For example, funds for educationally deprived children under the Elementary and Secondary Education Act are allocated to school districts on the basis of their share of children aged 5-17 who live in poor families. Head Start funds are also allocated to states by a formula that takes account of each state's share of children under age 18 in families receiving Aid to Families with Dependent Children (AFDC) and its share of children under age 6 in poor families. The share of poor people is also one factor in the formula for allocating Community Development Block Grant funds to cities and counties.

In this chapter we consider the relationship of a poverty measure to eligibility and benefit standards for government means-tested programs that

---

[1] The poverty guidelines are issued annually by the U.S. Department of Health and Human Services (HHS) by smoothing the official poverty thresholds for different-size families. The guidelines are higher than the thresholds for Alaska (by 25%) and Hawaii (by 15%).

provide assistance to individual families.[2] In particular, we consider the implications of the changes we propose in the current poverty measure for program eligibility and benefit determination. To put the issue in perspective, we review in general the types of programs that are designed to help low-income people and consider a few specific examples. Different categories of programs pose somewhat different questions for the potential role of one or another poverty measure. Appendix D provides details on all such federal programs as they existed through 1994. In Chapter 8, we focus on the possible relationship of the proposed poverty measure to benefit levels in the AFDC program, and we also address the relationship of that measure to state AFDC standards of need, which, in many states, exceed actual benefit levels.

RECOMMENDATION

We argue throughout this report that the proposed poverty measure is a marked improvement over the current measure for use as a statistical indicator, and we recommend its adoption for this purpose. We believe that the proposed measure also deserves serious consideration for use as an income eligibility standard in government assistance programs that currently determine eligibility or benefit amounts by comparing family resources to the poverty guidelines derived from the official thresholds. However, we do not flatly recommend that the proposed measure be adopted in place of the current measure for program use. Rather, we urge program agencies to carefully review the proposed measure to determine whether it is appropriate and whether it may need to be modified in one or more respects to better serve program objectives.

In their review, program agencies should consider the implications of the proposed measure in relation to the current measure. They should also keep in mind some important criteria for evaluating any measure of need. In particular, it is critical that the measure provide for consistency between the definition of family resources and the definition of the poverty threshold (or other need standard). This criterion is important for a statistical measure of poverty so that population groups are appropriately classified by poverty status; it is also important for program use so that program benefits are given to needy families.

As we have noted above, the current poverty measure fails this consistency criterion in several important respects, for example, by not excluding

---

[2] There are other questions about the role of a poverty measure and about the changes we propose to the current measure for fund allocation purposes that we do not address. Thus, our recommendation to adjust the official poverty thresholds for geographic area differences in the cost of housing has obvious implications for the distribution of program funds among jurisdictions. However, broadly speaking, the availability of reliable data for estimating poverty rates for small geographic units may be a more important concern for fund allocation than the properties of a specific poverty measure.

taxes from family resources even though the poverty thresholds were computed on an after-tax basis. Hence, some working families that pay taxes may be erroneously classified above the poverty line because their resources are defined as gross rather than net income. The proposed poverty measure embodies a definition of family resources as money and near-money disposable income that is consistent with the derivation of the poverty thresholds from expenditure data for such basic needs as food, clothing, and shelter. However, the proposed definition is considerably more demanding of data than the current definition: full implementation would require asking about in-kind benefits and several types of expenses as well as money income.

For such assistance programs as food stamps and AFDC, which make a very detailed determination of financial eligibility and benefit amounts, implementing the proposed definition of family resources would not complicate program administration. Indeed, that definition, in concept if not in detail, is quite similar to the definitions already in use in these programs. However, other assistance programs currently have fairly simple application procedures that obtain a crude measure of gross money income and compare it with the relevant poverty guideline to determine program eligibility. For these programs, to implement the proposed resource definition could pose a burden on both applicants and program administrators. We believe there are ways to simplify that definition for programs for which a simple application process is valued and there is a willingness to give up some precision in classifying applicants' eligibility status (see below).

With regard to the need standard component of the proposed poverty measure, program agencies should consider whether the cutoff for eligibility should be 100 percent of the guidelines or a multiple, as is now the case in many programs. Obviously, there are budget implications of this choice, particularly for those entitlement programs that use the guidelines and that must provide benefits for all applicants who meet the eligibility criteria.

In this regard, it is important for program agencies to be aware of the implication of the proposal to update the poverty thresholds each year for real changes in basic consumption rather than to update them only for price inflation. The thresholds developed under the procedure will probably increase more rapidly than thresholds that are updated for price inflation only, even though they are not likely to increase as fast as a purely relative set of poverty thresholds.

There are ways to address the budgetary consequences of using poverty thresholds that are updated in real terms for program purposes. For example, eligibility could be limited to families with resources below a fraction of the thresholds. This strategy is not a contradiction in terms. We have argued strongly that updating the poverty thresholds for real growth in spending on basic necessities makes a great deal of sense for a statistical measure. There is considerable evidence that poverty thresholds are relative to time and place, and a regular, automatic adjustment for real growth seems preferable to an adjustment that occurs spasmodically. However, the design of government assistance programs must take into account many factors, only one of which is a statistical standard of need. Other considerations, such as funding constraints and competing uses for scarce tax dollars, may dictate that assistance program benefits be set at a level below the statistical poverty thresholds.

> RECOMMENDATION 7.1. **Agencies responsible for federal assistance programs that use the poverty guidelines derived from the official poverty thresholds (or a multiple) to determine eligibility for benefits and services should consider the use of the panel's proposed measure. In their assessment, agencies should determine whether it may be necessary to modify the measure—for example, through a simpler definition of family resources or by linking eligibility less closely to the poverty thresholds because of possible budgetary constraints—to better serve program objectives.**

GOVERNMENT ASSISTANCE PROGRAMS

Overview

In 1994, 70 federal and federal-state programs were providing cash, in-kind benefits, or other types of services to families or individuals who were deemed needy on the basis of an explicit income test.[3] Table 7-1 summarizes the number and expenditures of these programs in fiscal 1992 (see Burke, 1993, and Appendix D for details).

Of the 70 programs, 27 (39%) have as one of their income eligibility criteria that income be compared with the poverty guidelines or some multiple of them; see Table 7-2. They run the gamut from small programs that spend only a few million dollars a year (e.g., Follow Through and Senior Companions) to two of the largest assistance programs, food stamps and Medicaid. Of these programs, 14 use the poverty guidelines (or a multiple) as the sole criterion of income eligibility; they account for 2 percent of expenditures by all assistance programs. Examples are the Maternal and Child Health Services Block Grant, Legal Services, and Foster Grandparents. The other 13 programs, which account for 56 percent of expenditures by all assistance programs, have several ways of determining income eligibility. For example, School Lunch and School Breakfast accord eligibility to children whose families already participate in AFDC or food stamps, and they also permit other

---

[3] Assistance programs typically have other requirements for eligibility besides a comparison of income with a need standard: for example, they may provide benefits only to people in certain age categories or have a limit on assets in addition to income or have other restrictions or requirements. Our discussion focuses on programs' definitions of and limits on income.

TABLE 7-1   Government Assistance Programs That Link Eligibility to Income, Fiscal 1992

Program Type	Programs		Expenditures	
	Number	Percent	Million $	Percent
Programs that link eligibility solely to the federal poverty guidelines	14	20.0	6,510	2.3
Programs that link eligibility to the federal poverty guidelines and also to participation in other programs (e.g., AFDC, SSI, or food stamps)	13	18.6	156,580	56.1
Programs that link eligibility to a percentage of the local area (or state) median income	12	17.1	21,302	7.6
Programs that have their own income eligibility standards (or that link eligibility to participation in another program)	31	44.3	94,583	33.9
Total	70	100.0	278,975	100.0

SOURCE: Derived from Burke (1993).

NOTES: Not included in the table are two assistance programs that are wholly supported by state and local funds: General Assistance (fiscal 1992 expenditures of $3,340 million) and General Assistance—medical care component (fiscal 1992 expenditures of $4,850 million). Also not included are eight programs that allocate benefits on some other basis (e.g., area of residence): Indian Health Services, Nutrition Program for the Elderly, State Legalization Impact Assistance Grants, Chapter 1 Migrant Education Program, Emergency Food and Shelter Program, Food Distribution Program on Indian Reservations, Migrant High School Equivalency Program, and College Assistance Migrant Program, which had total fiscal 1992 expenditures of $2,626 million. For details of the programs in each category, see Appendix D.

SSI, Supplemental Security Income.

children to qualify on the basis of comparing their family income to a multiple of the poverty guidelines. Programs authorized by the Job Training Partnership Act (e.g., Job Corps and Summer Youth Employment) accord eligibility to people already participating in AFDC or food stamps and permit other people to qualify on the basis of comparing their family income to 100 percent of the poverty guidelines or 70 percent of the lower living standard income level determined by the Department of Labor, whichever amount is higher.

The remaining 43 programs (61%) use some other income eligibility

TABLE 7-2 Government Assistance Programs That Link Eligibility or Benefits to the Current Poverty Measure, by Program Type and Poverty Cutoff for Eligibility, Fiscal 1992

Programs That Provide All-or-Nothing Service	Poverty Cutoff for Eligibility (%)
Commodity Supplemental Food Program	100 (for elderly people)
Community Services Block Grant	100; 125 at state option
Follow Through	100
Foster Grandparents	125
Head Start[a]	100
Job Corps[a]	100
Legal Services	125 (up to 187.5 for people with excessive medical or child care expenses)
Medicaid[a,b]	100 for some people; 133 for others (up to 185 at state discretion for others)
Senior Community Service Employment Program[a]	125
Senior Companions	100
Special Milk Program	130
Special Programs for Students with Disadvantaged Backgrounds (TRIO Programs)	150
Special Supplemental Nutrition Program for Women, Infants, and Children (WIC)	100 to 185 at state discretion
Summer Food Service Program for Children	185 (applies to service areas, not applicants)
Summer Youth Employment Program[a]	100
Training for Disadvantaged Adults and Youth[a]	100
Vocational Education Opportunities, Disadvantaged Activities[a]	100
Weatherization Assistance[a]	125

Programs That Relate Benefits to Income or Charge for Services on a Sliding Scale	Poverty Cutoff for Eligibility (%)
Child and Adult Care Food Program	130 for free meals; 185 for reduced price
Community Health Centers	100 for free care; sliding scale up to 200
Food Stamp Program[a,b]	130 (gross income); 100 (net income)
Low-Income Home Energy Assistance Program (LIHEAP)[a]	150
Maternal and Child Health Services Block Grant	100 for free care; sliding scale for others
Migrant Health Centers	100 for free care; sliding scale up to 200
School Breakfast Program[a,b]	130 for free meals; 185 for reduced price
School Lunch Program[a,b]	130 for free meals; 185 for reduced price
Title X Family Planning Services	100 for free care; sliding scale up to 250

SOURCE: Burke (1993).

[a]Program also accords eligibility on bases other than the poverty guidelines (e.g., children on AFDC are automatically eligible for Head Start); see Appendix D.

[b]Entitlement program: eligible applicants cannot be denied benefits.

criterion. Of these programs, 12 of them, which account for 8 percent of total expenditures, determine income eligibility on the basis of comparing household income to a percentage of state or local area median family income. Examples are Section 8 Low-Income Housing Assistance and Rural Housing Loans. Finally, 31 programs, which account for 34 percent of total expenditures, have their own income eligibility standards. Examples are AFDC, Supplemental Security Income (SSI), veterans' pensions, and Stafford Loans.

The 27 programs that link eligibility for some or all applicants to the poverty thresholds or guidelines differ on a number of dimensions. These, in turn, have implications for using the proposed poverty measure for eligibility determination. One dimension is how the benefits are related to income. Some programs have a poverty-based income test simply to determine eligibility and do not further condition benefits for eligible people on the amount of their income. In other words, these programs provide an all-or-nothing service (examples are Head Start and Legal Services). Other programs do condition benefits on the amount of an applicant's income. For example, the Food Stamp Program reduces the dollar amount of the coupons provided to recipients in direct relationship to their "countable" income. Such programs as Maternal and Child Health Services charge recipients for services on a sliding scale: some people pay nothing, others pay a fraction of the costs, and still others pay full costs, depending on broad income-to-poverty guideline categories.

A second dimension is the complexity of the method for measuring applicants' incomes. Programs that provide an all-or-nothing benefit often have a fairly simple application form that does not ask applicants for extensive detail about income sources. Many programs that charge recipients for services on a sliding scale are also in this category. In contrast, the Food Stamp Program, which calibrates benefits quite closely to income, includes an elaborate process to determine applicants' gross income and their net income after allowable deductions.

Another distinction is between entitlement and nonentitlement programs. Entitlement programs (e.g., Medicaid, food stamps, School Lunch, and School Breakfast) must provide benefits to all eligible applicants. However, many of the programs that link eligibility to the poverty guidelines (e.g., Head Start, Legal Services) are not entitlements. These programs do not guarantee to provide services to all eligible families; rather, legislatively set budget limits determine how many eligible people who apply for services will actually be assisted and how many will be put on a waiting list.

Finally, programs vary in whether they use 100 percent or a multiple of the poverty guidelines as the basis for determining eligibility (see Table 7-2). For example, Head Start has an income cutoff of 100 percent of the poverty guidelines, but Legal Services has a cutoff of 125 percent, and Special Programs for Students with Disadvantaged Backgrounds has a cutoff of 150 percent. School Lunch and School Breakfast provide free meals to children of families with incomes below 130 percent of the poverty guidelines and charge a reduced price for families with incomes between 130 and 185 percent of the guidelines. Community and Migrant Health Centers provide free medical care to people with incomes below 100 percent of the poverty guidelines and charge reduced fees on a sliding scale to people with incomes between 100 and 200 percent of the guidelines. The Title X Family Planning Services Program operates in a similar manner except that the cutoff for reduced fees is 250 rather than 200 percent of the poverty guidelines. States have discretion to set income eligibility limits for the Special Supplemental Nutrition Program for Women, Infants, and Children (WIC) at the level used by state or local agencies for free health care, so long as the level is between 100 and 185 percent of the poverty guidelines.

Determining Income Eligibility: Selected Programs

To determine how families' incomes are estimated for comparison with the poverty guidelines, we examined application procedures for selected programs.[4] In many cases—for example, for Community Health Centers and Title X Family Planning Services[5]—local centers or agencies have a good deal of discretion in how they determine income eligibility. In other cases, such as food stamps, federal regulations are very specific about the definitions and procedures used. As examples of current procedures and definitions, we summarize the income determination process for Head Start, school nutrition programs, WIC, and food stamps. From our analysis, we conclude that the proposed poverty measure is advantageous for program use in many respects, although it may need modification in some instances.

Head Start

Local Head Start agencies have discretion in determining income eligibility, although they must have on file documentation for participating families that certifies that they met the income eligibility criteria. Families participating in AFDC are automatically eligible for Head Start, and no additional verification or documentation of their income is required. AFDC families make up about one-half of Head Start participants; the remainder are largely working poor families. Head Start agencies typically ask to see paystubs for documentation of earnings. The income definition used is the same as for the current poverty measure, namely, gross money income.[6]

---

[4] For more complete program descriptions, see Appendix D.

[5] Information provided by Malvina Ford, Congressional Research Service.

[6] Information provided by Craig Turner, Head Start Bureau, Administration for Children and Families, U.S. Department of Health and Human Services.

School Nutrition Programs

For school nutrition programs administered by the U.S. Department of Agriculture (USDA)—School Lunch, School Breakfast, Special Milk Program—federal regulations are fairly specific, although states may institute additional policies that do not conflict with the federal requirements. Generally, schools are required to inform households of the availability of free or reduced-price school meals to those who meet eligibility requirements. Households already participating in food stamps or AFDC can be certified automatically through contact with the local food stamp and AFDC offices; other households must provide information on their previous month's income.[7]

A USDA manual (Food and Nutrition Service, 1991) specifies the types of income to be included and excluded. Federal law excludes various benefits from the calculation of income, such as food stamps and educational assistance received under means-tested programs (e.g., Pell Grants); and negative self-employment income is set to zero; otherwise, the definition of income is much the same as the gross money income definition used in the March Current Population Survey for the official poverty statistics.

The specific information requested from households is in the form of a grid, with each household member listed down the side and the following sources of income listed across the top: gross monthly earnings (before deductions) for the first and second job; combined monthly payments from welfare, child support, alimony; combined monthly payments from pensions, retirement, Social Security; other monthly income. From the information provided, the school computes total income and compares it with a multiple of the appropriate poverty guideline (130% for free meals, 185% for reduced-price meals). Finally, the school is responsible for conducting annually a verification of income for a sample of participating households.

WIC

State agencies that operate the WIC program may adopt the income eligibility criteria for reduced-price school meals (i.e., 185% of the poverty guidelines), and, if they do so, they must follow the definition of income used by the school nutrition programs. Alternatively, state WIC agencies may adopt the income eligibility criteria used by state or local agencies for free or reduced-price health care, so long as the income limit is not less than 100 percent and not more than 185 percent of the poverty guidelines. Under this alternative, state WIC agencies may use the income definition of the state or local health care agencies. However, the value of in-kind housing or other in-kind benefits must not be counted as income; likewise, the value of various pay-

---

[7] Households in special circumstances (e.g., those that have money from seasonal work) may project their anticipated annual income rather than reporting previous month's income.

ments or benefits provided under certain federal programs as specified by law (e.g., Pell Grants) must be excluded. The intent of the option of tying income eligibility to the limits used by state or local health care agencies is to encourage coordination of WIC with health services and to simplify the administrative burden of determining eligibility (Food and Nutrition Service, 1988a).

Food Stamps

Households that receive AFDC or SSI, and so have already been through an eligibility determination process, are generally automatically eligible for food stamps. Other households can receive food stamps if they meet certain income and asset requirements. Because the program has a short (monthly) accounting period, it applies an asset test that is designed to screen out applicants who have savings and other liquid assets on which they can draw to cover a temporary period of low income. The program also applies a gross and net income test that is similar in many respects to the proposed calculation of gross and disposable income for purposes of measuring poverty.

Gross income for the Food Stamp Program includes all kinds of money income, with a few exceptions (e.g., the Earned Income Tax Credit [EITC] is not counted). Net income for households without an elderly or disabled member is gross income minus: a standard deduction that does not vary by household size and is adjusted for inflation each October ($131 a month in fiscal 1994); 20 percent of any earned income (to allow for taxes and work expenses); out-of-pocket dependent care expenses, when necessary for work or training, up to $200 per month for each dependent under age 2 and up to $175 for other dependents; and shelter expenses that exceed 50 percent of counted income after all other deductions up to a legislatively set ceiling ($231 a month as of July 1994). Net income for households with an elderly or disabled member is gross income minus: the standard, earned income, and dependent care deductions noted above; shelter expenses that exceed 50 percent of counted income after all other deductions, with no ceiling; and out-of-pocket medical care expenditures for the elderly or disabled member that exceed $35 a month.[8] Gross and net income are compared with the current Department of Health and Human Services (HHS) poverty guideline appropriate for the family's size to determine eligibility. Households without elderly or disabled members must have gross monthly income below 130 percent of the HHS poverty guidelines and net monthly income below 100 percent of the poverty guidelines. Households with an elderly or disabled member need only meet the net income test.

To determine benefits, a different cutoff is used because the Food Stamp Program is intended to supplement families' resources for food consumption

---

[8] Different standard deductions and shelter expenses ceilings apply in Alaska and Hawaii.

only. Hence, the cutoff is the USDA Thrifty Food Plan (instead of the poverty guidelines), and the amount of food stamps that eligible applicants receive is the difference between 30 percent of their countable income and the Thrifty Food Plan value for their size family. As an example, if the Thrifty Food Plan value for a family is $400 a month and the family has $900 of countable income, the family will receive $100 in food stamps—$400 minus $300 (30% of $900). In effect, the Food Stamp Program expects that households will spend 30 percent of their net countable income on food, or roughly the amount that food represents of the official poverty thresholds (as originally developed); the program supplements families' food-consumption resources up to the level of the Thrifty Food Plan.

USING THE PROPOSED POVERTY MEASURE

In assessing whether and how to use the proposed poverty measure for determining income eligibility for benefits or services, program agencies must consider a number of issues. These issues relate to the thresholds, the family resource definition, and other aspects of the measure.

The Thresholds

We have recommended a method for deriving the poverty thresholds each year but not a specific threshold for the reference family of four with which to initate a new series of poverty statistics. If the proposed measure is adopted for statistical purposes and a specific initial threshold is designated by the U.S. Office of Management and Budget, agencies will need to assess the consequences for program costs and caseloads of any difference between a new threshold and the current poverty guideline for a four-person family.

If the new threshold is higher, its use as an eligibility standard for programs will likely produce a larger pool of potential applicants. For nonentitlement programs (i.e., programs that do not guarantee services or benefits to all eligible applicants), there are no budgetary consequences from an increase in the applicant pool. However, should the newly eligible people apply for benefits or services, such programs would have to lengthen their waiting lists unless budget ceilings are raised. For entitlement programs that use the guidelines, there would be a direct effect on caseloads and costs if the applicant pool increases and the newly eligible people apply for assistance.

Even if the new threshold is the same as the current threshold, changes in the family resource definition could still increase the pool of potential applicants. This could happen for programs that automatically accord eligibility to families receiving welfare benefits (e.g., AFDC, SSI, or food stamps) and also allow other families to qualify on the basis of comparing their income with the poverty guidelines. Because of such changes to the family resource definition as deducting taxes and work-related expenses from income, the applicant pool for these programs could include a higher number of families not now receiving public assistance (plus the same number of families who are receiving public assistance).

Given a particular initial threshold, there could be an effect on the distribution of the applicant pool by family size due to the differences between the proposed equivalence scale and the scale implicit in the current guidelines. We have argued that the proposed scale is an improvement over the current scale, so this effect would be appropriate in terms of targeting services to those types of families most in need.[9]

There might also be an effect on the size of the applicant pool in different areas of the country because of the recommended adjustment to the thresholds for geographic differences in housing costs. Depending on its magnitude, this effect could be temporarily disruptive to programs in various areas that were accustomed to higher or lower caseloads, but it should represent an improved overall targeting of services.

The use of poverty thresholds that are adjusted for geographic differences in the cost of housing raises some special issues for the Food Stamp Program. The use of such thresholds for eligibility determination should, as just noted, represent an improved targeting of program benefits.[10] For benefit determination, however, the assumption that households spend 30 percent of their income on food would need to be reexamined—otherwise, newly eligible households in more expensive areas would not, in fact, benefit from the program. For example, if the maximum benefit for a particular size household were $300 per month and the eligibility level for that size household were raised from $1,000 to $1,200 because of higher housing costs in the area, then a household with $1,100 of net countable income would be newly eligible but would receive no food stamp benefits (30% of its countable income would be $330—above the maximum benefit). For such a household to benefit, the assumed percentage of countable income available for food expenditures would need to be lowered. Alternatively, the maximum benefit could be raised (as is currently done for Alaska and Hawaii), if it is assumed that food as well as housing costs are higher in the area.

A major issue with the use of the proposed method for determining

---

[9] The proposed scale is an improvement over the scale implicit in the current poverty thresholds, which has many irregularities. It is also an improvement over the scale implicit in the poverty guidelines: that scale is smooth, but it assumes that children need as much as adults, and it also assumes that each family member beyond the first costs the same (i.e., that economies of scale do not increase for larger families; see Chapter 3).

[10] It would have to be decided whether to adopt state-specific thresholds—to reflect the state involvement in administering the program—or the recommended breakdown by geographic division and size of metropolitan area; see Chapter 8.

poverty thresholds is that the method will generate new thresholds each year that reflect real changes in expenditures on food, clothing, and shelter. (We propose the use of 3-year moving averages to derive each year's thresholds, which will guard against big changes from one year to the next—see Chapter 2.) In years in which there is an economic downturn, the thresholds may decrease in real terms. In most years, however, given economic growth, they are likely to increase in real terms—that is, to increase more than the rate of inflation.

Thresholds that rise in real terms will not *necessarily* result in a larger number or proportion of poor people compared with thresholds that are simply adjusted for price changes (like the official thresholds). (Similarly, thresholds that fall in real terms will not necessarily result in a smaller number or proportion of poor people compared with price-adjusted thresholds.) The outcome depends on a combination of factors, such as changes in government tax policies, that affect the distribution of income in the vicinity of the thresholds. However, it is *likely* that the use of thresholds developed by the proposed procedure will produce a larger pool of potential program applicants, which, could, in turn, produce higher program costs and caseloads (or longer waiting lists) compared with continued use of the poverty guidelines derived from the official thresholds.

Program agencies must consider their response to this likely consequence. One option would be to periodically reconsider the multiple of the thresholds that a program uses as the cutoff for eligibility (or the cutoff for partial payment by the applicant in the case of programs that charge on a sliding scale). For example, the School Lunch Program might, at some future date, decide, on cost grounds, that it would lower eligibility for free lunches from 130 percent to 100 percent of the poverty level.

Another option would be to use the proposed equivalence scale and geographic adjustments for housing costs but continue to update the initial threshold simply for price changes. This option is less attractive because it implies the continuance of two different poverty measures. It seems preferable to have one official measure and require decision makers to consider in a forthright manner the issues involved in determining the multiple—or fraction—of the official thresholds to use for program eligibility. In debating what multiple to choose, decision makers will necessarily have to acknowledge possibly competing goals, such as the desire to help people whose resources fall below a reasonable standard of need and the desire to contain program spending within specified limits.[11]

---

[11] Chapter 8 discusses a range of factors that affect decisions about program eligibility standards and benefit levels, with specific reference to AFDC.

The Family Resource Definition

Proper implementation of the proposed poverty measure requires not only using the revised thresholds, but also changing the definition of income to compare with those thresholds. As we have stressed throughout, a poverty measure is a package in which the two components—the budget or threshold concept and the definition of family resources—must be consistent. Although the initial poverty threshold for the proposed measure might well be set at a level close to the current threshold, it represents a different concept, namely, a basic budget for food, clothing, shelter, and a little more for other necessities. This budget explicitly excludes some kinds of expenses—such as taxes, work-related expenses, child support, and out-of-pocket medical care expenses—which are instead treated as deductions from income. The proposed definition of disposable income also includes the value of in-kind benefits. This change in definition has somewhat different implications for programs that currently have a fairly simple process for determining gross regular money income and programs that already collect extensive information with which to determine gross and net income.

Simplified Determination of Disposable Income

For programs that currently obtain a crude measure of gross money income, full implementation of the proposed disposable income definition would require collecting additional information from applicants about income and expenses. Hence, there could be increased administrative costs and an increased burden on applicants.

We are certainly not in a position to provide detailed guidance to federal and state program agencies to determine how best they might implement the proposed disposable income definition. However, we have some ideas for ways to do so that could reduce the added burden on program agencies and applicants. It is important to note that the approaches we suggest, while minimizing burden, may increase the chance of an error in classifying an applicant's eligibility status in comparison with an approach that asks very detailed questions about applicants' income and expenses. (The assumption, based on survey research results, is that asking more detailed questions will elicit more complete responses; see Appendix B.) However, programs that at present obtain a fairly crude and hence less burdensome measure of gross money income probably already experience some classification errors.

A simplified determination of disposable income might work as follows, by taking the School Lunch and School Breakfast Programs as examples. These programs currently provide automatic eligibility to AFDC and food stamp families and presumably would continue doing so. For other families, the program asks about monthly income by several broad categories, including earnings for up to two jobs. A possibility for obtaining after-tax income would be to ask for net pay after deductions for Social Security and payroll taxes. A drawback is that such monthly pay information probably would not reflect the EITC. Another alternative would be for the Food and Nutrition Service, with guidance from the Census Bureau, to provide schools with a simple formula for calculating payroll and net income taxes from information on gross earnings and family composition. The specifications could indicate an income level above which it would not be necessary to estimate taxes; in other words, there should be no need to go through the calculation for families clearly above the thresholds.

For child care costs and child support payments, it seems fairly straightforward to ask families if they pay for child care or child support and their typical monthly costs. The flat deduction for commuting and other work-related expenses would not require asking families for any added information. With regard to in-kind benefits, it would not be necessary to ask about food stamp income, because food stamp families are automatically eligible.[12] Families could be asked if they receive housing assistance, although the value of such assistance is difficult to determine, and it might be wise, for administrative ease, to ignore this source of income.[13] Finally, rather than asking families about last month's out-of-pocket medical costs, which might not be representative of their annual costs, it might be easier simply to ask whether they have public or private health insurance. The Food and Nutrition Service, with guidance from the Census Bureau, could provide schools with a formula for assigning average out-of-pocket expenses to applicants on the basis of their family composition (including ages of family members) and insurance coverage.

The process just described for determining disposable income would be more involved than the current process for determining gross money income. However, we think that a "cookbook" (which might be computerized) could be developed for state and local agencies that would provide a reasonably straightforward way to calculate disposable income with acceptable accuracy with only a few added questions being asked of applicants.

An alternative approach would be to develop a "menu" of poverty thresholds for different types of families—such as working families with and without child care expenses and with and without health insurance coverage—that are appropriate to compare with a *gross* money income definition of family resources. For example, the threshold for a working family of two adults and

---

[12] However, programs that rely solely on comparing income with the poverty guidelines to determine eligibility and do not accord automatic eligibility to welfare families would need to ask about food stamps and, perhaps, other sources of in-kind income.

[13] In fact, many public housing recipients are also receiving food stamps or AFDC and hence would not need to be queried about income. Data from the 1991 American Housing Survey showed that 54 percent of renters receiving housing assistance also received food stamps (Nelson and Redburn, 1994:Table 1).

two children that pays for child care and has health insurance could be based on the threshold that results from the panel's concept plus average amounts for such families for income and payroll taxes, child care expenses, and out-of-pocket medical care expenses.

We do not recommend this approach for the statistical measure of poverty for a number of reasons. It would require the development of a large number of thresholds that, even so, would not likely provide an accurate measure of poverty status for the many families that are not "average." However, we believe the use of this approach has merit to determine eligibility for assistance programs in which the goal is a reasonable estimate that minimizes burden on applicants and program staff.

To use Head Start as an example, families not on AFDC might be asked, as now, for gross money income and documentation of earnings. They might also be asked, on a simple yes-no basis, whether they pay child care or child support, whether they have health insurance, and whether they receive food stamps or live in public housing. Using this information, the Head Start agency could compare the family's gross money income to the appropriate threshold for that family's circumstances by consulting a menu of thresholds. The process would be similar to that performed now, except that the menu would contain thresholds that vary by factors (e.g, work status, presence of health insurance coverage, etc.) in addition to family type and geographic area. The Census Bureau could assist program agencies by developing the menu.

In sum, we believe that there are reasonable strategies for program agencies that want to use the proposed poverty measure but, at the same time, retain a relatively simple application process. Whatever the strategy adopted to implement the proposed measure (e.g., a "cookbook" or "menu" approach or some other strategy), its use should improve the targeting of services to needy people compared to the current measure.

Full Determination of Disposable Income

A number of assistance programs already obtain a great deal of information about applicants' resources in order to calculate gross and net income. The definition of net family income that is used in many of these programs is similar in broad outline, if not in specific details, to the proposed definition of family resources for the poverty measure. Hence, such programs as food stamps or AFDC would not find it difficult to use the proposed disposable income definition, although they should still consider the particulars of the definition and their appropriateness for program use.

As we have stressed previously, it is important that the concept underlying the eligibility cutoff for a program be consistent with the family resource definitions. For example, if a program's need standard makes no allowance for expenses required to earn income (e.g., taxes, child care, commuting costs), then the determination of countable income should subtract any such expenses that are incurred before comparing income with the eligibility cutoff.

In this regard, we note that poverty thresholds developed according to the proposed concept would be more appropriate in many ways for eligibility determination in the Food Stamp Program than would the current poverty guidelines. This program currently defines countable income to exclude child care expenses and an allowance for taxes and other work-related expenses, which is consistent with the proposed threshold concept (but not with the current guidelines). In addition, out-of-pocket medical care expenditures above a certain limit are excluded from income for the elderly and disabled.[14] In contrast, however, the fact that EITC benefits cannot be counted as income (by law) for purposes of food stamp eligibility introduces an element of inconsistency with the proposed concept. Again, we are not in a position to provide specific guidance for programs. We repeat that the need concept and the definition of countable income in a program should be consistent.

Other Issues

There are some other features of the proposed poverty measure that may or may not be suitable for program use. For example, the proposal is that need be measured on an annual basis, that asset values not be included in resources, and that the unit for measuring need be the family as defined by the Census Bureau. Program agencies may well have sound reasons for reaching some other decision on these aspects of program design.

Thus, some programs are intended to provide short-term assistance and hence use a shorter accounting period than a year: for example, the accounting period in food stamps and AFDC is 1 month. In order to ensure that people applying for benefits have used up their available resources and are genuinely in crisis, programs with short accounting periods typically limit the assets that applicants can have and still be eligible for assistance.

With regard to the assistance unit, programs differ in their target populations and hence often differ in their definition of an eligible unit—for example, the Food Stamp Program generally defines eligible units to be the entire household, whereas AFDC generally defines eligible units to be families consisting of dependent children and their parent(s)—a narrower definition of family than that used by the Census Bureau. These differences from the proposed statistical poverty measure are certainly appropriate in light of program objectives.

---

[14] Shelter costs in excess of 50 percent of income (up to a ceiling for households with no elderly or disabled members) are also deducted from income for purposes of food stamp eligibility. This provision benefits people who, whether they live in high-cost or low-cost areas, pay what is deemed an excessive amount for housing relative to their resources.

The Poverty Measure and AFDC

8

In addition to reviewing the statistical measure of poverty, the panel was asked to consider issues of benefit levels for government family assistance programs—in particular, a national minimum benefit standard for the Aid to Families with Dependent Children (AFDC) program. Currently, there are large differences in AFDC benefit standards across states, and no state provides benefits as generous as the official poverty thresholds.

Federal policy makers have several times considered enacting a uniform minimum benefit standard that would provide a nationwide floor for AFDC benefits. The congressional debate over the Family Support Act (FSA) of 1988 included proposals for a national minimum benefit, but they were not accepted, largely because of the sizable estimated budgetary costs to the government. The FSA did request a study of minimum benefit standards, however, and this chapter responds to that request. We considered conceptual and statistical issues involved in setting a national minimum benefit standard for AFDC, just as we considered such issues for the poverty line.

In our review, we focused on the nature of the relationship between program benefit levels (whether in AFDC or other cash and near-cash assistance programs) and a measure of poverty (whether ours or another), and we show why that relationship is indirect at best. We also considered the relationship of the proposed poverty measure to AFDC standards of need. AFDC is unique among cash and near-cash assistance programs in that the states are required to establish a standard of need but are not required to—and often do not—use this standard to determine actual benefits. (See Appendix D for details of the AFDC program.)

335

DETERMINING PROGRAM BENEFIT LEVELS

We recommend (in Chapter 7) that serious consideration be given to the use of the proposed poverty measure as an eligibility standard for programs that tie eligibility for benefits and services to the current poverty measure. It might seem a logical next step to suggest a direct relationship of the proposed poverty measure to program benefits. Certainly, the existence of a poverty threshold that makes reasonable adjustments for differences in family circumstances, including differences in the cost of living across regions of the country, creates an impetus for program benefits to be related to that threshold. However, there are many factors that properly enter into a determination of benefit levels, only one of which is a poverty threshold.

At present, there is wide variation in AFDC benefits across the 50 states and the District of Columbia, and, in most states, benefits are considerably below the official poverty threshold. As of January 1994, the states' median standard of need for a three-person family was 60 percent of the corresponding official poverty threshold, and the median maximum benefit was 38 percent of the poverty threshold.[1] The median of the maximum combined AFDC and food stamp benefit for the states was 69 percent of the poverty threshold. Looking across states, the maximum AFDC benefit for a three-person family in January 1994 varied from $923 per month in Alaska to $120 in Mississippi, with a median of $366, a mean of $396, and a coefficient of variation of 40 percent; see Table 8-1.[2] The maximum AFDC benefit ranged from $240 to $552 (25-58% of the poverty threshold) in about two-thirds of the states; eight states exceeded this range, and eight states fell below it.

The maximum combined AFDC and food stamp benefit for a three-person family exhibited somewhat less dispersion, varying from $1,208 in Alaska to $415 in Mississippi, with a median of $658, a mean of $675, and a coefficient of variation of 22 percent. Food stamps have this effect because of the program's benefit formula, which assumes that families will devote 30 percent of their countable income to food expenditures (see Chapter 7). Hence, an increase of $1 in AFDC benefits (or other countable income) decreases food stamp benefits by 30 cents, and a decrease of $1 in AFDC benefits (or other countable income) increases food stamp benefits by 30 cents. The maximum combined AFDC and food stamp benefit ranged from $528 to $822 (55-86% of the poverty threshold) in 39 states. Adjusting AFDC and food stamp benefit levels to take account of differences in the cost of living by state further reduces the variation, although only to a limited extent (see below).

---

[1] The three-person family (parent or caretaker and two children) is the usual reference family for AFDC.

[2] The coefficient of variation is the standard deviation of a distribution as a percentage of the mean value; the standard deviation is the value that when added to or subtracted from the mean includes about two-thirds of the observations (states in this case).

TABLE 8-1   AFDC Need Standards, Maximum AFDC Benefits, and Maximum Combined AFDC and Food Stamp Benefits for a Family of Three, January 1994

State	AFDC Need Standard	Maximum AFDC Benefit Dollar Value	Maximum AFDC Benefit Percent of Need	Maximum Combined AFDC/Food Stamp Benefit Dollar Value	Maximum Combined AFDC/Food Stamp Benefit Percent of Need
Alabama	673	164	24	459	68
Alaska	975	923	95	1,208	124
Arizona	964	347	36	639	66
Arkansas	705	204	29	499	71
California	715	607	85	821	115
Colorado	421	356	85	645	153
Connecticut	680	680	100	872	128
Delaware	338	338	100	633	187
District of Columbia	712	420	59	690	97
Florida	991	303	31	598	60
Georgia	424	280	66	575	136
Hawaii	1,140	712	62	1,134	99
Idaho	991	317	32	612	62
Illinois	890	367	41	658	74
Indiana	320	288	90	583	182
Iowa	849	426	50	694	82
Kansas	429	429	100	713	166
Kentucky	526	228	43	523	99
Louisiana	658	190	29	485	74
Maine	553	418	76	689	125
Maryland	507	366	72	661	130
Massachusetts	579	579	100	801	138
Michigan[a]	551	459	83	717	130
Minnesota	532	532	100	768	144
Mississippi	368	120	33	415	113
Missouri	846	292	35	587	69
Montana	511	401	78	677	132
Nebraska	364	364	100	651	179
Nevada	699	348	50	640	92
New Hampshire	1,648	550	33	781	47
New Jersey	985	424	43	700	71
New Mexico	357	357	100	646	181
New York[b]	577	577	100	816	141
North Carolina	544	272	50	567	104
North Dakota	409	409	100	682	167
Ohio	879	341	39	636	72
Oklahoma	471	324	69	619	131
Oregon	460	460	100	753	164
Pennsylvania	614	421	69	691	113

continued on next page

TABLE 8-1   *Continued*

| State | AFDC Need Standard | Maximum AFDC Benefit | | Maximum Combined AFDC/Food Stamp Benefit | |
		Dollar Value	Percent of Need	Dollar Value	Percent of Need
Rhode Island	554	554	100	822	148
South Carolina	440	200	45	495	113
South Dakota	491	417	85	688	140
Tennessee	426	185	43	480	113
Texas	574	184	32	479	83
Utah	552	414	75	686	124
Vermont	1,124	638	57	843	75
Virginia	393	354	90	644	164
Washington	1,158	546	47	804	69
West Virginia	497	249	50	544	109
Wisconsin	647	517	80	758	117
Wyoming	674	360	53	648	96
Mean	655	396	66	675	115
Median	574	366	66	658	113
Range	320–1,648	120–923	24–100	415–1,208	47–187
Coefficient of variation[c]	40.7%	39.5%	39.6%	21.8%	32.5%

SOURCE: U.S. House of Representatives (1994:366-367).

[a]The values apply to Wayne County.
[b]The values apply to New York City.
[c]The standard deviation of the distribution as a percentage of the mean value.

Proposals for AFDC Minimum Benefits: A Brief History

The original Aid to Dependent Children program, the predecessor to AFDC, was enacted in 1935 as part of the legislation that instituted a national Social Security system.[3]   It was designed to put on a sounder footing the states' programs to provide "mothers' pensions," but there was no intent to mandate a prominent role for the federal government.[4]   The legislation provided that the federal government would pay 33 percent of the program's costs, with a

---

[3] Peterson and Rom (1990:Chap. 4) is the main source for this historical review; see also U.S. Senate (1986).

[4] In contrast, it was argued in the case of Social Security that national standards were needed to protect working people, given the mobility of labor across state boundaries. Similarly, for unemployment insurance, it was argued that a nationally uniform payroll tax was needed to ensure that states could not gain an unfair business advantage by choosing not to provide unemployment compensation.

maximum federal payment of $6 a month for the first child and $4 for other children. In 1950 the program was amended to provide benefits to the mother herself (or another caretaker of a dependent child or children), and in 1962 the program was amended to provide benefits (at state discretion) to two-parent families in which both were unemployed. The original legislation required that the states pay one-third of the costs (i.e., it prohibited states from the common practice of laying off all their costs on local jurisdictions), and it made federal payments "conditional on passage and enforcement of mandatory State laws and on the submission of approved plans assuring minimum standards in investigation, amounts of grants, and administration" (*Congressional Record,* January 17, 1935:548).

Since one-half of the counties in the United States did not provide mothers' pensions at the time and there was wide variation in payments across counties within states, the legislation had the effect of reducing within-state variation in benefits. However, it had little effect on across-state variation, leaving broad discretion to the states to set need standards, payments, and eligibility rules. For example, states were allowed to keep their residency requirements, and most did so until the Supreme Court in 1969 ruled them to be unconstitutional.

Historically, reformers have followed three strategies to try to establish more uniform state policies with regard to AFDC benefits (see Peterson and Rom, 1990:99-100), focusing on the matching formula, a supplementary national program, and national minimum benefit standards.

The Matching Formula The federal matching percentage was raised from 33 to 50 percent in 1939, to be consistent with the percentage for programs to assist the needy elderly, blind, and disabled. The formula was changed several times more between 1944 and 1958. Finally, in 1965, states were given the option of switching to the matching formula adopted for the Medicaid program. This formula committed the federal government to paying at least 50 percent of the welfare benefit in every state and to paying a higher matching rate (up to 83%) in those states with lower per capita income. Currently, all states use the Medicaid matching formula for AFDC benefits. The matching percentages in fiscal 1994 varied from 50-55 percent in 19 states and the District of Columbia to 70-79 percent in 13 states (U.S. House of Representatives, 1994:Table 10-17).

The rationale for the changes in the matching formula included the desire to provide incentives for low-benefit states to raise their benefits. However, Peterson and Rom (1990) found that the differences in benefit levels across states remained essentially unchanged, with a coefficient of variation that ranged from 34 to 37 percent in each decade from the 1940s to the 1980s.

A Supplementary Program with a National Benefit Standard—Food Stamps Food assistance programs in the United States were initially very localized. Many communities did not participate in the food stamp (or commodity distribution) program, and eligibility standards varied widely among those that did. In 1970 the Food Stamp Program was effectively nationalized: a single national standard was adopted, which was higher than any then in use in the states; the Secretary of Agriculture was empowered to set national eligibility requirements; and stiff penalties could be imposed on states that did not operate a program in every county. In 1977 Congress eliminated all purchase requirements for food stamps, making them a simple supplement to cash assistance in inverse proportion to family income (as well as a benefit to working families not receiving cash assistance).

The effect of these changes was to reduce the variation across states in the combined value of AFDC and food stamp benefits. However, there was no incentive for low-benefit states to raise AFDC benefits per se; rather the provision that food stamp benefits increase (decrease) by 30 cents for every dollar decrease (increase) in cash benefits in effect rewarded states that kept cash benefits low and penalized states that increased them.

A National Minimum Benefit Standard for AFDC   The strategy of legislating a uniform minimum benefit standard for AFDC has never achieved legislative success. In an early discussion of needed reforms in public assistance programs, Leon Keyserling's Conference on Economic Progress (1959:58) urged that "minimum uniform standards among the States should be set by the Federal Government." In 1965, the Office of Economic Opportunity (OEO) proposed a negative income tax program with a single nationwide payment schedule as part of its first "national anti-poverty plan." As part of its second plan in 1966, OEO again proposed a negative income tax program with a single nationwide payment schedule; besides being available to all poor persons without regard to demographic category, this proposed program would have gradually replaced existing public assistance programs (including AFDC) by 1972. In that same year the Advisory Council on Public Welfare (1966:15,22,117) recommended a "minimum standard for public assistance payments below which no State may fall." It proposed (p. xii) that the "Federal Government . . . set nationwide standards, adjusted by objective criteria to varying costs and conditions among the States, and assume the total cost of their implementation above a stipulated State share."

In 1967 President Johnson proposed that states be required to pay 100 percent of their standard of need, but he did not propose any specific minimum benefit standard. The proposal was rejected in the House Ways and Means Committee. The President's Commission on Income Maintenance (1969:7) recommended a "universal income supplement program financed and administered by the Federal Government." Concerning benefit levels for this income supplement program, the Commission stated (p. 59) that "attempts to reflect different costs of living in different areas would involve many difficulties and so a uniform National supplement is recommended."

The Family Assistance Plan (FAP) put forward by the Nixon Administration in the late 1960s provided for two kinds of programs, each with national minimum benefit standards: a program for low-income elderly, blind, and disabled (which subsequently became the Supplemental Security Income [SSI] program), and a program for all families with dependent children, regardless of work status. The proposed FAP AFDC minimum benefit was $1,600 a year for a family of four (about 40% of the official poverty line at that time)—a level that would have raised benefits in 16 states. FAP passed the House in 1970 but died in the Senate: conservatives questioned the adequacy of the work incentives; liberals criticized the national minimum benefit as inadequate.

The Carter Administration's Better Jobs and Income Program, proposed as legislation in 1977, also included a national minimum benefit for a program that would have combined AFDC, SSI, and food stamps; the minimum was set at $4,200 for a family of four whose head could not be expected to work (about 70% of the poverty line). This proposal died in Congress. In 1979 a scaled-back plan was introduced that proposed a national minimum benefit for AFDC at about 75 percent of the poverty line. The House passed this plan with the minimum benefit lowered to 65 percent of the poverty line (which would have raised benefits in 13 states). This bill died in the Senate.

As noted above, proposals for a national minimum benefit were originally considered for the 1988 FSA. In 1987 the House Ways and Means Committee approved a minimum benefit standard, but opposition from southern Democrats on the grounds of increased costs to their states resulted in stripping this provision from the legislation. The FSA instead mandated a study of minimum benefit standards.

Issues in Program Benefit Design

Today, the de facto national minimum level of available benefits for AFDC recipients is the maximum food stamp allowance combined with the maximum AFDC benefit in the lowest benefit state. In January 1994, this amount was $415 per month for a three-person family, or 43 percent of the corresponding poverty threshold. Hence, the issue of a national minimum benefit standard for AFDC really comes down to an issue of raising this de facto standard. Arguments for adopting such a nationwide minimum benefit standard for AFDC have been made on the basis of equity: that low-income families with children should not be disadvantaged simply by reason of their state of residence. In addition, others have argued that differences in benefits encourage low-income families to migrate from low-benefit to high-benefit states. There have been studies of the migration effects of AFDC, but they suffer from serious data and methodological problems. The results suggest that there is an effect on the migration behavior of low-income families but that the effect, for a number of reasons, is quite weak (see below).

We considered the issue of a national minimum benefit standard in somewhat broader terms, asking the question of how or if the proposed poverty measure could or should be linked with benefit levels for a program such as AFDC or a combination of AFDC and other cash and near-cash assistance programs. We first broached this issue in Chapter 7, in which we discussed the possible use of the proposed poverty measure for programs that already relate eligibility to the current measure. We pointed out some of the reasons that program agencies might want to make the link less direct, for example, by setting eligibility cutoffs at a fraction of the poverty thresholds. Here we explore more fully the reasons that a program benefit standard could differ from a poverty standard and, more generally, why the design of an assistance program could deviate from the goal of helping everyone who is classified as poor.

A note on terminology: When we speak of a "benefit standard" in the context of AFDC, we mean what is referred to in that program as the "maximum benefit" in contrast to either the "need standard" or the "payment standard." A family must have gross income below 185 percent of the need standard to be eligible for AFDC; it must also have net or countable income below 100 percent of the payment standard. A number of states have a payment standard below their need standard, and some states cap the maximum benefit at a lower level than the payment standard (see below).

The measurement of poverty or need does not necessarily imply anything about the extent to which need can or should be alleviated through government assistance programs. There are five key issues that separate measurement of need and alleviation of need: budget constraints, both overall and from competing demands on funding resources; strategies and preferences for targeting program benefits; interactions among programs; behavioral responses to program incentives; and, finally, cost-sharing provisions for federal-state programs.

Budget Constraints

Scarce budget resources may well limit the extent to which benefit standards can approach the poverty threshold, particularly in entitlement programs, such as AFDC, that must provide benefits to all eligible applicants. Both globally and in the United States, the areas with the greatest poverty are typically the areas that can least afford high benefits. For example, in some African countries, such a high proportion of the population is poor (by any standard) that very few resources are available internally to alleviate poverty.

For AFDC, the states with low benefit standards tend to be the states with higher poverty rates and with lower per capita incomes and, hence, with less ability to provide assistance to their needy families. Thus, maximum benefits in January 1990 were negatively correlated with the 1989 state poverty rate (correlation coefficient, −.55) and positively correlated with the 1989 state per capita income (correlation coefficient, .67).[5] However, there is considerable variation in benefit levels among the states that is not explained by differences in income. Peterson and Rom (1989) and Plotnick and Winters (1985) show that differences in AFDC benefits across states relate to a variety of political, ethnic, and economic differences.

For the nation as a whole, it would be hard to argue that the United States lacks sufficient revenue-generating ability to provide assistance to families below the poverty level. But the country's funding resources are not unlimited, and there are many demands on them. Assistance programs must compete with all other uses of taxpayers' funds.

Targeting Strategies and Preferences

In order to maximize the effectiveness of limited funds and achieve other policy goals, there may be reasons to target assistance payments to particular groups, even though simple measurement of need would not necessarily identify them as unique. For example, because of the long-term social cost of children growing up in economic deprivation, it may be sensible to concentrate assistance dollars on poor families with children, even though other groups have need that is just as great.

There are many examples of targeting in current programs. The Earned Income Tax Credit (EITC) was originally targeted to working poor families with children and was recently expanded to cover childless workers as well (see Appendix D). Food stamps offers another example of targeting, in that the program is designed to provide a more secure safety net for the elderly and disabled than for other people. This feature operates through the definition of countable income, which permits more generous deductions for households with elderly and disabled members in determining eligibility and benefits. Also, there is a higher asset limit for households with an elderly member (see Appendix D).

Another approach would be to concentrate scarce assistance dollars on the poorest families (the "worst off" among the poor), even though helping the families closest to the poverty line (the "best off" among the poor) would achieve the fastest reduction in measured need. In other words, although the strategy of helping the poorest poor will not produce as large a reduction in measured need per dollar spent as helping other poor people, it may be the best strategy to reduce poverty.

---

[5] The correlations were carried out by using data on AFDC benefits from U.S. House of Representatives (1990:553-555) and data on state poverty rates and per capita incomes from the 1990 census (Bureau of the Census, 1993d:Tables 733, 741).

Program Interactions

The existence of multiple assistance programs can affect the level of the benefit standard that makes sense for any one of them. For example, AFDC interacts with food stamps and public housing, and it makes little sense to think of an AFDC benefit standard in isolation from these programs (or in isolation from such programs as the EITC and enforcement of child support). However, given the different ways in which eligibility and benefits are calculated, it is not easy to determine an appropriate adjustment to AFDC benefit levels to take account of program interactions.

In the case of AFDC and food stamps, for example, one could certainly argue for excluding food costs from the AFDC benefit standard because of the almost universal provision of food stamps (and school meals) to AFDC families. As noted above, it would also be to a state's financial benefit to reduce its AFDC benefit standard by as much as the value of the Thrifty Food Plan because the Food Stamp Program will provide higher benefits than otherwise would have been the case. However, only in the case of states with very low AFDC benefit standards will the Food Stamp Program in fact make up the entire difference for recipients. This occurs because the program assumes that, after deductions, 30 percent of countable income including AFDC benefits is available for food consumption and, hence, reduces food stamp benefits accordingly. As a hypothetical example, consider a state that wants to provide combined AFDC and food stamp benefits at the level of the official poverty threshold. The deductions in the Food Stamp Program make it difficult to calculate by how much the state should reduce its AFDC benefit standard, but it can be demonstrated that not to reduce the AFDC standard at all may overcompensate recipients by as much as 10 percent relative to the poverty threshold, while to reduce the AFDC standard by the full amount of the Thrifty Food Plan may undercompensate recipients by as much as 17 percent.[6]

Program interactions virtually dictate that designers of assistance programs use complicated models to evaluate likely program effects. Some models are designed to point out odd interactions of such program features as maximum benefit levels and tax rates on other income by estimating the benefit package

---

[6] The first bound is obtained as follows: assume the AFDC benefit standard is $991 per month, or 100 percent of the poverty guideline for a family of three in 1993 (no state actually paid this amount). Then a family with the maximum $991 benefit from AFDC and the standard and excess shelter deductions for food stamps would have $653 of countable food stamp income and would receive $99 in food stamps (the Thrifty Food Plan value of $295 minus 30% of $653), for a total combined benefit of $991 plus $99, or $1,090 (110% of the poverty guideline). To obtain the other result, assume that the same state reduced its benefit standard to $696 by subtracting the entire value of the Thrifty Food Plan. Then a family with the maximum $696 AFDC benefit but *only* the standard food stamp deduction would have $565 in countable food stamp income and would receive $125 in food stamps ($295 minus 30% of $565), for a total combined benefit of $696 plus $125, or $821 (83% of the poverty guideline).

that would accrue to a specific type of family at a particular income level. Other models use microsimulation techniques operating on large-scale household databases to project the effects on program costs and caseloads of specified program features, given the distribution of the population and estimates of the likelihood of participation and other behavioral effects (see Citro and Hanushek, 1991; Lewis and Michel, 1990).

Program Incentives

Human beings participate in programs, and programs undeniably affect their behavior. Some effects are intended, others are unintended; some effects are positive, others are negative.

Some programs have an explicit goal of providing a positive incentive: for example, the federal government subsidizes student loans to encourage more young people to obtain the economic and other benefits of a college education. As another example, the Special Supplemental Nutrition Program for Women, Infants, and Children (WIC) seeks out poor pregnant women, mothers, and children to provide food supplements with the goal of healthier pregnancies, healthier babies, and, ultimately, healthier children and adults.

Other programs have a primary goal of providing income support to needy people. Such cash and near-cash assistance programs as AFDC and food stamps must contend with the fact that economic support has negative incentive effects to the extent that recipients are encouraged to rely on the program and not take steps to become self-supporting. Research on AFDC has examined incentive effects in the areas of work effort, family structure, and migration.

Work Effects Both economic theory and empirical research indicate that such programs as AFDC adversely affect the work choices of the eligible population. These programs provide a "guaranteed" base income to those who do not work; the resulting "income effect" allows individuals to work less. These programs also impose taxes on earned income. Since workers' net wages are now lower, the "substitution effect" encourages them to decrease the number of hours worked as it is relatively less expensive for them to do so. The combination of these provisions results in an unambiguous decrease in the aggregate number of hours of market work by the eligible low-income population.[7]

Extensive research has been undertaken to estimate the magnitude of the

_____

[7] In theory, there is an alternative explanation: it is possible that the primary effect of extra program dollars for low-income families is to induce them to underreport their earned (or other) income. That is, rather than decreasing work hours, they may decrease reporting of work hours (or switch to work where it is easier to evade official notice). However, there is no empirical evidence on this point.

reduction in work resulting from the disincentives embedded in assistance programs (see Danziger, Haveman, and Plotnick, 1981, and Moffitt, 1992, for extensive literature reviews on the subject). Although evidence shows that AFDC reduces the number of hours worked by single mothers, the estimates of those reductions vary among studies—from 1 to 10 hours per week. Moffitt (1992), in his review of the literature, concludes that "there is still considerable uncertainty regarding the magnitude of the effects."

Moffitt (1992) points out that there is very little research on the effects of in-kind assistance on labor supply.[8] He also notes the importance of exploring the effects of multiple assistance programs; however, these effects are difficult to model, and little work has been done in the area.

Family Structure Decisions Much of the literature on family structure focuses on whether AFDC encourages the formation of single-parent families headed by women. Since benefits are targeted to mothers with children and no spouse present, they may provide incentives to delay marriage or remarriage, to obtain a divorce, or to have children outside of marriage. Early work looking at the effect of AFDC on the increase in female-headed families is extremely mixed (see the summary in Groeneveld, Hannan, and Tuma, 1983). Studies in the 1980s, however, show more consistent evidence of an effect (see Danziger et al., 1982; Ellwood and Bane, 1985; Hoffman and Duncan, 1988; Moffitt, 1992). There is also some evidence of an effect of AFDC benefit levels on the probability that a female head lives independently rather than in a larger family (see Ellwood and Bane, 1985; Hutchens, Jakubson, and Schwartz, 1989).

Extensive research has been done on the effect of AFDC on illegitimacy. The work has studied whether the existence of public assistance increases the chances that babies will be born to unmarried women since a woman no longer needs a husband to help support a child. The work has also considered whether the existence of public assistance increases the likelihood that a woman will have a child in order to become eligible for benefits at all or have another child in order to receive additional benefits. The evidence on this issue in the literature is inconclusive: some studies find effects for some groups (e.g., white or black teenagers), and others find no effects for the same groups (see Duncan and Hoffman, 1990; Ellwood and Bane, 1985; An, Haveman, and Wolfe, 1991; Lundburg and Plotnick, 1990; Plotnick, 1990).

Migration Effects The extent to which the wide variation in AFDC benefit levels across states influences patterns of interstate migration is of

---

[8] See Fraker and Moffitt (1988) on the disincentive effects of the Food Stamp Program on the labor supply of female heads. Blank (1989), Moffitt and Wolfe (1990), and Winkler (1989) have analyzed the labor supply effects of the Medicaid program on the Medicaid-eligible population.

particular relevance to the issue of a nationwide minimum benefit standard. Hence, we considered it in some detail.

Substantial cross-state differentials in AFDC benefits have existed since the inception of the AFDC program, but they have created greater policy concern since residency requirements were ruled unconstitutional in 1969. In particular, policy makers (particularly in high-benefit states) have worried that their states attract welfare recipients, thereby increasing the burden on taxpayers. A simple comparison of the expected income available to AFDC-eligible families in high- and low-benefit states clearly indicates that such families can receive more income in a high-benefit state, which should create an incentive for them to relocate. Since the same states have generally remained high- or low-benefit states, if such migration occurs, it should have been steadily occurring in about the same regional patterns throughout the past 25 years. There are, however, at least three reasons why such an effect might be small or not exist at all.

First, moving costs money. Not only are there actual transportation costs associated with moving, but families that migrate will often have to pay a security deposit for a new apartment, experience some transitional time during which they are neither working nor on AFDC, and bear the myriad of costs associated with relocation to a new city and residence. Low-income families may be least able to bear these moving costs.

Second, families—and particularly low-income women—may lack information about their income opportunities in distant state locations. States do not generally advertise their AFDC benefit levels, and unless women have other sources of information (such as friends or relatives in another location), they may have only a hazy idea about alternative benefit levels.

Third, relocation decisions are affected by many things other than income expectations. In particular, especially for low-income women with children, there may be substantial nonmonetary costs to moving. The presence of family and friends in their current location may provide many benefits: friends and family can provide free baby-sitting services, can be a source of shared resources in hard economic times, and can be an important source of psychological support. In addition, women with children might be quite risk-averse about relocating their children to an unknown low-income neighborhood, with concerns about school, crime, and gangs. For many women, these nonmonetary costs might be large enough that they completely swamp any differences in expected income levels.

These arguments indicate that the expected effects of AFDC benefit levels on migration behavior among low-income women with children are probably small, at least in part because this is a population that one would expect to be less mobile than many others. On the margin, however, one may still expect that AFDC benefits would have a positive effect on migration probabilities.

In order to measure the size of any welfare-induced migration, one ideally would have longitudinal data that track family location decisions. The data would also contain information on women's expectations and their economic opportunities in alternative locations, including not only what they know about alternative AFDC benefit levels in different locations, but also what they know about wage and employment opportunities. The need to have control variables available on non-AFDC economic opportunities is particularly important, since state AFDC benefit levels are positively correlated with state income and wage levels. (This is not surprising, given that only high income states can afford to pay high AFDC benefits and that only states with high wage levels can pay high AFDC benefits without creating large work disincentives.) Finally, the data would contain information on whether women have friends, family, or any other source of support or contacts within alternative state locations. (For example, knowing if a woman or her parents have ever lived in another state would be one way of controlling for the non-monetary costs of choosing a different location.)

Unfortunately, a national data set with such information does not exist. The empirical research has been based on much more limited data, and, as a result, the quality of most the analyses is suspect (see Moffitt, 1992, for a review of the literature). Despite the problems, however, two conclusions are warranted: migration rates among AFDC recipients are quite low, and there is a small positive effect of AFDC benefits on the probability of migrating to (or not migrating out of) a high-benefit state (see, e.g., Blank, 1988; Clark, 1988, 1990, 1992; Gramlich and Laren, 1984; however, Peterson and Rom, 1989, find larger effects). The results are convincing not because any one of the studies is very well done, but because studies done in different ways with very different types of errors all point in the same direction.

The research suggests that welfare-induced migration should be a second-order concern for policy makers. For states that have large populations very close to each other, large benefit differences may indeed induce a migration flow. However, on average, the effects of AFDC benefits on migration are small and movement among the AFDC population is infrequent.

The fact that different states have had long-term AFDC benefit differentials that are very large and have been very large for many years is perhaps further evidence that migration effects are hard to discern in the data. Although states may talk about this problem, high-benefit states have not been concerned enough about it (with a few exceptions) to cut their benefits relative to other states.

There is a lot that is not known about migration effects. There is little or no evidence on the propensity to use AFDC by recent migrants in comparison with natives in a state; on the comparative duration of their AFDC spells if they do become recipients; or on the effects of AFDC benefits on inducing families not currently eligible for AFDC to migrate to a state (i.e., whether people think about "potential safety net" issues). In addition, the growing number of foreign immigrants into the United States may be affected differently by this issue than are native-born U.S. residents.

Summary Overall, it is clear that cash and near-cash assistance programs have negative effects on such behaviors as work effort, although the effects may often be small. These incentive effects can cause a disjuncture between measured need and the amount of assistance program dollars required to alleviate that need. That is, if people who are provided benefits that are intended to move them out of poverty respond in such ways as working less, the net effect will be to leave them in poverty and to require even more funds to move them out of poverty. Because of such behavioral effects, it is misleading to describe the aggregate "poverty gap" (i.e., the difference between the poverty line and a family's resources, aggregated over all families) as the dollar amount that the government would have to spend to eliminate poverty. Because of behavioral responses, an expenditure that should decrease the poverty gap to zero will almost surely fall short. Moreover, the incentive problem is even broader in that program benefits (whether from public assistance programs or social insurance programs, such as unemployment compensation) may lead to reduced work by beneficiaries, even though the poverty gap or other poverty statistic is not affected.

Yet a decision not to provide any type of assistance because there may be some undesired behavioral responses on the part of some program participants is extreme. Such programs as AFDC have their success stories as well as their problems, and, as noted above, behavioral effects, when present, are often small. More fundamentally, there are groups in need—such as children—who are not responsible for their situations but who will suffer if benefits are curtailed.

A program designer, then, faces the very difficult task of specifying benefit levels and other program provisions so as to assist needy people but in a manner that does not encourage behaviors that increase program costs or may otherwise be viewed as dysfunctional and, if possible, that encourages functional behaviors. The task is made more difficult by the fact that research findings on incentive effects are often incomplete or inconclusive.[9] There is also the problem that other aspects of the environment may undercut efforts to provide incentives for increased self-support: for example, there may not be jobs available in the private sector for welfare recipients.

Issues of program incentives have been at the center of policy debate for AFDC, which is directed to families whom the public would like to see increasingly responsible for their own support. Consequently, there has been considerable experimentation with changes in benefit levels and formulas for

---

[9] Indeed, as Citro and Hanushek (1991) note, a major weakness of models that policy analysts use to estimate the likely effects of changes in benefit levels and others features of program design is that the models are not able to properly account for behavioral responses.

calculating disposable income to try to develop effective incentives for recipients to become self-supporting through work and to encourage family stability and better parenting. To date, results show limited effects on such behaviors as work effort from changes in benefit levels and the tax rate on earnings. The evidence is not yet in on more recent state initiatives, such as not increasing benefits when another child is born or reducing benefits if parents do not stay in school or fail to have their children vaccinated. It is important, moreover, to note that other programs besides AFDC raise concerns about incentives. For example, assistance programs for retired or disabled people, such as Social Security and SSI, have negative effects on work effort (see Hurd, 1990; Quinn, Burkhauser, and Myers, 1990; Rust and Phelan, 1993; Wise, 1992).

Federal-State Cost Sharing

In the United States, federal-state cost-sharing provisions have important effects—not always intended—on program benefit levels and the possibilities for changing those levels. For AFDC, the federal government historically has tried to provide incentives to low-income, low-benefit states to raise benefits by picking up a higher share of assistance program costs in these states. However, there has been little effect on states' behavior: low-benefit states have generally opted to minimize their own budget outlays rather than to raise benefits, and, hence, the variation in benefits across states has remained high (see Peterson and Rom, 1990). Similarly, states have taken advantage of the fact that the Food Stamp Program, for which benefits are funded entirely by the federal government, will partly make up for lower AFDC benefit standards.

The current situation in which low-income, low-benefit states receive higher rates of federal reimbursement makes it difficult to devise a politically palatable scheme for raising AFDC benefits to some national minimum standard. A review of one such proposal by the Congressional Budget Office (CBO) (1989a), the Partnership Act of 1987 (introduced in the 100th Congress as S. 862 but never enacted), starkly illuminates the problems.

The Partnership Act proposed to expand the federal role in financing AFDC and Medicaid and to pay for these expansions by eliminating a number of grant-in-aid programs (e.g., Community Services Block Grants and Urban Mass Transit Research). The act provided for a national minimum AFDC benefit standard that, when combined with food stamps, would ultimately reach 90 percent of the federal poverty line for families with no other income. At the same time, the federal matching rate for AFDC benefits up to the minimum standard would be raised to 90 percent.

The evaluation of the federal and state costs of this proposal found that it was not cost-neutral overall as it was intended to be. Rather, if the program had been fully phased in by 1994, CBO (1989a) estimated net costs to the federal government of $38 billion and net savings to the states of $22 billion, for a net increase in federal-state government expenditures of $16 billion. More important, CBO found that the effects would be very uneven across states: states in the South would actually incur net costs rather than savings, and savings would be highest for wealthier states. Low-income, low-benefit states would have to pay more than better-off, more generous states to bring their benefits up to the federal minimum AFDC standard; moreover, those states, with their already higher matching percentages, would gain less from the increased federal matching rate than better-off states. Hence, there would be little incentive for low-income, low-benefit states to support this type of proposal.

Of course, there are other ways in which to combine a national minimum benefit standard for AFDC with a provision for federal-state cost sharing. However, the current structure of the program makes it difficult to devise a scheme that does not increase overall program costs or that does not disadvantage some states relative to others.

Summary

This brief review of some key factors that enter into the design of assistance programs—funding constraints, considerations of the target population, program interactions, incentive effects, and federal-state cost-sharing provisions—makes it clear why it is difficult to link poverty thresholds directly to benefits. To those who are involved in evaluating and designing government assistance programs, our observations will come as no surprise and indeed may seem obvious. Yet we believe it is worth underscoring the point that measuring need, by determining how many people have resources below a reasonable poverty standard, is different from determining the proper societal response to that need.

Many factors properly enter into a determination of program benefit standards, including judgments about the extent to which society is prepared to allocate scarce resources to supporting low-income people and the mix of goals that society wants government assistance programs to serve. The critical role of such judgments is the reason that a panel such as ours, chosen for expertise in measurement issues, cannot make recommendations about appropriate benefit levels for specific assistance programs. Ultimately, the determination of appropriate programs and policies to alleviate poverty involves political choices—namely, the consideration of competing public objectives against the constraints of scarce public resources within the framework of a nation's social and political climate and belief system.

However, the fact that we do not make a recommendation about national minimum benefit standards for AFDC (or other programs) should not be taken to mean that there is no argument for such a benefit standard. On one hand, it is clear that the states differ in their preferences for spending on public assistance, and these preferences should be given weight in any national policy making. On the other hand, there are equity problems in providing needy families with very different levels of public support on the basis of where they happen to live when their economic problems arise. From this perspective, while the proposed poverty measure (or any standard of need) cannot be used by itself to determine benefit levels, it does have a role to play in the policy debate.

DETERMINING STATE
AFDC STANDARDS OF NEED

In most government assistance programs, the benefit standard (i.e., the maximum amount of benefits provided to people with no other income) and the need standard are one and the same: people who are eligible because their countable income falls below the benefit standard are in turn entitled to receive benefits up to the amount of the standard.[10] As noted above, the standard for a particular program reflects judgments about a variety of factors, including appropriate levels of need, constraints on available funds, and the desire to provide positive incentives to recipients.

AFDC is unique in that federal legislation requires each state to establish a standard of need for families with children who have no other means of support, and, in a separate process, to determine a payment standard, which may be lower than the need standard.[11] Both the need standard and the payment standard restrict eligibility for benefits (see below). Furthermore, states may set a maximum benefit amount that is below both the standard of need and the payment standard.

Recommendation

One might surmise that the need standard, as distinct from the payment standard or maximum benefit, is supposed to represent a type of poverty concept. In this case, one might want to consider the use of the proposed poverty measure as the standard.[12] The use of the proposed measure would reduce the current wide disparity in need standards among the states, while recognizing geographic cost-of-living differences. However, it is not clear that the states have typically interpreted the need standard as a poverty concept. Indeed, the role of the need standard in the AFDC program seems

---

[10] Strictly speaking, this statement applies to cash benefit programs (e.g., SSI, veterans' pensions, etc.). Near-cash programs (e.g., food stamps and assisted housing) have a benefit standard that falls below the eligibility standard because the benefit pertains to a single commodity.

[11] See Appendix D for details of the AFDC program.

[12] As discussed below, 14 states link their need standard to the current poverty guidelines.

murky at best, given that states can, and often do, set benefit standards that fall below their need standards.

Since the provision for separately determined need standards exists in the AFDC program, however, we believe it useful to consider the issues involved in the possible use of the proposed poverty measure by the states for this purpose. We begin by describing the basic regulatory framework within which AFDC has operated. We then describe methods of setting need standards that were used in the 1970s and 1980s, current differences in standards and equivalence scales among the states and their relationship to the current poverty line, and trends in need standards and maximum benefits over time. Finally, we discuss the potential relevance of the proposed poverty measure to AFDC need standards. We conclude by encouraging the states to give serious consideration to linking their AFDC need standard to the proposed poverty measure. On balance, that measure would be advantageous for this purpose, although it may need to be modified in some respects.

RECOMMENDATION 8.1. **The states should consider linking their need standard for the Aid to Families with Dependent Children program to the panel's proposed poverty measure and whether it may be necessary to modify this measure to better serve program objectives.**

Program Regulations

AFDC is a state-administered program with funding provided by both the states and the federal government through a matching provision (see Appendix D). In order to qualify for federal funding, a state must establish a standard of need that defines in monetary amounts the basic needs the state wishes to recognize as appropriate for an assistance standard of living—although neither the components of the standard nor the methods for setting the standard are prescribed by federal law or regulation. The state must apply this standard uniformly and statewide in determining financial eligibility for assistance, but it may vary the standard to account for family size or composition, area cost-of-living differentials, or other factors.

States may adopt lower payment standards and maximum benefit amounts than their need standards by such methods as paying a percentage of the difference between the family's income and the need standard, paying a percentage of the need standard, or capping benefits at a specified amount. Recently, a number of states have altered their benefit provisions to satisfy budget constraints and to try to induce recipients to adopt preferred behaviors. As examples, some states no longer provide an additional benefit for an additional child or they condition benefit amounts on such actions as the recipient's obtaining immunization shots for his or her children.[13]

---

[13] See Wiseman (1993) for a list of these kinds of changes in payment standards for which states had waivers from the federal government approved or pending in 1992.

Over the years, amendments to the law, court decisions, and federal regulations have formally reaffirmed the states' autonomy in deciding AFDC benefit levels. In particular, the 1967 amendments to the Social Security Act affirmed the right of states to set benefit maximums and to apply "ratable reductions" in order to set benefits lower than the standard of need. The 1967 amendments included a provision to require states to update their need standard to reflect cost-of-living increases since the standard was adopted; however, states were not required to pay benefits consistent with these increases (for an account of the results of this provision, see Rabin, 1970).

Although the states have very wide latitude in setting their need standard and benefit levels, federal regulations have always been more specific about the resource side of the ledger for determining AFDC eligibility and benefits (see U.S. House of Representatives, 1994:327-331; Solomon and Neisner, 1993). Currently, to receive AFDC payments, a family must pass two income tests. First, the family's gross income cannot be higher than 185 percent of the state's need standard and the family's net or countable income must not exceed 100 percent of the need standard or payment standard, whichever is lower.[14]

Standard Setting in the 1970s

In 1980, Urban Systems Research & Engineering, Inc. (USR&E) completed a study for the Social Security Administration of AFDC standard setting practices, which included a survey of all 50 states and the District of Columbia and case studies of 11 states. USR&E was critical of state practices with regard to standard setting. In part, this criticism stemmed from the viewpoint expressed in the USR&E study that a standard must be "normative" or "absolute," in the sense that an expert standard of need should be developed for each budget component—independent of expenditure patterns—and then priced out. But as we discuss throughout this report, there are other types of poverty or need standards that merit serious consideration, with advantages and disadvantages. However, USR&E seems justifiably to have concluded that relatively few states in the 1970s were following good standard setting practices, in the sense that they developed their need standard as the result of a well-documented, carefully worked-out process or periodically reviewed their standard to determine whether it should be updated or redefined.

USR&E classified the methods originally used by the states to derive their need standard; see Table 8-2.

Market Basket Pricing Studies "The market basket approach, which involves the specification and pricing of every component of need, is the traditional method for conceiving and measuring absolute need, and historically it

---

[14] See Appendix D for details on changes to these percentages over time and on other provisions of AFDC with regard to countable income and assets.

TABLE 8-2 State Approaches to Setting AFDC Need Standards in the 1970s and 1980s

Standard Setting Method	Used in 1970s	Used in 1980s
Local market basket pricing study	Alabama	
	California	
	Colorado	Colorado
	Connecticut	
	Delaware	
		District of Columbia
	Florida	
	Hawaii	
	Idaho	Idaho
	Illinois	
	Indiana	
		Iowa
	Kentucky	
		Louisiana
	Massachusetts	Massachusetts
	Minnesota	
		Missouri
		Montana
	Nebraska	Nebraska
	New Jersey	
	Oklahoma	Oklahoma
	Oregon	Oregon
	Pennsylvania	
	South Carolina	
	South Dakota	
		Utah
		Vermont
	Washington	Washington
Expenditure survey (of AFDC recipients)	New Mexico	
	North Carolina	
	Ohio	
	Tennessee	
	Texas	
	Virginia	
BLS lower level budget (as is or modified)	Maine	Maine
	Maryland	
	New York	New York
		North Carolina
		Pennsylvania
		Tennessee
	Utah	
	Wisconsin	Wisconsin
Multiplier or expenditure ratio		Illinois
	Montana	
		Wyoming
Combination	Georgia	
	Iowa	

continued on next page

TABLE 8-2 *Continued*

Standard Setting Method	Used in 1970s	Used in 1980s
Combination—*continued*	Kansas Michigan Vermont West Virginia	
Legislative determination		Maryland Michigan North Dakota
Average payment		New Hampshire New Jersey Rhode Island
Poverty guidelines (as is or modified)		Alabama Arizona Arkansas Delaware Florida Georgia Hawaii Indiana Kentucky Mississippi Nevada New Mexico Ohio South Carolina
Arbitrary or not available	Alaska Arizona Arkansas District of Columbia Louisiana Mississippi Missouri Nevada New Hampshire North Dakota Rhode Island Wyoming	Alaska California (N.A.) Connecticut Kansas Minnesota (N.A.) South Dakota Texas (N.A.) Virginia West Virginia

SOURCE: Data from Urban Systems Research & Engineering (1980:Exhibits 1 and 2); Larin and Porter (1992:xii).

has been the most popular basis for AFDC need standards" (Urban Systems Research & Engineering, 1980:8); 21 states reported using this approach. However, only three states had standards that were based on pricing studies conducted in the last 10 years (i.e., in 1969-1979), and only one state had updated its standard regularly on the basis of repeated pricing studies to account for cost-of-living increases. USR&E criticized (perhaps too harshly) the practice in the more recent market basket studies of using expenditure surveys to determine the shelter component of the need standard rather than developing a normative standard for shelter and then pricing it out.

Expenditure Surveys   Six states reported basing their standard on expenditure surveys that were limited to AFDC recipients.   USR&E properly criticized this approach as tautological, in that the population for determining the "standard" was based on current program participants.

Lower Level Budget   Five states reported adapting the lower level family budget of the Bureau of Labor Statistics (BLS) as the basis for their need standards, and all of these states had done so as of 1969 or later. USR&E noted correctly that the BLS budgets represented a combination of normative standards and actual expenditure patterns. The states using the BLS lower level budget generally deleted categories they deemed "inappropriate," either on judgmental grounds (e.g., alcoholic beverages) or on grounds that other programs covered the expenditure (e.g., medical care). However, only two of the five states had regularly updated their need standard.

Other   One state used a multiplier approach similar to the Orshansky method for deriving the poverty line; six states used a combination of methods; and twelve states used completely arbitrary methods or methods that could not be ascertained in the USR&E survey.

Standard Setting in the 1980s

The Congressional Research Service regularly tracks changes in the level of the states' need standards and benefit levels (see, e.g., Solomon, 1991; Solomon and Neisner, 1993), but little information was obtained about standard setting practices in the 1980s until recently. In 1992, the Center on Budget and Policy Priorities completed a study for the Administration on Children and Families of AFDC standard setting practices in the late 1980s. This report (Larin and Porter, 1992) was prepared to fulfill the requirement in the 1988 Family Support Act that the states evaluate their AFDC need standard at least once every 3 years and report the results to the Secretary of the Department of Health and Human Services (HHS).

In early 1991 HHS sent the states a questionnaire asking for information on how each state's need standard in effect as of October 1, 1990, was developed, the relationship between the state's need standard and benefit levels, and any changes in the need standard over the preceding 3 years. The Center on Budget and Policy Priorities analyzed the questionnaire responses (California, Minnesota, and Texas did not respond).

Larin and Porter (1992:5) conclude, as did USR&E in its earlier study, that "the majority of states cannot demonstrate that their need standards represent an amount of money necessary to purchase basic necessities." Larin and Porter document and evaluate six types of methods for setting AFDC need standards by the states in effect as of 1990 (see Table 8-2):

Federal Poverty Guidelines   Fourteen states reported relating their need standard in some way to the HHS poverty guidelines.[15] Of these, four states reported using the HHS poverty guidelines as is. Ten states modified the guidelines in such ways as subtracting the cost of the Thrifty Food Plan, subtracting average food stamp and Medicaid benefits, subtracting the cost of "nonessential commodities," setting their need standard as a percentage of the guidelines, or allowing their need standard to decline as a percentage of the guidelines because of not adjusting for inflation.

BLS Lower Level Budget or Living Standard   Six states reported using the BLS lower level budget or living standard—last published in 1982 and developed with expenditure data from the early 1960s—as the basis for their need standards. (Another state was considering the use of a modified lower level budget for its need standard, and the welfare department in another state develops a modified lower level budget as guidance for the state legislature.) Two of the six states modified the BLS standard (e.g., by omitting men's haircuts, household supplies, and occupational costs, as well as making changes to other components of the lower level budget). These states have priced the various budget components by using BLS data or conducting local price surveys; however, none of them has adjusted the standard to keep pace with inflation.

Local Market Basket Surveys   Fourteen states reported basing their need standard on local market basket surveys, but many of these states have not conducted such a survey recently.

Expenditure Ratio (or Multiplier Method)   One state reported using Consumer Expenditure Survey (CEX) data to determine a ratio of all expenditures, other than housing, to apply to the cost of the Thrifty Food Plan. Housing standards were calculated separately on the basis of the actual housing costs of AFDC recipients, with three different standards used for different regions of the state. Another state reported a similar type of method, but developed its multiplier on the basis of CEX data for the lowest quintile of the household income distribution.

---

[15] The HHS poverty guidelines represent a smoothed version of the official poverty thresholds.

Legislative Determination   Three states reported that need standards are set by their legislatures on the basis of budgetary considerations.

Average Payment   Three states reported that they developed need standards in the early 1970s that represented average AFDC payment levels by family size. (AFDC benefits at that time were determined on a discretionary basis by caseworkers according to the particular circumstances of each recipient family.)

Unknown Methods   Six states "are unable to document how their need standards were originally constructed, either because records are incomplete or lost or because their standards seem to have been set arbitrarily with no reference to living costs" (Larin and Porter, 1992:17).

Comparing Larin and Porter (1992) with USR&E (1980), one finds that many states reported using a different method in 1990 than in 1980; see Table 8-2. Only 10 states appear to have used the same method in both decades: Maine, New York, and Wisconsin consistently reported using a variation of the BLS lower level budget, and Colorado, Idaho, Massachusetts, Nebraska, Oklahoma, Oregon, and Washington consistently reported using the market basket pricing method.[16] Perhaps the most important change is that 14 states now relate their need standard explicitly to the HHS poverty guidelines.

Differences Among States

Differences in Need Standards and Benefits

As noted above, AFDC need standards vary widely among the states (see Table 8-1). In January 1994, the need standards for the 50 states and the District of Columbia varied from $1,648 per month in New Hampshire to $320 in Indiana, with a median value of $574, a mean value of $655, and a coefficient of variation of 41 percent. The maximum AFDC benefit exhibited almost as much dispersion, although the addition of food stamps reduced the dispersion somewhat.

In a historical analysis of AFDC benefits, Peterson and Rom (1990:Table 1-1) found that a high degree of variation in benefit levels has always characterized the states. They determined that the coefficient of variation ranged

---

[16] Inferences about standard setting methods across decades cannot be made with certainty. USR&E and Larin and Porter provide conflicting accounts for some states: for example, Arizona is reported as "unknown method" in USR&E, but in Larin and Porter, Arizona is reported as having previously used a variant of the BLS lower level budget and as currently using the HHS poverty guidelines. Similarly, Missouri is reported as "unknown method" in USR&E, but in Larin and Porter, Missouri is reported as having conducted market basket pricing studies in 1969 and 1975. Also, the "average payment" method that Larin and Porter say that several states adopted in the early 1970s is not one of the methods identified in the USR&E study.

between 32 and 35 percent for the average monthly AFDC payment for 1940-1990 and between 34 and 37 percent for the maximum benefit for a four-person family for 1960-1990. The coefficient of variation was smaller for the maximum combined AFDC and food stamp benefit, ranging between 16 and 21 percent for a four-person family for 1970-1990.

In looking at the relationship of the maximum AFDC benefit to the need standard in January 1994 (see Table 8-1), 11 states paid a maximum benefit that represented 100 percent of their need standard; 23 states paid between 50 and 99 percent of their need standard (the median state paid 66 percent of its need standard); and the remaining 17 states paid less than 50 percent of their need standard, including 6 states that paid less than 33 percent of their need standard.

In looking at the adequacy of AFDC need standards and benefits against the official poverty threshold, 8 states had need standards in January 1994 that were at or above the 1993 official average weighted poverty threshold for a family of three, and 12 states had need standards that were between 70 and 99 percent of the poverty level; see Table 8-3. The remainder had need standards that were below 70 percent of the poverty level. In no state did the maximum AFDC benefit exceed the poverty level, and in only two states did the maximum benefit exceed 70 percent of the poverty level. With the addition of food stamps, the maximum combined benefit exceeded the poverty level in 2 states and was between 70 and 99 percent of the poverty level in 22 states.

In looking at the disparities in AFDC need standards and benefit levels, one obvious question is whether they are related to differences in needs and costs of living across states. We constructed an index of the adjustments by state to a national poverty threshold that would result from taking account of differences in the cost of housing. We analyzed 1990 census data to determine cost-of-housing index values by state (relative to a national value of 1.00) and then adjusted each index value downwards by a factor reflecting the proportion that shelter costs (including utilities) represent of the proposed poverty thresholds. (The methodology was the same that we used to determine adjusted cost-of-housing index values by region and size of metropolitan area for the statistical poverty measure; see Chapter 3). We also constructed an index of state median family income from 1990 census tabulations (Bureau of the Census, no date(b)) relative to 1.00 for the average median family income across the states. Not surprisingly, the index of state-adjusted poverty thresholds shows less variation than does the index of median family income; see Table 8-4. The state-adjusted poverty threshold index values range from 24 percent above to 15 percent below the national average, with a coefficient of variation of 10 percent.[17] The median family income index values range from

---

[17] The coefficient of variation of 10 percent for the state-adjusted poverty threshold index is similar to that of 8 percent for a state cost-of-living index developed by Peterson and Rom

TABLE 8-3 AFDC Need Standards, Maximum AFDC Benefits, and Maximum Combined AFDC and Food Stamp Benefits for a Family of Three, as a Percentage of the 1993 Weighted Average Monthly Poverty Threshold, January 1994

| State | Percent of Poverty Threshold | | |
	AFDC Need Standard	Maximum AFDC Benefit	Maximum Combined AFDC/Food Stamp Benefit
Alabama	70	17	48
Alaska	81	77	101
Arizona	100	36	67
Arkansas	73	21	52
California	74	63	86
Colorado	44	37	67
Connecticut	71	71	91
Delaware	35	35	66
District of Columbia	74	44	72
Florida	103	32	62
Georgia	44	29	60
Hawaii	103	64	103
Idaho	103	33	64
Illinois	93	38	69
Indiana	33	30	61
Iowa	88	44	72
Kansas	45	45	74
Kentucky	55	24	54
Louisiana	69	20	51
Maine	58	44	72
Maryland	53	38	69
Massachusetts	60	60	83
Michigan[a]	57	48	75
Minnesota	55	55	80
Mississippi	38	13	43
Missouri	88	30	61
Montana	53	42	71
Nebraska	38	38	68
Nevada	73	36	67
New Hampshire	172	57	81
New Jersey	103	44	73
New Mexico	37	37	67
New York[b]	60	60	85
North Carolina	57	28	59
North Dakota	43	43	71
Ohio	92	36	66
Oklahoma	49	34	64
Oregon	48	48	78
Pennsylvania	64	44	72
Rhode Island	58	58	86

continued on next page

TABLE 8-3 *Continued*

State	Percent of Poverty Threshold		
	AFDC Need Standard	Maximum AFDC Benefit	Maximum Combined AFDC/Food Stamp Benefit
South Carolina	46	21	52
South Dakota	51	43	72
Tennessee	44	19	50
Texas	60	19	50
Utah	58	43	71
Vermont	117	68	88
Virginia	41	37	67
Washington	121	57	84
West Virginia	52	26	57
Wisconsin	67	54	79
Wyoming	70	38	68
Mean	67	41	70
Median	60	38	69
Range	35–172	13–77	43–103
Coefficient of variation[c]	39.9%	36.4%	18.6%

SOURCE: U.S. House of Representatives (1994:366-367).

NOTE: The 1993 weighted average monthly poverty threshold for a family of three was $960 (the Census Bureau's annual figure of $11,521, divided by 12); this threshold was increased by 25 percent for Alaska and by 15 percent for Hawaii (as is done for the poverty guidelines but not the official thresholds).

[a]The values apply to Wayne County.
[b]The values apply to New York City.
[c]The standard deviation of the distribution as a percentage of the mean value.

43 percent above to 29 percent below the national average with a coefficient of variation of 17 percent.

We then divided each state's AFDC need standard, maximum benefit, and combined maximum AFDC and food stamp benefit as of January 1994 by the appropriate state-adjusted poverty threshold index value and the appropriate median family income index value.[18] If differences in the cost of living

(1990:Table 1-2). Their index averaged cost-of-living indicators for 1985 developed by the American Chamber of Commerce Researchers Association for all the cities in each state, weighted by city population size.

[18] State median family income (or a state-adjusted poverty threshold) could have changed between the 1990 census and January 1994; however, the results of the same set of calculations using January 1991 values for AFDC need standards, maximum benefits, and combined maximum AFDC and food stamp benefits were very similar to those reported for the January 1994 values.

TABLE 8-4   State Median Family Income and State-Adjusted Poverty Thresholds under the Panel's Proposed Measure

State	Index for State Median Family Income	Index for State-Adjusted Poverty Thresholds with the Proposed Measure
Alabama	0.835	0.881
Alaska	1.355	1.102
Arizona	0.936	1.017
Arkansas	0.739	0.873
California	1.180	1.178
Colorado	1.046	0.973
Connecticut	1.431	1.188
Delaware	1.172	1.066
District of Columbia	1.055	1.112
Florida	0.937	1.049
Georgia	0.976	0.993
Hawaii	1.256	1.243
Idaho	0.858	0.862
Illinois	1.126	1.020
Indiana	0.992	0.949
Iowa	0.921	0.903
Kansas	0.959	0.926
Kentucky	0.787	0.874
Louisiana	0.766	0.902
Maine	0.943	1.029
Maryland	1.310	1.106
Massachusetts	1.291	1.191
Michigan	1.066	0.998
Minnesota	1.074	1.023
Mississippi	0.712	0.853
Missouri	0.927	0.929
Montana	0.816	0.865
Nebraska	0.920	0.908
Nevada	1.043	1.078
New Hampshire	1.211	1.122
New Jersey	1.385	1.202
New Mexico	0.804	0.922
New York	1.156	1.078
North Carolina	0.918	0.940
North Dakota	0.836	0.872
Ohio	1.000	0.955
Oklahoma	0.831	0.883
Oregon	0.941	0.964
Pennsylvania	1.014	0.987
Rhode Island	1.140	1.099
South Carolina	0.897	0.936
South Dakota	0.804	0.872
Tennessee	0.860	0.920

continued on next page

TABLE 8-4 *Continued*

State	Index for State Median Family Income	Index for State-Adjusted Poverty Thresholds with the Proposed Measure
Texas	0.919	0.963
Utah	0.967	0.900
Vermont	1.012	1.060
Virginia	1.112	1.023
Washington	1.071	1.011
West Virginia	0.745	0.846
Wisconsin	1.021	0.965
Wyoming	0.937	0.863
U.S. average	1.000	1.000
Range	0.712–1.431	0.846–1.243
Coefficient of variation[a]	17.3%	10.3%

NOTE: See text and Chapter 3 for explanation of construction of the indexes.

[a]The standard deviation of a distribution as a percentage of the mean value.

across states (as proxied by cost-of-housing differences in the poverty threshold) are the only reason for the differences in need standards and benefit levels, then the calculation with state-adjusted poverty threshold index values should result in the same (or close to the same) dollar amounts of the need standard and maximum benefit in all states. In other words, the amounts in high-cost, high-benefit states would decrease to the mean and the amounts in low-cost, low-benefit states would increase to the mean. The same reasoning applies to the calculation with state median family income index values.

These patterns do not occur. There is only a modest effect on the variation across states in AFDC need standards when differences in the cost of living or median family income are taken out of the dollar amounts: the coefficient of variation is reduced from 41 percent to 37 percent; see Table 8-5. For maximum AFDC benefits and maximum combined AFDC and food stamp benefits, there is a somewhat greater reduction in the variation across states: the coefficient of variation for maximum AFDC benefits is reduced from 40 percent to 29-33 percent, and the coefficient of variation for maximum combined AFDC and food stamp benefits is reduced from 22 percent to 15-16 percent. However, even in the case of maximum combined AFDC and food stamp benefits, significant variation remains that cannot be explained by differences in cost of living or income levels across the states.

TABLE 8-5 Mean and Distribution of State AFDC Need Standards, Maximum AFDC Benefits, and Maximum Combined AFDC and Food Stamp Benefits for a Family of Three, as Reported by the States and as Adjusted for Differences in Income and Cost of Housing, January 1994, in Dollars

| | | As Adjusted by an Index for | |
Statistic	As Reported	State Median Family Income	State-Adjusted Poverty Threshold[a]
AFDC Need Standards			
Mean	655	658	657
Range	320–1,648	288–1,361	317–1,469
Standard deviation[b]	267	240	242
Coefficient of variation[c]	40.7%	36.5%	36.8%
AFDC Maximum Benefits			
Mean	396	389	394
Range	120–923	169–681	141–838
Standard deviation	156	113	130
Coefficient of variation	39.5%	29.2%	33.1%
AFDC and Food Stamp Maximum Benefits			
Mean	675	677	679
Range	415–1,208	505–892	521–1,096
Standard deviation	147	98	111
Coefficient of variation	21.8%	14.5%	16.3%

NOTE: Data derived from Tables 8-1 and 8-4; see text for description of calculations.

[a]The state-adjusted poverty threshold takes account of state differences in cost of housing adjusted for the share that shelter costs (including utilities) represent in the panel's proposed poverty budget.

[b]The value that when added to or subtracted from the mean includes about two-thirds of the observations (states).

[c]The standard deviation as a percentage of the mean value.

Differences in Equivalence Scales

Equivalence scales—the proportion by which benefits to the AFDC unit are increased for each added child—also vary across states; see Table 8-6.[19] Data are available on the maximum AFDC benefit by family size as of January 1994 for the 50 states and the District of Columbia, ranging from the basic two-person unit (parent or other caretaker and child) through the six-person unit

---

[19] As noted above, some states do not currently pay benefits for additional children beyond the first or second, as an intended deterrent to continued childbearing on the part of AFDC recipients.

TABLE 8-6   Equivalence Scale Implicit in Maximum AFDC Benefits for Two-Person Through Six-Person Families, January 1994

State	Second Child (3-Person Family)	Third Child (4-Person Family)	Fourth Child (5-Person Family)	Fifth Child (6-Person Family)	Average, Added Child
	Amount Added to Two-Person (One-Adult/One-Child) Benefit (1.00) for Each Added Child				
Alabama	.197	.219	.226	.197	.210
Alaska	.124	.124	.124	.124	.124
Arizona	.262	.258	.258	.262	.260
Arkansas	.259	.265	.241	.278	.261
California	.239	.237	.206	.208	.222
Colorado	.271	.271	.286	.279	.277
Connecticut	.239	.204	.184	.193	.205
Delaware	.252	.256	.252	.256	.254
District of Columbia	.273	.282	.236	.315	.277
Florida	.257	.253	.257	.253	.255
Georgia	.191	.213	.204	.136	.186
Hawaii	.260	.260	.260	.260	.260
Idaho	.263	.259	.263	.259	.261
Illinois	.369	.175	.265	.224	.258
Indiana	.258	.253	.258	.253	.255
Iowa	.180	.191	.147	.172	.172
Kansas	.219	.193	.173	.173	.190
Kentucky	.163	.291	.245	.219	.230
Louisiana	.377	.319	.312	.283	.322
Maine	.340	.346	.340	.343	.342
Maryland	.280	.262	.245	.178	.241
Massachusetts	.191	.183	.189	.193	.189
Michigan	.237	.280	.259	.358	.284
Minnesota	.217	.204	.174	.174	.192
Mississippi	.250	.250	.250	.250	.250
Missouri	.248	.214	.197	.184	.210
Montana	.261	.261	.261	.261	.261
Nebraska	.242	.242	.242	.242	.242
Nevada	.208	.208	.208	.205	.207
New Hampshire	.143	.131	.125	.168	.142
New Jersey	.317	.199	.199	.199	.228
New Mexico	.261	.261	.258	.261	.261
New York	.233	.235	.241	.179	.222
North Carolina	.153	.106	.114	.106	.120
North Dakota	.228	.276	.204	.177	.221
Ohio	.222	.287	.258	.201	.242
Oklahoma	.291	.311	.271	.271	.286
Oregon	.165	.266	.241	.241	.228
Pennsylvania	.276	.282	.282	.242	.270
Rhode Island	.234	.174	.174	.200	.195

TABLE 8-6 *Continued*

| State | Amount Added to Two-Person (One-Adult/One-Child) Benefit (1.00) for Each Added Child | | | | |
	Second Child (3-Person Family)	Third Child (4-Person Family)	Fourth Child (5-Person Family)	Fifth Child (6-Person Family)	Average, Added Child
South Carolina	.258	.252	.258	.252	.255
South Dakota	.133	.128	.130	.130	.130
Tennessee	.303	.289	.268	.289	.287
Texas	.165	.234	.158	.241	.199
Utah	.247	.211	.202	.169	.207
Vermont	.190	.147	.162	.104	.151
Virginia	.204	.190	.265	.102	.190
Washington	.241	.218	.223	.230	.228
West Virginia	.239	.313	.239	.264	.264
Wisconsin	.175	.227	.207	.132	.185
Wyoming	.125	.094	.188	.188	.148
Mean	.234	.231	.224	.217	.227
Median	.239	.242	.241	.219	.228
Range	.124–.377	.094–.346	.114–.340	.102–.358	.120–.342
Coefficient of variation[a]	24.0%	24.2%	22.0%	27.1%	21.5%
Current poverty measure	.169	.307	.229	.197	.226
Panel's proposed equivalence scale— alternative 1[b]	.295	.275	.256	.248	.269
Panel's proposed equivalence scale— alternative 2[c]	.255	.227	.206	.199	.222

NOTE: Data calculated from U.S. House of Representatives (1994:368-369) for each state; calculated from Bureau of the Census (1993c:Table A) for the current poverty measure.

[a]The standard deviation of a distribution as a percentage of the mean value.
[b]Scale economy factor of 0.75.
[c]Scale economy factor of 0.65.

(basic unit plus four added children). At one extreme, Louisiana increases its $138 benefit for the basic two-person unit by 32 percent on average ($44) for each additional child. At the other extreme, Alaska increases its much higher benefit of $821 for the basic unit by only 12 percent ($102) for each additional child. The median value that is added on average to the basic unit benefit for each added child is 23 percent.[20]

In looking at the shape of the equivalence scales for AFDC benefits, five states have a regular pattern whereby, within 1 or 2 percentage points, they add the same amount to the basic unit benefit for each additional child; 10 other states have a regular pattern within 6 percentage points. Ten states have a declining pattern, whereby they add progressively less for each child after the second or third. In contrast, 10 states add more for the third and fourth child than for either the second or fifth. Finally, 16 states have erratic patterns. For instance, they may add more for the third and fifth children than for the second and fourth. In this, they resemble the equivalence scale implicit in the current U.S. poverty measure, in which the second child adds 17 percent to the two-person (one-adult/one-child) poverty threshold, the third child adds 31 percent, the fourth child adds 23 percent, and the fifth child adds 20 percent.[21]

The type of equivalence scale that we recommend for the poverty measure would increase the benefit for a one-adult/one-child family the most for the second child, with declining percentages for each additional child to reflect household economies of scale. Depending on the value of the scale economy factor, our proposed equivalence scale would add an average of 27 percent (using a factor of 0.75) or an average of 22 percent (using a factor of 0.65) to the basic unit benefit for each additional child.

Trends in Need Standards and Benefits

Looking at trends over the last two decades, it appears that relatively few states have increased their need standard or maximum benefit to keep up with inflation. Relatively few states have statutes that require them to adjust their standards for inflation, and even those states that have such requirements do not always heed them in periods of budget stringency. As of 1988, seven states had statutory requirements for adjusting their need standard to keep up with inflation, one state had a requirement to update its benefit level, and three

---

[20] Note that the ratios of the benefit for an added child to the benefit for the basic AFDC unit are not comparable to equivalence scales expressed in terms of a one-person family or household. Such scales can be constructed for January 1994 from U.S. House of Representatives (1994:368-369).

[21] The average value added per child to the U.S. poverty threshold for the two-person (one-adult/one-child) family is 23 percent, the same as the median value for the 50 states and the District of Columbia.

states had requirements to update both their need standard and their benefit levels; only one state apparently had a requirement to periodically reevaluate the need standard itself (Center on Social Welfare Policy and Law, 1988).

In the 1970s, inflation rose significantly—by 111 percent (as measured by the CPI-U). Yet only four states increased the value of their need standard in real dollar terms during this period, and the median state saw its need standard decline by 38 percent (in real terms); see Table 8-7. The decline in real terms in the value of the maximum benefit in the median state was somewhat less— 26 percent; see Table 8-8. As a result, the number of states paying "full need" doubled over the period (from 14 to 29 states), and the number paying 70 percent or more of need increased from 33 to 44 states.

In the 1980s, inflation moderated—increasing by 63 percent—and 26 states increased the value of their need standard to keep up with or exceed the rate of inflation. In the median state the need standard remained constant in real dollar terms. Many states updated their need standard after the passage of the 1981 Omnibus Budget Reconciliation Act, which included a provision that families could not be eligible for AFDC benefits if their gross income exceeded 150 percent (later raised to 185 percent) of the state need standard. In this way, states were able to avoid denying eligibility to families with earnings who would otherwise have been above the gross income cutoff although below the net income cutoff after allowable deductions. However, states did not necessarily update their benefit level to match: for example, Alabama doubled its need standard between 1980 and 1985 but did not raise its maximum benefit (see U.S. House of Representatives, 1991:601-605). Indeed, in the median state the maximum benefit declined by 22 percent. From 1980 to 1991 the number of states paying full need dropped from 29 to 16, and the number paying 70 percent or more of need dropped from 44 to 27 states.

In looking at the whole time span, the need standard declined in real terms in the median state by 33 percent from 1970 to 1991, and the maximum benefit declined in real terms by 38 percent.[22] One consequence of declining AFDC benefits over the period was that food stamps (which are indexed yearly for inflation) accounted for an increasing proportion of the combined AFDC and food stamps benefit. This change reduced the financial burden on the states, since the federal government pays the full cost of food stamps.

Conclusions

Clearly, a persistent characteristic of the AFDC program has been the great variation in need standards (and benefit levels) among the states—variation

---

[22] The median state's need standard remained approximately constant in real terms from January 1991 to January 1994, while the median state's maximum AFDC benefit continued to decline (see U.S. House of Representatives, 1994:Tables 10-13, 10-14).

TABLE 8-7 AFDC Need Standards for a Family of Three, July 1970, July 1980, and January 1991, in Constant (January 1991) Dollars

State	AFDC Need Standard (in January 1991 dollars)			Percentage Change		
	July 1970	July 1980	Jan. 1991	1970–1980	1980–1991	1970–1991
Alabama	635	313	603	−51	93	−5
Alaska	1,208	745	891	−38	20	−26
Arizona	731	380	621	−48	63	−15
Arkansas	514	381	705	−26	85	37
California	1,211	782	694	−35	−11	−43
Colorado	666	473	421	−29	−11	−37
Connecticut	976	774	680	−21	−12	−30
Delaware	845	434	338	−49	−22	−60
District of Columbia	790	642	712	−19	11	−10
Florida	652	318	880	−51	177	35
Georgia	611	315	424	−48	35	−31
Hawaii	780	763	1,012	−2	33	30
Idaho	821	605	554	−26	−8	−33
Illinois	800	469	811	−41	73	1
Indiana	938	500	320	−47	−36	−66
Iowa	852	587	497	−31	−15	−42
Kansas	838	562	409	−33	−27	−51
Kentucky	718	306	526	−57	72	−27
Louisiana	593	655	658	10	0	11
Maine	956	676	652	−29	−4	−32
Maryland	859	440	562	−49	28	−35
Massachusetts	925	618	539	−33	−13	−42
Michigan[a]	756	693	586	−8	−15	−22
Minnesota	883	680	532	−23	−22	−40
Mississippi	697	359	368	−48	3	−47
Missouri	983	509	312	−48	−39	−68
Montana	762	422	453	−45	7	−41
Nebraska	969	505	364	−48	−28	−62
Nevada	928	465	550	−50	18	−41
New Hampshire	904	564	516	−38	−9	−43
New Jersey	1,042	587	424	−44	−28	−59
New Mexico	576	359	310	−38	−14	−46
New York[b]	963	642	577	−33	−10	−40
North Carolina	580	313	544	−46	74	−6
North Dakota	800	544	401	−32	−26	−50
Ohio	714	564	776	−21	38	9
Oklahoma	618	460	471	−26	2	−24
Oregon	790	460	444	−42	−3	−44
Pennsylvania	914	541	614	−41	13	−33
Rhode Island	790	554	554	−30	0	−30
South Carolina	559	305	440	−45	44	−21
South Dakota	911	523	385	−43	−26	−58
Tennessee	618	292	412	−53	41	−33

TABLE 8-7 *Continued*

State	AFDC Need Standard (in January 1991 dollars)			Percentage Change		
	July 1970	July 1980	Jan. 1991	1970–1980	1980–1991	1970–1991
Texas	683	253	574	−63	127	−16
Utah	769	782	537	2	−31	−30
Vermont	990	1,092	1,029	10	−6	4
Virginia	828	561	393	−32	−30	−53
Washington	890	747	983	−16	32	10
West Virginia	759	448	497	−41	11	−35
Wisconsin	738	851	647	15	−24	−12
Wyoming	849	513	674	−40	31	−21
Mean	807	536	566	−34	13	−28
Median	800	513	544	−38	0	−33
Range	514–1,211	253–1,092	310–1,029	(−63)–15	(−39)–177	(−68)–37
Coefficient of variation[c]	18.9%	31.7%	31.3%	51.8%	337.3%	88.7%

NOTES: Data calculated from U.S. House of Representatives (1991:602-605). The adjustment to constant January 1991 dollars was made using the values for the urban Consumer Price Index (CPI-U).

[a]The values apply to Wayne County.
[b]The values apply to New York City.
[c]The standard deviation of a distribution as a percentage of the mean value.

that considerably exceeds estimated differences in the cost of living across states. Another characteristic has been the absence in many states of systematic procedures for setting and periodically revising the AFDC need standard.

A fundamental question is whether the concept of a separate need standard makes sense: most assistance programs do not distinguish between a need standard and the maximum benefit the program will pay to participants with no other source of support. Limits on gross as well as countable income in these programs (e.g., SSI) are set as a function of the benefit standard, and such a practice could be followed in AFDC as well.

Urban Systems Research & Engineering (1980:22) argued that the AFDC need standard serves the useful function of a goal or benchmark and that need standards are not an exercise in futility:

> *The systematic derivation and conscientious maintenance of normative standards of need can lead not only to higher need standards, but also to higher payment levels than would be achieved in the absence of any commitment to a realistic benchmark of adequacy* [emphasis in original].

TABLE 8-8 AFDC Maximum Benefits for a Family of Three, July 1970, July 1980, and January 1991, in Constant (January 1991) Dollars

State	July 1970 Max. AFDC Ben.	July 1970 Percent of Need Std.	July 1980 Max. AFDC Ben.	July 1980 Percent of Need Std.	January 1991 Max. AFDC Ben.	January 1991 Percent of Need Std.	Percentage Change 1970–1980	Percentage Change 1980–1991	Percentage Change 1970–1991
Alabama	224	35	192	61	124	21	−14	−35	−45
Alaska	1,132	94	745	100	891	100	−34	−20	−21
Arizona	476	65	329	87	293	47	−31	−11	−38
Arkansas	307	60	262	69	204	29	−15	−22	−34
California	642	53	771	99	694	100	20	−10	8
Colorado	666	100	473	100	356	85	−29	−25	−47
Connecticut	976	100	774	100	680	100	−21	−12	−30
Delaware	552	65	434	100	338	100	−21	−22	−39
District of Columbia	673	85	466	73	428	60	−31	−8	−36
Florida	393	60	318	100	294	33	−19	−8	−25
Georgia	369	60	267	85	280	66	−28	5	−24
Hawaii	780	100	763	100	632	62	−2	−17	−19
Idaho	728	89	526	87	317	57	−28	−40	−56
Illinois	800	100	469	100	367	45	−41	−22	−54
Indiana	414	44	416	83	288	90	0	−31	−30
Iowa	693	81	587	100	426	86	−15	−27	−39
Kansas	766	91	562	100	409	100	−27	−27	−47
Kentucky	507	71	306	100	228	43	−40	−25	−55
Louisiana	304	51	248	38	190	29	−18	−23	−37
Maine	466	49	456	68	453	69	−2	−1	−3
Maryland	559	65	440	100	406	72	−21	−8	−27
Massachusetts	925	100	618	100	539	100	−33	−13	−42
Michigan[a]	756	100	693	100	525	90	−8	−24	−31
Minnesota	883	100	680	100	532	100	−23	−22	−40
Mississippi	193	28	156	43	120	33	−19	−23	−38
Missouri	359	37	404	80	292	94	13	−28	−19
Montana	697	91	422	100	370	82	−39	−12	−47

Nebraska	590	61	505	100	364	100	−14	−28	−38
Nevada	417	45	427	92	330	60	2	−23	−21
New Hampshire	904	100	564	100	516	100	−38	−9	−43
New Jersey	1,042	100	587	100	424	100	−44	−28	−59
New Mexico	514	89	359	100	310	100	−30	−14	−40
New York[b]	963	100	642	100	577	100	−33	−10	−40
North Carolina	500	86	313	100	272	50	−37	−13	−46
North Dakota	735	92	544	100	401	100	−26	−26	−45
Ohio	555	78	429	76	334	43	−22	−22	−40
Oklahoma	524	85	460	100	341	72	−12	−26	−35
Oregon	635	80	460	100	444	100	−28	−3	−30
Pennsylvania	914	100	541	100	421	69	−41	−22	−54
Rhode Island	790	100	554	100	554	100	−30	0	−30
South Carolina	293	52	210	69	210	48	−28	0	−28
South Dakota	911	100	523	100	385	100	−43	−26	−58
Tennessee	386	62	199	68	195	47	−48	−2	−49
Texas	511	75	189	75	184	32	−63	−3	−64
Utah	604	79	587	75	402	75	−3	−32	−33
Vermont	921	93	802	73	679	66	−13	−15	−26
Virginia	776	94	505	90	354	90	−35	−30	−54
Washington	890	100	747	100	531	54	−16	−29	−40
West Virginia	393	52	336	75	249	50	−15	−26	−37
Wisconsin	635	86	724	85	517	80	14	−29	−19
Wyoming	735	87	513	100	360	53	−30	−30	−51
Mean	635	78	480	89	393	72	−23	−18	−37
Median	635	85	469	100	367	72	−26	−22	−38
Range	193–1,132	28–100	157–807	38–100	120–891	21–100	(−63)–20	(−40)–20	(−64)–8
Coefficient of variation[c]	35.5%	27.0%	35.6%	17.3%	39.5%	34.7%	71.4%	65.2%	37.1%

NOTES: Data calculated from U.S. House of Representatives (1991:602–605). The adjustment to constant January 1991 dollars was made using the CPI-U.

[a] The values apply to Wayne County.
[b] The values apply to New York City.
[c] The standard deviation of a distribution as a percentage of the mean value.

USR&E based this argument on the behavior of the subset of states that either made a conscientious effort during the 1970s to set normative standards or, although not having recently established a systematically derived need standard, had committed themselves to maintaining the value of their need standard in real terms. These states as a group increased both their need standard and their benefit level more than other states in the 1969-1979 period. However, it seems to us as likely or more likely that a common set of factors (e.g., a more supportive attitude toward welfare programs) explains the propensity to raise both need and benefit standards in some states rather than that higher need standards in and of themselves cause states to raise their benefits.

We do not offer a recommendation about the merits of having a separate need standard in the AFDC program, although we are among those who find the concept of questionable utility. Welfare policy is currently the subject of intense debate, and the AFDC program as it has operated historically may likely change in significant ways, perhaps rendering moot the issue of the soundness or adequacy of the need standard for the existing program. However, given that current law requires states to set need standards (and allows them to have lower benefit standards), our concern is whether it makes sense for states to adopt the proposed poverty measure in place of their own standard.

A recent development in standard setting practices with relevance to this issue is that, in the past decade, 14 states have explicitly geared their need standard to the current poverty guidelines, which derive from the official thresholds. In many of these states, the link is more theoretical than actual, in that the need standard, either by law or regulation or because of failure to adjust for inflation, is a small fraction of the poverty guidelines. In other states, the definition of the poverty guidelines has been altered to exclude some types of consumption. Overall, however, a growing number of states are finding it convenient to link their AFDC need standard to the poverty guidelines in some fashion.

We recommend that states that tie their AFDC need standard to the current poverty measure consider the use of the proposed measure instead, and we encourage all of the states to make a similar assessment. The Family Support Act requires states to review their need standard every 3 years and report to HHS. We note that HHS could request the states to complete an assessment that considers the possible use of the proposed poverty measure for inclusion in their next regular reports.

An important element of such a review is an assessment of the implications of the proposed measure—both the thresholds and the definition of family resources—in relation to a state's current need standard (whether the poverty guidelines or its own standard) and the rules for determining gross and net income. Also important to consider is whether the proposed measure may need to be modified in one or more respects to be more suitable for program purposes. Finally, it is important to keep in mind the need for consistency between the thresholds and the resource definition in whatever measure a state uses.

Comparative Advantage of the Proposed Poverty Measure

The use of the proposed threshold concept to set state need standards of AFDC would represent an improvement over the current measure in several respects. One improvement relates to the equivalence scale by which the reference family poverty threshold is adjusted to take account of different needs for different types of families: the proposed scale is more reasonable than that embedded in the official thresholds.

Another improvement is that the proposed threshold concept incorporates geographic variation in housing costs. For the statistical measure of poverty, we recommended that the thresholds vary by nine regions and several categories of size of metropolitan area within region (see Chapter 3). States may want to use thresholds that are specific to their state as a whole, and it is certainly feasible to develop such thresholds from decennial census data (see Table 8-4). Alternatively, states may want to have thresholds that vary by size of metropolitan area (or other geographic unit) within the state, and it is also feasible to develop such thresholds from census data. We caution against making further distinctions, particularly for small metropolitan or other areas, as the sample sizes underlying the estimates can become uncomfortably small. Thus, for many metropolitan areas under about 125,000 population, there are only 200-300 cases of housing units in the 1990 decennial census data with the specified characteristics that are used to estimate geographic differences in housing costs. The Census Bureau and Bureau of Labor Statistics could assist the states by constructing thresholds by state and by substate area and by providing estimates of the sampling error underlying the geographic indexes. The states could then determine whether there is enough intrastate variation and whether the estimates of that variation are sufficiently reliable to warrant using several different thresholds.

Finally, an important improvement is that we propose a consistent budget concept and definition of family resources. Moreover, the proposed resource definition is more congruent with the income definition in the AFDC program than is the current gross money income definition, so it would be more consistent to use the proposed threshold concept in place of the current concept. For example, the AFDC definition of countable income deducts child care and other work expenses. It does not deduct out-of-pocket medical care expenditures, but AFDC recipients are automatically eligible for Medicaid, which limits their out-of-pocket expenditures (although the generosity of the program varies among states). There are also some inconsistencies. For example, the EITC and a few other sources of income may not be counted as income in the AFDC program. Also, in-kind benefits are not counted as income (see further discussion below). Overall, however, the income definition in concept (if not necessarily in the specific details, such as the amount allowed for child care or work expenses) is quite consistent with the budget concept that underlies the proposed poverty thresholds and definition of family resources.

Problematic Aspects of the Proposed Poverty Measure

Program Interactions   One issue that arises with the use of the proposed threshold concept (or the current concept, for that matter) is that AFDC is not the only program of basic consumption support for low-income families. Specifically, such programs as food stamps, school meals, public housing, and home energy assistance provide important components of consumption for many AFDC families—kinds of consumption that are included in the need concepts that underlie both the current poverty measure and the proposed alternative.

Currently, a few of the states that tie their need standard to the HHS poverty guidelines attempt to take account of interaction effects with other assistance programs by subtracting food or food and medical care costs from the guidelines in order to form their AFDC need standard. However, such adjustments are not necessarily appropriate, even when the need standard would otherwise equal the poverty thresholds.[23]

With regard to medical care, the official poverty thresholds arguably do not include medical expenses that would be covered by Medicaid or other health insurance; the proposed thresholds do not include such expenses either (see Chapter 4). Hence, to subtract Medicaid from the poverty guidelines—or from thresholds developed under the proposed measure—is to assume that such benefits are fungible and can be used for other needed goods, when this is not generally the case.

There is a clearer case for subtracting food stamps from the poverty thresholds to form AFDC need standards, particularly since food stamps are not counted as income for computing AFDC benefits. However, as we noted earlier, the way in which food stamp benefits are computed—specifically, the assumption that 30 percent of countable income (including AFDC benefits) will be available for food consumption—means that it is not straightforward to determine an appropriate adjustment. To subtract the entire value of the Thrifty Food Plan from the poverty thresholds would likely result in too great

---

[23] Logically, such adjustments should not even be considered when the need standard is set at a fraction of the poverty thresholds, as is the case in a number of states. See Larin and Porter (1992) for a discussion of the problems in adjusting the current poverty guidelines to try to account for program interactions.

a reduction in the AFDC need standard; how much less than that amount might be appropriate is open to question.

Clearly, the issue of program interactions is a very difficult one. It may make most sense for the states to think of the AFDC need standard as a global standard, and then address program interaction questions in determining AFDC benefit levels.

Implications of Updating for Costs and Caseloads Another important issue with the possible use of the proposed poverty measure to determine AFDC need standards concerns the proposed procedure for updating the thresholds. As we have stressed, thresholds developed under that procedure will reflect real increases in basic consumption, not just price changes. The use of thresholds updated in this manner offers the advantage that states would not have to periodically evaluate their need standard for real changes in living standards. Although few states have historically sought to revise their standard on any regular basis, there are some exceptions, and the Family Support Act now requires states to evaluate their need standard at least once every 3 years and to report the results to HHS.

However, with the proposed procedure, the states would face concerns about possibly larger caseloads and higher costs compared with the use of the current poverty guidelines (see Chapter 7). One way in which the need standard is linked to eligibility for AFDC—and, hence, potentially to caseloads and the costs associated with changes in caseloads—is through federal law. The effects of this link may be relatively minor because the tie, strictly speaking, is only to gross income. Families with gross incomes that do not exceed 185 percent of the need standard may be eligible, but only if their *net* income does not exceed the payment standard. Hence, in states that do not raise their payment standard, increases in the need standard that result from the use of the proposed procedure will not necessarily add to caseloads or costs.[24]

More important effects on costs and caseloads may stem from the links that state laws provide between the need standards and the determination of net income eligibility and benefits. These links are more or less direct, depending on which of several methods a state uses to calculate eligibility and benefits; for some examples of how changes in need standards can affect families' eligibility status and benefits depending on the method used by the state, see Figure 8-1.

---

[24] The adoption of higher need standards could cause some families with very high deductions from gross income to become eligible, but the number is likely to be small. There is evidence that states do not necessarily worry about increased costs from raising their need standard, from their reactions to federal legislation in the early 1980s that limited eligibility to families with gross income below 150 percent of the need standard (subsequently increased to 185%). Many states, including those with low benefits, raised their need standards but not their benefit levels. This response allowed previously eligible families with high deductions to continue to be eligible but limited any increase in their benefits.

EXAMPLE A: STATE PAYS 100 PERCENT OF DIFFERENCE BETWEEN NEED STANDARD AND COUNTABLE INCOME An increase in the need standard affects the number of eligible families and translates dollar for dollar into an increase in benefits.

FAMILY 1: *Countable income of $450 per month*
    If need standard is $400 per month, family will be ineligible.
    If need standard is increased by $100 per month, family will be eligible for
        $50 benefit ($500 − $450).
FAMILY 2: *Countable income of $350 per month*
    If need standard is $400 per month, family will be eligible for $50 benefit
        ($400 − $350).
    If need standard is increased by $100 per month, family will be eligible for
        a benefit increase of $100 per month ($500 − $350 = $150).

EXAMPLE B: STATE PAYS FRACTION (50%) OF DIFFERENCE BETWEEN NEED STANDARD AND COUNTABLE INCOME An increase in the need standard affects the number of eligible families but increases benefits only fractionally.

FAMILY 1: *Countable income of $450 per month*
    If need standard is $400 per month, family will be ineligible.
    If need standard is increased by $100 per month, family will be eligible for
        $25 benefit (($500 − $450) x 0.50).
FAMILY 2: *Countable income of $350 per month*
    If need standard is $400 per month, family will be eligible for $25 benefit
        (($400 − $350) x 0.50).
    If need standard is increased by $100 per month, family will be eligible for
        a benefit increase of $50 per month (($500 − $350) x 0.50 = $75).

FIGURE 8-1 AFDC eligibility and benefits of hypothetical families in states with different eligibility and benefit determination methods.

• Example A: A state pays the full difference between the need standard and countable income. In this case, the need standard (which determines gross income eligibility) is the same as the payment standard (which determines net or countable income eligibility), and both are the same as the maximum benefit paid to families with no other income. The link of the need standard to eligibility and benefit levels and hence to caseloads and costs is most obvious in these cases: an increase in the need standard allows families with higher net (as well as gross) incomes to become eligible and, for a given level of countable income, provides a higher level of benefits.

• Example B: A state pays a fraction of the difference between the need standard and countable income. In this case, the need standard and the payment standard are the same, but the maximum benefit is lower. Here, there is a direct link of the need standard to eligibility, which means a link to caseloads and the costs associated with changes in caseloads. However, the

---

EXAMPLE C: STATE PAYS DIFFERENCE BETWEEN FRACTION (50%) OF NEED STANDARD AND COUNTABLE INCOME An increase in the need standard only fractionally increases the number of eligible families as well as the amount of benefits.

FAMILY 1: *Countable income of $450 per month*
  If need standard is $800 per month, family will be ineligible ($800 x 0.50 = $400, which is <$450).
  If need standard is increased by $100 per month, family will still be ineligible ($900 x 0.50 = $450, which equals $450).
FAMILY 2: *Countable income of $350 per month*
  If need standard is $800 per month, family will be eligible for $50 benefit (($800 x 0.50) – $350 = $50).
  If need standard is increased by $100 per month, family will be eligible for a benefit increase of $50 per month (($900 x 0.50) – $350 = $100).

EXAMPLE D: STATE PAYS 100 PERCENT OF DIFFERENCE BETWEEN NEED STANDARD AND COUNTABLE INCOME SUBJECT TO A MAXIMUM BENEFIT An increase in the need standard affects neither the number of eligible families nor benefits unless the maximum benefit is also increased.

FAMILY 1: *Countable income of $450 per month.*
  If need standard is $400 per month and maximum benefit is $375 per month, family will be ineligible.
  If need standard is increased by $100 per month but maximum benefit is unchanged, family will still be ineligible.
FAMILY 2: *Countable income of $350 per month*
  If need standard is $400 per month and maximum benefit is $375 per month, family will be eligible for $25 benefit ($375 – $350).
  If need standard is increased by $100 per month but maximum benefit is unchanged, family will still be eligible for $25 benefit.

---

link to benefits per case is attenuated because eligible families with a given level of countable income will receive only a fraction of an increase in the need standard.

• Example C: A state pays a fraction of the need standard itself. In this case, the need standard exceeds both the payment standard and the maximum benefit. Here, the link of the need standard to both eligibility and benefits is attenuated.

• Example D: A state uses one of the three methods listed above to make an initial determination of eligibility and benefits, but then imposes a maximum benefit that is lower than both its need and its payment standards. In this state, increases in the need standard have no effect, practically speaking, on either eligibility or benefit amounts unless the maximum benefit is also increased.

Clearly, each state will need to analyze the possible implications for program costs and caseloads of basing its need standard on poverty thresholds that are developed under the proposed updating procedure. Given the differences among states in methods for determining eligibility and benefits, the states may well come to different conclusions.

Effects of Updating on Program Incentives   Some states that have a maximum benefit below their need standard provide higher benefits to families with other income, such as earnings or child support, through a "fill-the-gap" method of calculating benefits. The details of this method vary across states, but the essence is that families are allowed to retain other income without having their AFDC benefit reduced, so long as the total of their benefit and other income does not exceed the need standard (see Larin and Porter, 1992:App).

To illustrate, consider a state with a need (and payment) standard and maximum payment of $400 per month (i.e., the state pays 100% of need). In this state, a newly eligible family that has $200 of earnings will receive only $200 in AFDC, as the family's earnings will be subtracted in full from the need standard. But in another state, one that has a maximum benefit of $400 per month but a need (and payment) standard of $600 per month and that allows families to fill the gap, the same family will receive an AFDC benefit of $400 because the family's $200 in earnings will be subtracted from the (higher) need standard.

The fill-the-gap approach to benefit calculation is a way to provide incentives to working families. Hence, states that want to provide such incentives may find it attractive to base their need standard on poverty thresholds that are developed under the proposed updating procedure.

Summary

We have offered a number of reasons that the use of the proposed poverty measure by the states for their AFDC need standard could be advantageous and some areas of concern, principally involving possible effects on program costs and caseloads. We do not want our discussion of budgetary implications to be misinterpreted. We do not intend to argue against the adoption of need standards for the AFDC program that are updated in real terms; indeed, from the perspective of the low-income population, there is much to recommend such a step by the states. However, assistance programs must balance a number of objectives and contend with a number of constraints. We urge that program designers fully evaluate all of the ramifications before deciding to adopt for program purposes a measure that is proposed for statistical purposes.

For the AFDC need standard, it is important to note that the states, under current law, have considerable latitude with which to attenuate the link of the need standard to eligibility and benefits, by such strategies as setting the payment standard at a fraction of the need standard. Hence, considerations of possible adverse consequences for program costs and caseloads should perhaps weigh less heavily than the advantages of using the proposed poverty measure to set AFDC standards of need.

In conclusion, we believe that, on balance, the use of the proposed poverty concept for the purpose of determining AFDC need standards would be beneficial, even if individual states set their need (or benefit) standard at different fractions of the poverty threshold. Use of the poverty thresholds that are developed under the proposed procedure would be generally consistent with the AFDC definition of income and would recognize important interstate differences in living costs within a common framework that would provide a benchmark for evaluating the adequacy of eligibility levels across states.

APPENDICES

Dissent

John F. Cogan

Poverty statistics are the primary indicator of living conditions among people at the economic spectrum's lower end. These data are among the most important and the most politically sensitive data published by the U.S. government. That the method used to measure poverty has remained unchanged since its inception, despite well-recognized conceptual and methodological problems, is testimony to this sensitivity. In this environment, only a report firmly grounded in science can produce the kind of agreement among government officials that would lead to improvements in measuring poverty. The major recommendations and conclusions for changing the measurement of poverty by the Panel on Poverty and Family Assistance are not based on scientific evidence. They lie well outside the National Research Council's stated mission "to deliver science advice" to the government. Therefore, I have chosen to dissent.

There are parts of the report for which the panel should be commended. The sections that address problems with the current measure, alternative poverty concepts, and measuring poverty across families of different sizes are particularly illuminating. More analyses based on the scientific literature would have improved the report. Social science research has developed a vast body of scientific knowledge about issues relating to the measurement of poverty. Indeed, many panel members have been important contributors to this knowledge base. There exist, for example, well-developed studies for constructing efficient, meaningful indices to account for geographical differences in living costs. This literature identifies sampling procedures that can be applied to maximize the informational content of surveys at minimum cost and to develop appropriate weighting schemes to create a consumption bundle that reflects true differences in living costs. There is also a rich literature on statistical properties of alternative imputation procedures that would be required to incorporate in-kind benefits and taxes into measures of family resources. To some people, these contributions may not be eye-catching; they may not be newsworthy; but they are scientific.

Instead of focusing on these areas where science can make a contribution, the report is devoted to recommendations and conclusions that are driven by value judgments. According to the report, the poverty line should be raised from its current level, it should rise faster than inflation over time, and fewer resources should be counted when determining whether a family's income is above or below the poverty line. These recommendations are not scientific judgments. They are value judgments made by scientists—with a particular point of view. In essence, the panel has mostly eschewed the role of scientific panel and has instead assumed the role of a government policy maker. By so doing, the panel has not served well either the policy community or the scientific community. Although it can be difficult to establish a precise boundary between where science ends and policy making begins, this panel has ventured far afield in a desire to make a difference. Instead of using strong scientific research to produce recommendations that would compel a particular policy approach, the panel has made recommendations with little scientific bases.

My dissent focuses on four major recommendations and conclusions: measuring the poverty line, choosing a range for the poverty line, updating the poverty line, and accounting for medical care in measuring family resources. This dissent is not intended to be a comprehensive critique of the panel report. Although there is considerably more in the report that I find objectionable, to avoid obscuring the central reason for my dissent, I do not address objections that are not germane to it.

MEASURING THE POVERTY LINE

The report recommends a new method for measuring the poverty line:

> The poverty threshold should represent a budget for food, clothing, and shelter (including utilities) and a small additional amount to allow for other needs . . .

I focus first on this seemingly noncontroversial recommendation because it illustrates the lack of scientific basis that permeates the report's major recommendations for changing the measurement of poverty.

My objection to this recommendation is that the choice of particular commodities is not based on science. The choice may appear to be quite reasonable, and the panel may be correct when it argues that these commodities "represent basic living needs with which no one would quarrel." But what scientific basis exists for concluding that food, clothing, and shelter are basic needs and health care or personal care services are not? Is it a scientific proposition that designer tennis shoes are a basic need but that the services of primary care physicians are not? What scientific basis exists for concluding that *all* types of food, clothing, and shelter, rather than only a subset, are basic needs? The report provides no answers to these questions. It does not attempt to establish a scientific basis nor does it present scientific evidence to support its choices.

The panel's primary rationale is that "the United States has major assistance programs to provide food and housing . . . [and] clothing allowances historically were separately identified grants under Aid to Families with Dependent Children." This argument is faulty on several accounts. First, given the broad array of government-provided benefits, the same argument could be used to support the inclusion of any number of other commodities as basic needs. Health care, education, transportation, and laundry services are all currently provided by the federal government to the poor. Second, the fact that the government provided medical care to the poor on an entitlement basis long before it established entitlements for either food or housing assistance might suggest that medical care is every bit as basic a need as the former set of commodities. Also, the fact that the U.S. government spends an increasingly substantial proportion of its budget to provide medical insurance for the low-income population is a strong indication that medical care is viewed as a priority commodity.

The foregoing should not be taken to mean, however, that scientific study has no role in this choice. Scientific analysis can play a significant role by evaluating methods to improve the quality of existing consumption data. It can establish criteria for evaluating the statistical accuracy of alternative poverty budgets. It can evaluate alternative sampling methodologies to improve a survey's ability to count certain groups, such as the homeless. Scientific analysis can ascertain living conditions of families at different income levels so that policy officials can determine the levels of income that should qualify as poverty.

UPDATING THE POVERTY LINE

The panel report recommends updating the poverty line annually by the growth rate in the median level of expenditures on food, clothing, and shelter, rather than by the Consumer Price Index as is the current practice. If adopted, the recommendation would fundamentally change the concept of poverty from an absolute standard to a relative standard. Under the recommended method, the poverty line would rise about 8 percent faster per year than under the current method.

This recommendation, like the previously discussed one, cannot be deduced from any set of scientific principles, facts, or arguments. Any updating method, be it one to ensure an absolute poverty threshold, a relative threshold, or one that falls somewhere in between, is a policy choice, not a scientific one. But unlike the previously discussed recommendation, this one would have a substantial impact on the level of poverty over time.

At various points, the report forthrightly states that many of its recommendations are not made on the basis of scientific evidence alone, that they also involve the value judgments of panel members. But this recommendation is all judgment and no science. The choice of how rapidly the poverty line should rise over time derives from society's values. Judgments about these values are more properly made by elected officials charged with translating societal values into law rather than in reports issued by scientific bodies.

CHOOSING A RANGE FOR THE POVERTY LINE

The report's introduction argues correctly that the choice of a poverty threshold is not a scientific one. The panel then concludes that the appropriate range for the poverty line is between $13,700 and $15,900 for a family of four.[1] This range is between 14 and 33 percent higher than the comparable current poverty line. In terms of consumption of the three basic needs—food, clothing, and shelter—40 to 55 percent of four-person families consume less than this amount. The report attempts to create an impression that this range lies within the scientific community's consensus about where the poverty line should be drawn. The policy-making community should be aware that there is no consensus within the scientific community. Furthermore, even if there were, it should carry no more weight among policy makers than a consensus among theoretical physicists that they prefer tofu to beef burgers.

Choosing a poverty line or a range for that line is a policy maker's job, not the job of a scientific panel. Scientific expertise can inform policy makers' choices. For example, this expertise can be brought to bear on measuring and assessing living conditions at or near alternative poverty lines. Unfortunately, the report provides no information on the level of economic deprivation among persons at any of the poverty levels discussed.

MEASURING FAMILY RESOURCES:
THE ISSUE OF MEDICAL CARE

For measuring family resources, the report recommends that out-of-pocket expenditures for medical care be subtracted from a family's income. This recommendation is troubling. It assumes that all medical care expenditures are

---

[1] The report is vague about why the panel chose to label its range a conclusion instead of a recommendation. However, the distinction is immaterial since there is no scientific basis for recommending or concluding that a particular range is appropriate.

nondiscretionary. Within the field of economic science, the assumption that all medical care expenses are nondiscretionary runs contrary to three decades of economic research. From the early work of Pauly (1968) and Grossman (1972) to later work by Newhouse (1993) and others, economists have viewed health as an economic good, responsive to both income and price changes. This consumer choice approach has dominated economic analysis of health care and a greatly enhanced analysis of health care expenditures. Although this research does not offer any firm conclusions about how health care should be treated in the context of poverty measurement, its basic premise is at odds with the panel's rationale.

The panel's recommendation is based on an approach suggested in a 1985 conference paper by David Ellwood and Larry Summers. In the decade since that paper was presented, there has not been, to my knowledge, a single critical evaluation or discussion of it in any major peer reviewed scientific economics journal. The paper's merits aside, its approach has not undergone the kind of assessment that science requires before a scientific consensus is reached.

The report argues that deducting out-of-pocket expenses removes medical care entirely from the calculation of poverty. The argument is not correct, as the following example illustrates. Consider two healthy families—the Smith family and the Jones family. Suppose the Smith family has an income that is $2,000 higher than the Jones's. The Smith family purchases a $3,000 health insurance plan while the Jones family purchases no health insurance. Both families are fortunate enough to have no additional out-of-pocket health expenditures during the year. According to the report's recommended treatment, the Smith family would be poorer than the Jones family. And it would be so only because it chose to spend its higher income on health insurance.

The panel also argues that, by excluding medical care from its list of basic goods, its treatment is consistent. However, for two reasons, this argument is less than satisfactory. First, the 15 to 25 percent add-on to the poverty threshold "for other needed expenditures" can be construed as building in an amount for medical care. In fact, the dollar value of this percentage—$1,800 to $3,200—is more than one-half the actuarial value of Medicaid for the noninstitutionalized population and close to the cost of a typical private insurance plan. Second, the panel could have obtained the same range for the poverty threshold by including medical care as a fourth basic commodity and basing the threshold on the 20th instead of the 30th percentile of the consumption distribution.

One final point about the panel's treatment of in-kind benefits is in order. Much of the impetus for changing the way in which resources are counted comes from the fact that the current method ignores the value of billions of dollars in noncash benefits for food, housing, and medical care that are spent on low-income families. The reader will be surprised to see that the panel, after making adjustments to countable income, concludes that families living near the current poverty line have fewer countable resources than they would have under the current poverty measure.

CONCLUSION

I dissent because the report's recommendations—to choose three particular commodities upon which to base the calculation of poverty and to exclude other commodities; to establish a normative range of values within which the poverty line should fall; to increase the poverty line over time to account for perceived improvements in the standard of living; and to exclude medical expenses from family resources—are the outcome of highly subjective judgments. These are judgments that do not result from scientific inquiry and, therefore, in my opinion, are improperly placed in this report.

I do not believe that this report will be the basis for improving the measurement of poverty because its recommendations are not based on scientific evidence. To my disappointment, the panel has missed an extraordinary opportunity to enlighten and inform government officials about problems of measuring poverty and about the solutions to those problems.

REFERENCES

Grossman, M.
   1972   On the concept of health capital and the demand for health. *Journal of Political Economy* 80(March/April):223-255.
Newhouse, Joseph P.
   1972   *Free for All? Lessons from the RAND Health Insurance Experiment.* Cambridge, Mass.: Harvard University Press.
Pauly, M.V.
   1968   The economics of moral hazard: Comment. *American Economic Review* 58: 535.

Data Sources for Measuring Poverty

This appendix provides information on the major features of four continuing surveys that provide data relevant to measuring poverty and economic well-being: the Consumer Expenditure Survey (CEX), the Current Population Survey (CPS) March income supplement, the Panel Study of Income Dynamics (PSID), and the Survey of Income and Program Participation (SIPP). The appendix also provides detailed comparisons of the features and quality of the March CPS and SIPP. The March CPS is the current source of the nation's official income and poverty statistics; we recommend that SIPP become the official source instead (see Chapter 5). (The report of the Panel to Evaluate SIPP made the same recommendation; see Citro and Kalton, 1993:8).

MAJOR FEATURES OF THE CEX, MARCH CPS, PSID, AND SIPP

Consumer Expenditure Survey

The CEX is sponsored by the Bureau of Labor Statistics (BLS) and conducted by the Census Bureau, with a current budget of about $12 million per year. Historically, surveys of expenditures by consumers (with varying names and formats) were fielded at roughly 10- to 15-year intervals from 1901 to 1950. The 1950 survey was the first one to be officially designated the Consumer Expenditure Survey. The 1950 and 1960-1961 surveys used annual recall for expenditures. In 1972-1973, the current design of a quarterly Interview Survey and a two-week Diary Survey was introduced. In 1980 the CEX became a continuing survey. Its major uses are to provide the market basket for the Consumer Price Index and to provide data for analysis of expenditures in relation to demographic and other characteristics. (For information on the CEX, see Bureau of Labor Statistics, no date; Jacobs and Shipp, 1990.)

Design and Use

The Interview Survey includes a sample of 6,800 consumer units (of which about 5,000 are used for quarterly estimates), interviewed in person at 3-month intervals. Households are in the sample for five quarters (the first interview has a 1-month recall and is used for bounding purposes and to collect an inventory of durable goods). There are monthly rotation groups: each month, one-fifth of the sample is new and one-fifth is completing its fifth and final interview. Household response rates to the Interview Survey have averaged about 85 percent since 1980. There appears to be little time-in-sample bias in the survey, but considerable recall error: for example, apparel expenditures reported for the first month prior to the interview are 124 percent of the monthly mean, while those reported for the third month prior to the interview are only 76 percent of the mean (Silberstein, 1989).

The Diary Survey includes a sample of 6,000 consumer units, each of which records daily expenditures for 2 weeks. Interviews are spread out over the year. Interviewers make three visits to each unit: an initial visit to drop off the first-week diary, a second visit to drop off the second-week diary and pick up the first-week diary, and a third visit to pick up the second-week diary. Household response rates to the Diary Survey have ranged from about 85 to 90 percent.

The CEX covers the U.S. civilian noninstitutionalized population, including military in civilian housing, students in university or college housing, and group homes. (The 1982-1983 interviews excluded the rural population because of budget cuts.) The reporting unit is the consumer unit, defined as one of the following: a single person living alone or sharing a household with others but financially independent; family (household members related by blood, marriage, or adoption); two or more persons living together who share responsibility for two of three major expenses—food, housing, and other expenses. The respondent is any member of the consumer unit aged 16 or older with most knowledge of the unit's finances. People who leave a sampled address are not followed.

In its publications, BLS makes use of data from both the Interview and the Diary Surveys to develop a total picture of expenditures. Comparisons with data from the National Income and Product Accounts (NIPA) indicate that the CEX estimates for some categories are quite complete; these include rent, utilities, fuels, and public services; vehicle purchases; and gasoline and motor oil. But for other categories the CEX estimates fall considerably short: for example, from information provided by BLS, the ratios of CEX to NIPA estimates from 1987 to 1990 were only about 0.70 for food, 0.75 for household furnishings and equipment, 0.60 for apparel and services, and 0.60 for public transportation (see also Bosworth, Burtless, and Sabelhaus, 1991; Gieseman, 1987; Slesnick, 1991a).[1]

Researchers who analyze expenditure data typically work with the Interview Survey, from which users can construct annual data on expenditures and income. (The Interview and Diary Survey samples are independent, so there is no way to actually link the microrecords.) However, some proportion of consumer units in the sample for the Interview Survey do not have observations for all four quarters because of dropping out of the survey or moving away from the sampled address. (The sample, technically, is one of addresses. Consumer units that move from the sampled address are not followed, but, instead, the new occupants are interviewed.) Also, because of the rotation design, a large proportion of observations with complete information must have their data adjusted in some manner in order to obtain calendar-year estimates.

Content of the Interview Survey

- *Demographic characteristics*
- *Work experience* Information is obtained for consumer unit members aged 14 and over on work experience and job characteristics in the previous quarter and in the prior 12 months (the latter information is obtained at the second and fifth interviews).
- *Detailed expenditures* Detailed quarterly data (per each payment or bill) are obtained for expenditure categories that comprise an estimated 60-70 percent of total expenditures, including rent, facilities, and services for rented living quarters (including housing assistance subsidies); payments on mortgages, lump sum home equity loans, and line of credit home equity loans; ownership costs (extra payments on mortgage principal, ground rent, cooperative or condominium fees); telephone expenses; utilities and fuels; construction, repairs, alterations, and maintenance of property; purchases of appliances, household equipment, and other selected items; household equipment repairs, service contracts, and furniture repair and reupholstering; purchases of home furnishings and related household items; purchases of clothing; purchases of infants' clothing, watches, jewelry, and hairpieces; purchases of sewing materials; payments for leased vehicles; purchases of vehicles; disposals of vehicles; vehicle maintenance and repair; vehicle equipment, parts, and accessories; licensing, registration, and inspection of vehicles; other vehicle operating expenses; premiums for other than health insurance; premiums for health insurance; coverage by Medicare and Medicaid; medical and health expenditures

---

[1] However, the NIPA and CEX data are not strictly comparable.

and reimbursements; educational expenses paid by the consumer unit and by others (including for nursery school and day care centers); trips by type of expense for each trip completed during the quarter; reimbursements for trip expenses; local overnight stays; and gifts of commodities for people outside the family.

• *Global (or usual) expenditures* Global (or usual) expenditures are obtained for categories that comprise an additional estimated 20-25 percent of total expenditures, including quarterly amounts for subscriptions, memberships, books, and entertainment expenses; quarterly amounts for miscellaneous items (e.g., funerals, catered affairs, accounting fees, home services, including babysitting and in-home child care, pets and pet expenses, alimony, child support, charitable contributions); usual weekly expenses for supermarkets and specialty food stores; usual monthly expenses for liquor and food away from home; quarterly benefits from food stamps (and months received) and other meals provided free; quarterly amounts for selected services and goods (e.g., laundromats); usual weekly expenses for tobacco products; and usual monthly expenses for haircuts for men and women members of the consumer unit.

• *Expenditures in last 12 months* Data on expenditures in the prior 12 months are obtained at the fifth interview for occupational expenses (e.g., union dues) and contributions, including alimony, child support, college expenses for students attending school away from home, gifts to people outside the consumer unit, contributions to charities, contributions to religious organizations, contributions to educational organizations, political contributions, and other contributions.

• *Real assets* An inventory of major household appliances and features of the dwelling unit, together with descriptions of each owned property, are obtained at the first interview, and changes in ownership of property and mortgages are obtained each quarter. The rental value of owned home and the value of owned home are obtained.

• *Financial assets* Data obtained include current credit balances (e.g., credit cards, credit unions, bank loans); credit balances a year ago; finance charges paid in the prior 12 months (e.g., on revolving credit cards, late payments to doctors); changes in financial assets, comparing value last month and 1 year ago (e.g., savings accounts, checking accounts, savings bonds, securities); purchases and sales of stocks, bonds, or mutual funds in the prior 12 months; investments to or withdrawals from own business or farm in the prior 12 months; amounts owed currently and 1 year ago by others to someone in the consumer unit; and settlements during past year on insurance policies. All of these items are obtained at the fifth interview; current credit balances are also obtained at the second interview.

• *Income in the prior 12 months* Data on income for the prior 12 months are obtained at the second and fifth interviews. Sources obtained for each consumer unit member aged 14 and over include wages or salary, nonfarm self-employment income, farm self-employment income, Social Security or railroad retirement, and Supplemental Security Income (SSI). Sources obtained for the consumer unit as a whole include worker's compensation and veterans' benefits; public assistance; interest on savings accounts and bonds; regular income from dividends, royalties, and estates and trusts; income from pensions or annuities from private and public sources; net income or loss from roomers or boarders; net income or loss from rental property; income from alimony, child support, and regular contributions from persons outside the consumer unit; lump-sum payments; money from the sale of household furnishings or other belongings; other money income (e.g., scholarships, foster care payments); and refunds (e.g., from federal income tax or insurance policies).

• *Taxes* Data are obtained at the second and fifth interviews on tax deductions from the last paycheck of each consumer unit member aged 14 and over (federal income tax, state and local income tax, and Social Security payroll tax and deductions for pensions). Data are also obtained for the prior 12 months on payments by the consumer unit as a whole for additional federal income tax (beyond that withheld from earnings), additional state and local taxes, property taxes not reported elsewhere, and other taxes not reported elsewhere. Sales taxes are calculated from information provided for individual expenditures and are included in the component expenditures.

CPS March Income Supplement

The CPS is a continuing survey, begun in the 1940s. Income questions were first asked in 1945 (for income year 1944).[2] Since 1956 the income questions have been part of the supplement each March; since 1970 the March supplement has also included questions on work experience in the prior year. (Supplements in other months cover such topics as voting behavior, educational enrollment, and fertility and marital history.) BLS sponsors the core of the CPS, which is designed to provide monthly unemployment rates. The Census Bureau conducts the survey and sponsors the March income supplement. The total budget for the CPS is about $28 million per year, of which about $2 million to $3 million is for the March supplement. (For information on the March CPS, see Bureau of the Census, 1992b; and Citro, 1991.)

Design

The CPS has a rotating design. Households are in the sample for 4 months, out of the sample for 8 months, and in again for 4 months. Hence, there is 50

---

[2] Since about 1960, however, the income data for 1944 and 1945 and the nonfarm income data for 1946 have been omitted from the Census Bureau's P-60 series money income reports.

percent overlap in the sample for poverty estimates from year to year. The sample size is about 60,000 households.

The sample covers the U.S. civilian noninstitutionalized population. The March supplement also includes military in civilian housing and an additional sample of 2,500 housing units that had contained at least one adult of Hispanic origin as of the preceding November interview. The reporting unit is the household, with unrelated individuals and families also identified. The respondent is each household member aged 15 and older, but proxy responses are readily accepted. Interviews are in person for the first month and then by telephone to the extent possible. People who leave a sampled address are not followed. (Response rates and other aspects of data quality are reviewed below.)

A major redesign of the CPS was recently implemented (see Cohany, Polivka, and Rothgeb, 1994). The redesign includes respecification of the sample design on the basis of information from the 1990 census about the geographic distribution and other characteristics of the population, changing the data collection mode to computer-assisted personal interviewing and computer-assisted telephone interviewing (CAPI/CATI), and making important wording changes to the core questions on labor force participation. No changes were made to the March income supplement (except to put the questionnaire into a CAPI/CATI format), but the responses may be affected by one or more aspects of the redesign of the core survey.

Content

The content of the core CPS interview includes

- demographic characteristics; and
- labor force participation, hours worked, reason for part-time work, reason for temporary absence from job, industry and occupation in prior week, job search behavior in the previous 4 weeks if not working and when last worked, usual hours and usual earnings, union membership, reason left last job, and reasons for looking for work (for selected rotation groups).

The content of the March supplement includes

- labor force participation and job history in the prior calendar year for each household member aged 15 or older;
- annual income for the prior calendar year for each household member aged 15 or older by detailed source—about 30 types of regular cash income are identified separately, including wages and salaries, net self-employment income, Social Security for oneself or a spouse, Social Security for one's children, railroad retirement, unemployment compensation, veterans' compensation, black lung payments, disability payments, SSI, Aid to Families with Dependent Children (AFDC), other welfare, child support, alimony, private

pension, federal civilian pension, military pension, state or local government pension, annuity income, income from estates and trusts, other retirement or disability or survivor payments, money from relatives or friends, interest income, dividends, net rental income, income from individual retirement accounts, Pell Grants, other educational financial aid, other cash income;
  • participation in noncash benefit programs, including energy assistance, food stamps, public housing, and school lunch; and
  • health insurance coverage.

Panel Study of Income Dynamics

The PSID is a continuing panel survey of a cohort of families, begun in 1968. The survey is sponsored and conducted by the University of Michigan Survey Research Center (SRC). Since 1983 the National Science Foundation has been the principal funder, with substantial continuing support from the Office of the Assistant Secretary for Planning and Evaluation in the U.S. Department of Health and Human Services. (The survey was originally funded by the Office of Economic Opportunity; other agencies that have provided funds include the U.S. Departments of Labor and Agriculture, the National Institute of Child Health and Human Development, the National Institute on Aging, and the Ford, Sloan, and Rockefeller foundations.) The current annual budget is about $2.6 million, which includes direct and overhead costs for the core survey only, not including separately funded supplements. (For information on the PSID, see Hill, 1992; Survey Research Center, 1989.)

Design

The sample comprises three components: (1) 2,900 families interviewed in 1968 from the SRC national sampling frame, representative of the civilian, noninstitutionalized population; (2) 1,900 low-income families with heads under age 60 who were interviewed in 1968 from the 1966-1967 Survey of Economic Opportunity (SEO); and (3) 2,000 Hispanic families added in 1990. Currently, 9,000 families (including original sample families and the subsequent families of their members) are interviewed once each year. The reporting unit is the family, defined as one of the following: a single person living alone or sharing a household with other nonrelatives; a family of members related by blood, marriage, or adoption; an unmarried couple living together in what appears to be a fairly permanent arrangement. The respondent is the family head, usually the adult male head if there is one. Interviews are conducted annually and, since 1973, mostly by telephone (92%). Original sample members who leave to form separate family units are followed (including children born to original sample members), and information is obtained about the coresidents in their new families. Sample members who are institutionalized are tracked and interviewed subsequently if they return to a family setting.

The PSID experienced a large sample loss—24 percent—at the initial interview in 1968, but additional sample loss dropped to 8 percent of the eligible families at the second interview, and it was only 1-2 percent at each interview thereafter (Survey Research Center, 1989:Table 2a). The initial large sample loss was partly due to the PSID sample design, which originally included a national probability sample of about 2,900 families and a sample of about 1,900 low-income families drawn from the sample used for the 1967 SEO. Several factors increased the nonresponse from the SEO sample, including the requirement by the Census Bureau that SEO families sign a release allowing their names to be given to the PSID (Hill, 1992).

The extent to which attrition introduces bias into estimates from the PSID is not clear. Several studies in the 1980s found that, although cumulative sample loss was over 50 percent (52% by 1980 and 58% by 1985), there was no evidence that attrition correlated with individual characteristics in a way that would produce biased estimates. For example, Becketti et al. (1988:490) found no evidence that attrition "has any effect on estimates of the parameters of the earnings equations that we studied." Duncan, Juster, and Morgan (1984) also found that response rates were just as high in the PSID among families in the lowest income decile as in the middle or upper income deciles (see also Curtin, Juster, and Morgan, 1989, and other studies cited in Hill, 1992). However, Duncan and Rodgers (1991) found bigger differences in poverty rates for white children between the PSID and the March CPS in 1981-1986 than in 1967-1971 (the PSID rates were lower in both periods). They attribute the finding to the fact that, as of 1986 (before the addition in 1990 of a new Hispanic sample), the PSID represented only about one-third of the Hispanic children reported in the CPS while it represented all non-Hispanic white and black children.

One indicator of data quality is that about 95 percent of heads and spouses provide "adequate responses" for labor and asset income so that the responses do not have to be edited. The percentage of adequate responses has been in the range 94-98 percent over the life of the survey (Survey Research Center, 1989:Table 5).

Content

The PSID collects the most detailed information about family heads and, since the late 1970s, about wives and cohabitors. The core content includes

- demographic characteristics;
- employment information—current and employment history in past year;
- income sources and amounts for the head for the past calendar year

(including which months received) from wages or salaries; bonuses, overtime, tips, or commissions; professional trade or practice; farming or market gardening; roomers or boarders; extra jobs; rent; dividends, interest, trust funds, or royalties; AFDC; SSI; other welfare; Social Security (including separately listed amounts for other family members); veterans' benefits; other retirement pay, pensions, or annuities; unemployment compensation; worker's compensation; alimony; child support; help from relatives; and anything else;

• income sources and amounts for the spouse for the past calendar year (including which months received) from earnings; unemployment compensation; worker's compensation; and interest, welfare, pensions, child support, or any other source (with each source to be separately listed);

• income sources and amounts for other individual family members aged 16 and over for the past calendar year (including which months received) from earnings from first and second jobs; and any other income such as pensions, welfare, interest, gifts, or anything else (with each source to be separately listed);[3]

• income earned by individual family members under aged 16 and family lump-sum income (e.g., inheritance or insurance settlements) in past calendar year;

• public assistance—food stamps (amount in past calendar year and specific months in which received), housing subsidies, energy assistance, and Medicaid or other welfare medical services;

• estimate of federal taxes paid (based on information about income, exemptions, dependents living outside the household, whether itemized, mortgage interest payments, and property taxes);

• housing, including current value, remaining mortgage principal, monthly mortgage payment for owned home, monthly rent, and annual utility costs;

• estimate of annual food costs (in home and away from home) from reports of average weekly expenditures;

• financial assistance to people living elsewhere;

• housework time;

• geographic mobility;

• socioeconomic background;

• health, religion, and military service; and

• county-level data (unemployment rate, wage rate for unskilled workers, labor market demand conditions).

Event histories (dated to the month) are recorded for demographic, employment, and poverty characteristics. Supplemental topics have included

---

[3] It is difficult to assign a value to the number of income sources collected in the PSID, because of the question format for family members other than the head, which asks for particular sources to be named without going through a specified list.

achievement motivation, attitudes, child care, cognitive ability, commuting to work, disability and illness, do-it-yourself activities, extended family and kinship ties, fertility and family planning, financial situation and health of parents, food stamp and SSI eligibility, fringe benefits, hospitalization, housework, housing and neighborhood characteristics, housing utilities, impact of inflation, inheritances, job training, retirement plans and experiences, retrospective histories, saving behavior, smoking and exercise, spells of unemployment and time out of the labor force, time and money help with emergencies, time use, and wealth. In 1990, there were some links to Medicare records.

Survey of Income and Program Participation

SIPP is a continuing panel survey, begun in 1983, that is sponsored and conducted by the Bureau of the Census. The current annual budget is about $30 million to $32 million. (For information on SIPP, see Citro and Kalton, 1993; and Jabine, King, and Petroni, 1990.)

Design

The current design introduces a new sample panel each February. Each sample of households (panel) is interviewed every 4 months for 32 months (or 2.67 years); because of budget restrictions, some panels have had fewer than eight interview waves.[4] There are monthly rotation groups. Until 1992 interviews were in person to the extent possible; beginning in February 1992 the first and sixth interviews have been in person with the rest by telephone. Under this design, three panels are in the field in most months of each year. (For information about response rates and other aspects of data quality, see below.)

The sample covers the U.S. civilian noninstitutionalized population and members of the armed forces living off post or with their families on post. Sample size has varied from 12,500 to 23,500 households per panel; 20,000 households is the current design target. The reporting unit is the household, with unrelated individuals and families also identified. The respondent is each household member aged 15 and older; proxy responses are accepted if necessary. Original sample members aged 15 and older who move to new households are followed and information is obtained about the coresidents in their new households. Sample members who are institutionalized are tracked and interviewed subsequently if they return to a household setting.

The proposed redesign of SIPP recommended by the Panel to Evaluate SIPP calls for introducing a new panel every 2 years instead of every year; interviewing each panel at 4-month intervals for 48 months (12 waves) instead

---

[4] The 1993 panel will be extended for a total of 10 years, with annual interviews after the first 3 years of interviews every 4 months.

of 32 months (8 waves); and increasing the sample size per panel from 20,000 to 27,000 households. Under this design, two panels would be in the field each year (see Citro and Kalton, 1993). The redesign of SIPP proposed by the Census Bureau Senior Management Redesign Team calls for introducing a new panel every 4 years (i.e., with no overlap across panels); interviewing each panel at 4-month intervals for 48 months; and increasing the sample size per panel to 50,000 households.

The redesign of SIPP will be fully implemented in the 1996 panel, with a dress rehearsal in 1995. In addition to extending the length and increasing the sample size of each panel, features of the redesign include new samples drawn on the basis of information from the 1990 census, switching the data collection mode to CAPI/CATI, and changes in selected questionnaire items based on recommendations from the Panel to Evaluate SIPP and others. The new sample design for SIPP will also include an oversample of addresses in which the residents were below the poverty level in 1989, based on information from the 1990 census; proxy characteristics, such as housing tenure and family type, will be used for oversampling addresses for which the census long-form information on poverty status is not available.

Content

The content of the current SIPP core interview includes

- demographic characteristics;
- monthly information on labor force participation, job characteristics, and earnings;
- monthly information on public and private health insurance coverage; and
- monthly information on detailed sources and amounts of income from public and private transfer payments; information—monthly for the most part—on noncash benefits (food stamps, school lunch, etc.); and information for the 4-month period on income from assets. In total, about 65 separate sources of cash income are identified for each household member aged 15 and over, together with benefits from seven in-kind programs—for a few sources annual amounts are obtained in topical modules (see Citro and Kalton, 1993:Tables 3-1, 3-2).

Data are also collected in topical modules, which are asked once or twice in each panel, on a wide range of subjects, including

- annual income and income taxes;
- educational financing and enrollment;
- eligibility for selected programs (including expenditures on shelter, out-of-pocket medical care costs, and dependent care);
- employee benefits (1984 panel only);

- housing costs and finance;
- individual retirement accounts;
- personal history (fertility, marital status, migration, welfare recipiency, and other topics); and
- wealth (property, retirement expectations and pension plan coverage, assets and liabilities).

In addition, each panel includes a topical module with variable content designed to respond to the needs of policy analysis agencies. Topics covered to date have included characteristics of job from which retired, child care, child support, disability status of children, energy use, extended measures of well-being, functional activities, health status and utilization of health care, home health care, household relationships, housing costs and finance, job offers and reservation wage, long-term care, pension plan coverage, retirement plans, support for nonhousehold members, training, work expenses, and work schedule (see Citro and Kalton, 1993:Table 3-13).

Summary Comparisons

In evaluating the usefulness of a survey for measuring poverty, it is important to consider several characteristics: sample size and design; the amount of detail for data on income, taxes, assets, and expenditures; and the quality of the information. Table B-1 summarizes some key characteristics of the CEX, March CPS, PSID, and SIPP; the next section discusses in more detail the quality of the income data. (The last section provides a detailed comparison of the March CPS and SIPP.)

The surveys range in size from 5,000 consumer units (CEX) to 60,000 households (March CPS). The CEX, March CPS, and PSID collect income data for a number of separate cash and in-kind sources for the previous calendar year or the 12 months prior to interview waves, with some differences among the three; the SIPP obtains income data at each 4-month wave, with monthly reporting for most sources. All the surveys, except the March CPS, collect information with which to determine a variety of taxes. The CEX and SIPP obtain detailed information on asset holdings; the PSID ascertains home value and equity; the March CPS does not ask about assets except to obtain income flows. Finally, all the surveys, except the March CPS, obtain regular information on such expenditures as food and shelter; the CEX obtains extensive expenditure information.

Quality of Income Data

A detailed comparison of data quality across the four surveys is beyond the scope of this appendix, but some rough aggregate comparisons for income reporting can be made.

All four surveys clearly experience net underreporting of income.[5] The very rough comparisons of aggregate incomes for the population as a whole suggest that the March CPS captures about 90 percent of the regular cash income estimated by independent sources (Bureau of the Census, 1989a:Table A2; 1992b:Table C-1) and that the CEX (Interview Survey) in turn captures about 90 percent of the income reported in the March CPS (Cutler and Katz, 1991:Table A2). Aggregate income amounts for SIPP and the March CPS are virtually the same (Jabine, King, and Petroni, 1990:Table 10.8): SIPP obtains higher reports of nonearnings income (by about 6%), but somewhat lower reports of earnings (by about 2%) compared with the March CPS. The assumption is that some people are reporting net rather than gross earnings to SIPP. If SIPP obtained as complete reporting of earnings as the March CPS, it would capture 1-2 additional percentage points of regular income.

In inferring from comparisons of poverty rates across the surveys, it appears that income underreporting at the lower end of the distribution is most problematic in the CEX, followed by the March CPS, with the PSID and SIPP obtaining more complete reporting. Thus, in the period 1984-1991, poverty rates based on before-tax cash income from the CEX were higher than the rates from the March CPS, which, in turn, were higher than those from SIPP (see Table 5-12). Duncan and Rodgers (1991) find that poverty rates in the PSID are below those in the March CPS and comparable to those in SIPP. Duncan, Smeeding, and Rodgers (1992:Table 1) consistently find a smaller percentage of families with incomes below $15,000 in the PSID than in the March CPS; the difference ranged from 0.4 to 3.0 percentage points in the period 1967-1988. (As noted above, PSID estimates of low-income families do not appear biased by differential attrition, although underrepresentation of Hispanics may account for some of the CPS-PSID diffference.)

The evidence suggests that the greater the emphasis on income reporting in a survey, the lower is the estimated poverty rate. Thus, the less complete income reporting at the lower end of the distribution in the March CPS relative to SIPP is probably partly due to the fact that the March CPS is a supplement to a survey in which the major emphasis is on collecting monthly labor force information. Income reporting is probably particularly poor in the CEX Interview Survey also partly because the CEX is an expenditure survey, not an income survey. The secondary role of income data is evident in many aspects of the Interview Survey design and questionnaire content. Thus, income is asked for the preceding 12 months, rather than quarterly; only a few major income sources are asked separately for each adult member of the

---

[5] Net underreporting is a combination of underreports and overreports of income. For specific income types, classification errors also occur. Inferences of net underreporting, obtained from comparing survey estimates with those from the National Income and Product Accounts, other independent sources, or other surveys, must be made with care, as differences in definitions and processing procedures can affect the validity of the comparisons.

TABLE B-1 Summary Comparisons of CEX, March CPS, PSID, and SIPP

Feature	Consumer Expenditure Survey (Interview)	CPS (March Income Supplement)	Panel Study of Income Dynamics	Survey of Income and Program Participation
Sample Size and Design	5,000 consumer units; each unit in sample for 5 quarters; rotation group design; quarterly interviews	60,000 households; each household in sample for 8 months over 2-year period; rotation group design; monthly interviews (income supplement once per year)	9,000 families; overrepresents low-income families; continuing panel with annual interviews	40,000 households (50,000 proposed); new panel each February (every 4 years proposed); each original sample adult in panel for 32 months (48 months proposed); interviews every 4 months
Income Data	Annual data for 12 months prior to 2nd and 5th interviews; 5 sources for individuals, 11 sources for consumer unit; major in-kind benefits	Data for prior calendar year for about 35 cash and in-kind sources	Data for prior calendar year for about 25 cash and in-kind sources with specific months received	Data for about 70 cash and in-kind sources at each 4-month wave, with monthly reporting for most sources
Tax Data	Information to determine federal, state, and local income taxes; payroll taxes; property taxes; sales taxes	None	Information to determine federal and state income taxes; payroll taxes; property taxes	Information to determine federal, state, and local income taxes; payroll taxes; property taxes

consumer unit; and the total number of sources asked about is considerably smaller than in the other surveys. Experience gained in the Income Survey Development Program (ISDP—the predecessor to SIPP) and SIPP itself suggests that each of these factors hampers complete income reporting.[6]

---

[6] Experiments in the ISDP found that a "short" income form produced less complete reporting than the "long" form subsequently used in SIPP and that asking a single respondent about

TABLE B-1 *Continued*

Feature	Consumer Expenditure Survey (Interview)	CPS (March Income Supplement)	Panel Study of Income Dynamics	Survey of Income and Program Participation
Asset Holdings Data[a]	Detailed inventory of property holdings and household appliances; information at 5th interview on credit balances for current month and 1 year ago; information on financial asset holdings currently and 1 year ago	None, except ascertains home ownership	Regularly, information about home value and mortgage debt; occasionally, information about saving behavior and wealth	Detailed inventory of real and financial assets and liabilities once each panel; more frequent measures for assets relevant for assistance programs
Expenditure Data	Detailed quarterly data for expenditures estimated to account for 60–70% of total expenditures; global (or usual) quarterly data for expenditures estimated to account for another 20–25% of total	None	Monthly rent or mortgage costs; annual utility costs; average weekly food costs; child support payments	Information once or twice each panel on last month's out-of-pocket medical care costs, shelter costs (mortgage or rent and utilities), dependent care costs, and child support payments

[a]All four surveys obtain data on income flows from assets.

One problem in estimating poverty from income surveys is that they often show people with zero or very low income amounts that are not credible. As a result, analysts often find that people with very low incomes are not substantially worse off than people with higher income levels on such measures as ownership of vehicles, air conditioning, and number of bathrooms in their

income receipt by other members of the household produced less complete reporting than asking each member about his or her own income (Ycas and Lininger, 1983:27). Also, no imputations are performed in the CEX for missing income information.

homes. Presumably, findings of this sort stem from such phenomena as self-employed people who report zero income or losses on a business accounting basis but who have adequate cash flow for their own needs. Or some of these people may be students or others with low cash income but access to assets or other resources. Or some people may simply underreport their income, particularly if it is from "off-the-books" sources.

Scattered evidence suggests that SIPP may have fewer reporting problems of this sort, perhaps because SIPP takes more of a cash-flow approach to reporting of self-employment income. For example, in 1984, the proportion of people with income-to-poverty ratios of less than 50 percent was 38 percent of the total poverty population in the March CPS but only 29 percent in SIPP (Bureau of the Census, 1986:Table 6; Radbill and Short, 1992:Table 1). Also, SIPP data for 1984 (Radbill and Short, 1992:Table 10) showed steeper relationships of income-to-poverty ratio categories with such well-being measures as home and vehicle ownership than did the 1980 census data analyzed by Christopher Jencks (private communication). For example, home ownership ratios were as follows from the two data sources:

Unit's Income Level Relative to Poverty	Home Ownership Ratios	
	1980 Census	1984 SIPP
Income less than zero	.80	.19
Zero or positive income up to 0.50 of poverty	.38-.41	.19
Income 0.50-0.99 of poverty	.38-.46	.33
Income 1.00-1.99 of poverty	.50-.62	.49
Income 2.00 or more of poverty	.78	.65-.84

THE MARCH CPS AND SIPP COMPARED

This section provides a more detailed comparison of the March CPS income supplement and SIPP, focusing on the adequacy of information from each survey that is relevant to measuring poverty. It also discusses the ability of each survey to construct poverty measures with shorter or longer than annual accounting periods, to construct poverty measures for states, and to construct other measures related to poverty (e.g., measures of access to material goods or access to health care along the lines of work by Mayer and Jencks, 1993). Finally, it offers some comparisons of the quality of income reporting in the two surveys.

Categories of Information

Taxes The March CPS income supplement asks no questions about any type of tax payment. Currently, for use in its experimental poverty estimates, the Census Bureau models federal income taxes, state income taxes, and payroll taxes and imputes annual tax payment amounts to the CPS records (see Bureau of the Census, 1992a; Nelson and Green, 1986).

Generally, SIPP includes twice for each panel (in the summer or fall period) a topical module that asks about tax payments for the previous year. Questions on tax filing status, number of exemptions, type of form filed (joint, single, etc.), and schedules filed (e.g., Schedule A) are answered by more than 90 percent of respondents. However, questions on adjusted gross income, itemized deductions, tax credits, and net tax liability have high nonresponse rates, primarily because respondents are asked to produce their tax forms and use them as the basis for answers to these questions, but only about one-third do so. In addition, there are nonresponse rates of 7 to 14 percent for specific items for those people who do use their tax forms to respond (Bureau of the Census, no date(a)). The Census Bureau has work in progress to develop a tax estimation model for SIPP similar to the one used for the March CPS. The SIPP tax information, even with quality problems, should help in the development of a reliable model.

Nonmedical In-Kind Benefits The March CPS asks about the benefits a household received the previous year from the School Lunch Program (how many children in the household received free or reduced-price lunches during previous year); housing assistance (whether living in public housing or receiving rent subsidy); the Food Stamp Program (how many people were covered in prior year, how many months stamps were received, and the total value of stamps for the prior year); and energy assistance (how much money was received since previous October).

SIPP obtains considerably more detailed information: monthly information on recipiency and benefit amounts for food stamps and the Special Supplemental Nutrition Program for Women, Infants, and Children (WIC); information every 4 months about energy assistance, school lunch, and school breakfast; and information twice a panel about public housing and subsidized housing.

Medical Benefits/Costs The March CPS asks which household members were covered during the previous year by Medicare; Medicaid; Civilian Health and Medical Programs of the Uniformed Services (CHAMPUS), Civilian Health and Medical Programs for the Veterans' Administration (CHAMPVA), or military health care; and private health insurance. For the last, questions are asked about whether the coverage was in a plan in one's own name offered by a current or former employer or union; whether the employer or union paid for all or some of the costs; and who else in the household was covered under the plan. Separate questions are also asked about how many children under age 15 were covered during the prior year by Medicare or Medicaid, another health insurance plan, or by the insurance plan of someone not residing in the household.

SIPP obtains considerably more detailed information, distinguishing among coverage provided by the following programs: Medicare, Medicaid, CHAMPUS, CHAMPVA, military health insurance, current employer or union health insurance, former employer health insurance, and other health insurance. Coverage is ascertained every 4 months for Medicare and every month for the other programs. SIPP also determines which children in the household are covered under Medicaid or other health insurance.

With regard to out-of-pocket medical insurance and medical care costs, the March CPS obtains no information. SIPP asks each panel once about last month's unreimbursed medical care costs.

Child Care and Other Work Expenses   The March CPS asks no questions about child care arrangements or costs or other work expenses. (Occasionally, supplements in other months have included questions on child care arrangements and costs.)

SIPP obtains information once each panel on last month's dependent care costs incurred to enable a household member to be employed. All panels to date have also included a module on child care that asks detailed information about child care arrangements and costs. The 1984-1987 panels included a module on work expenses, including commuting and other costs.

Child Support Payments   The March CPS asks no questions about children outside the household or about payments to support such children.

All SIPP panels to date have included a detailed module on child support.

Asset Holdings   The March CPS asks no questions about the value of asset holdings or liabilities, but information is obtained on whether the house is owned or being bought or is rented. Questions are also asked on total income in the prior year from interest on investments (e.g., savings accounts, certificates of deposit); dividends from stocks and mutual funds; and net income from rent (including income from rented property, roomers or boarders, and royalties).

SIPP obtains detailed information on asset ownership (and income flows) every 4 months. SIPP also obtains a detailed balance sheet of financial and property assets once each panel, and some assets are valued twice a panel (see Citro and Kalton, 1993:Table 3-2).

Nonresponse rates are low for the core asset ownership questions, for example, about 1 percent for savings accounts and stocks; but they are generally high for the questions on 4-month income flows, for example, 30-35 percent for interest and 30 percent for reinvested dividends (Jabine, King, and Petroni, 1990:Table 5.5). After imputation for nonresponse, SIPP obtains an estimated 80 percent of the dividend income reported to the Internal Revenue Service (IRS; compared with 61% in the March CPS) and an estimated

65 percent of reported interest income (compared with 79% in the March CPS, which uses an improved imputation procedure). The March CPS estimate of interest income using the old imputation procedure was only 62 percent of the IRS estimate. Both SIPP and the March CPS fall much farther short of dividend and interest income aggregates when the comparison is made to the National Income and Product Accounts (NIPA); however, the NIPA estimates require extensive adjustments, which may not be complete, for comparability with household survey estimates (see Jabine, King, and Petroni, 1990:Table 10.3)

Nonresponse rates to the questions on value of asset holdings in the topical modules are also very high, although lower than were experienced in the ISDP: 35-40 percent for value of own business, market value of stocks and mutual fund shares, and debt on these assets. After imputation, SIPP obtains higher estimates of equity in homes and motor vehicles in comparison with estimates of the Federal Reserve Board because of somewhat higher estimates of gross value and considerably lower estimates of debt in SIPP, but it obtains considerably lower estimates of equity in noncorporate business, value of financial assets, and consumer debt (see Eargle, 1990:Table D-2).[7]

Ability to Support Other Estimates

Shorter or Longer Term Measures The March CPS provides annual measures of income and poverty. Almost no information is available with which to construct longer term measures. (Because of the rotation group design, one-half of the sample for one year's March supplement is in the sample for the next year's March supplement; hence, it could be possible to construct measures of poverty status over 2 years for this subsample.) Only very limited information is available with which to construct shorter term measures: information is obtained about months of receipt of food stamps and AFDC and about weeks worked, weeks unemployed, and weeks out of the labor force in the prior year.

SIPP, because of its monthly (or 4-month) income information, can be used to construct poverty measures for months, quarters, or other periods

---

[7] SIPP is not alone in experiencing quality problems with the collection of asset data. A number of panel surveys provide estimates of wealth that fall short of those from the Survey of Consumer Finances, a complete survey of household wealth that includes a household sample together with a sample of high-income households drawn from the IRS Statistics of Income file who agree to participate (see Curtin, Juster, and Morgan; 1989; Juster and Kuester, 1991). Recently, the Health and Retirement Study achieved more complete reporting of asset values by a technique called "bracketing," in which holders of an asset who don't know or refuse to provide a value are asked if the value is above a certain amount; if yes, whether it is above another (higher) amount, and so on. High rates of response are obtained by this method, although the response categories are very broad (Juster and Suzman, 1993:16-20).

shorter than a year. Under the current design, SIPP can provide limited longer term measures: for example, transitions in poverty status from one year to the next or estimates of the proportion entering poverty in the first year of a panel who are still poor 1 year or 1-1/2 years later. Under the proposed redesign to extend the length of each panel, SIPP would be able to support longer term measures with accounting periods of up to 4 years. (The 1993 SIPP Panel will be extended to cover a 10-year period, with annual interviews beginning after the first 3 years of interviews every 4 months.)

State Estimates   The CPS sample size and design make it possible to analyze poverty for geographic areas as well as population groups. The Census Bureau recently published state poverty rates (Bureau of the Census, 1992c:Table B). Standard errors for yearly estimates were small for large states (e.g., less than 5% for California and New York in 1991) but high for small states (e.g., 20% for Delaware and New Hampshire in 1991). Standard errors were smaller for 3-year average poverty rates (e.g., 3.5% for California and 15% for New Hampshire).

SIPP is less able to provide reasonably reliable state poverty estimates with the current sample size of about 40,000 households (based on combining two panels) and a design that does not disproportionately sample smaller states. The redesign will increase the sample size to 50,000–55,000 households, but it still may not provide as reliable state estimates as does the March CPS. The proposed oversampling of low-income households in SIPP, beginning with the 1996 panel by using information from the 1990 census, may increase the reliability of the data for detailed poverty analysis.

Related Measures   The March CPS does not obtain information that would enable the development of alternative measures of economic well-being, such as an index of access to material goods or an index of health status and access to health care.

SIPP also does not regularly obtain information that would permit the development of measures of access to a wide range of material goods. However, it does ascertain twice in each panel ownership of the residence and of a vacation home or undeveloped lot, together with information on the make, model, and year of each car, van, or truck owned by someone in the household and whether the household owns a motorcycle, boat, recreational, or other vehicle. Occasionally, a topical module has obtained additional information. For example, Wave 4 of the 1984 SIPP panel asked about housing conditions, including use of a list of consumer durables—range, oven, refrigerator, freezer, washer, dryer, dishwasher, black-and-white television, color television, air conditioning (see Radbill and Short, 1992:Table 10). Wave 6 of the 1991 SIPP panel and Wave 3 of the 1992 panel included a module on extended measures of well-being. This module has questions on consumer durables (e.g., whether the family has a clothes washer or dryer); living conditions (e.g., whether the house is in good repair and the neighborhood is safe); ability to meet expenses for basic needs (e..g, whether the family was ever evicted for nonpayment of rent); and sources of help (e.g., how much help you could expect to get from family living nearby if you were sick).

SIPP has often obtained information on health status and access to health care in topical modules. For example, Wave 3 of the 1984 panel asked about self-reported health status, days in last 4 months sick in bed, number of doctor visits in the last 12 months, and number of hospital nights in the last 12 months.

Quality of Income Data

A key issue in assessing the adequacy of the March CPS or the SIPP for measuring poverty is the quality of the estimates. Although some research on data quality has been done for the March CPS and considerably more research has been done for SIPP, it is not possible at this time to provide an estimate of the total error in the poverty or other income statistics from either survey. There is some comparative information available on what might be termed internal indicators of quality, such as population coverage ratios and household and item response rates, that may indicate potential problems in survey estimates. There is also some limited comparative information on aggregate statistics from the two surveys, such as the percentage of total income of various types that is captured, compared with independent sources. Such comparisons do not identify underlying components of error and must be made with care, given different definitions and procedures between the two surveys and between the surveys and other sources.

Despite limitations, the available information on data quality (discussed below) shows clearly that there is reason to be concerned about the quality of income and poverty statistics from both SIPP and the March CPS. Some indicators, such as item nonresponse rates and amounts of Social Security and other income types collected, in comparison with independent estimates, favor SIPP, while other indicators, such as household nonresponse rates and amount of wages and salaries collected, in comparison with independent estimates, favor the March CPS. Overall, however, SIPP appears to be doing a somewhat better job of measuring income, particularly at the lower end of the income distribution. SIPP's more frequent interviews and detailed probing for receipt of different income sources appear to be identifying more recipients of many income types than the March CPS, although the dollar amounts reported are not always more complete in SIPP than in the CPS. Perhaps more important, SIPP is arguably in a better position to take steps to improve income quality, because of its focus on income and program participation, whereas the March CPS is necessarily constrained as an appendage to a labor force survey. Indeed, no changes to the March income supplement were even considered as part of the recent redesign of the main CPS (except those changes, such as the sample redesign and the introduction of CAPI/CATI, that apply to the entire survey), and the research program on data quality is limited. SIPP will undergo a major redesign to improve the usefulness of the data (notably the extension of each panel to 48 months), which will likely include changes and improvements to the questionnaire. SIPP also has an active research program to investigate and improve data quality (see Jabine, King, and Petroni, 1990).

Population Undercoverage

It is well known that household surveys rarely cover the population as well as the decennial census (see Shapiro and Bettin, 1992; Shapiro and Kostanich, 1988). SIPP and the March CPS are no exception. Thus, even after adjustment for survey nonresponse, the SIPP data for March 1984 covered only 85 percent of black men and 91-93 percent of all other people when compared with census-based population estimates, while the March 1984 CPS covered only 84 percent of black men and 90-94 percent of all others. By age, black men in the 20-39 age categories were generally the worst covered. Coverage ratios were even worse in March 1986 for black men for both SIPP and the March CPS—80 and 82 percent, respectively (Jabine, King and Petroni, 1990:Tables 10.12, 10.13). More recent data indicate that the situation has not improved: the March 1992 CPS covered only 79 percent of black men, 87 percent of black women, and 90-95 percent of white and Hispanic men and women (Coder, 1992a:Table C-1).[8]

The Census Bureau uses ratio-estimation procedures to adjust SIPP and March CPS survey weights for population undercoverage. The weights are adjusted so that the population estimated from the surveys agrees with the updated decennial census-based population estimates by age, sex, race, and Hispanic origin. SIPP weights are also adjusted to agree with the March CPS weights by household type. However, these ratio adjustments do not correct all coverage errors. First, they do not correct for the undercount in the decennial census itself: although it is minimal in total—net undercount was estimated to be between 1 and 2 percent of the population in 1980 and

---

[8] Other household surveys, including the Consumer Expenditure Survey, also exhibit population undercoverage (see Shapiro and Bettin, 1992). Recent work indicates that population undercoverage in surveys may not be as high as previously believed, relative to the decennial census, when comparisons are made that exclude census *overcounts* (see Shapiro, Diffendal, and Cantor, 1993). However, survey undercoverage rates remain high: for example, the undercoverage rate for black males was 89 percent in the February, May, August, and November 1990 CPS, when compared with a 1990 census estimate adjusted for overcounts (versus 84% when compared with an unadjusted estimate). Moreover, these rates do not include the undercount in the census itself relative to demographic estimates of the population.

1990—it is substantial for some population groups. In 1980, an estimated 9-10 percent of black children under age 5 were missed, as were about 15 percent of middle-aged black men (Fay, Passel, and Robinson, 1988:Tables 3.2, 3.3; Robinson, 1990). (The decision was recently made to use census-based population estimates that are adjusted for the census undercount as weighting controls for the CPS and SIPP.)

Second, the ratio adjustments do not correct for characteristics other than age, sex, and ethnic origin on which the undercovered population might be expected to differ from the covered population. Fay (1989) analyzed within-household undercoverage in the CPS relative to the decennial census, using a 1980 CPS-census match. His results are suggestive of ways in which weighting adjustments do not adequately compensate for household survey undercoverage. For example, he finds that about one-fourth of adult black men who are counted in the census but not in the CPS are household heads, whose households should be categorized as married-couple households in the CPS but instead are categorized as households headed by unmarried women.

The correlates of undercoverage (besides age, race, and sex) are not definitely established. However, analysis of the 1980 census postenumeration survey and of other survey, administrative records, and ethnographic data suggests that undercount rates are higher for the following groups: household members other than the head, spouse, and children of the head; unmarried people; people living alone or in very large households; and people residing in central cities of large metropolitan areas (see Citro and Cohen, 1985; Fein, 1989). In addition, there is evidence that the rate of undercount increases as household income decreases.

Overall, these tentative findings suggest that minorities, unattached people, and low-income people are at much greater risk of not being covered in household surveys than other people and, hence, that undercoverage affects SIPP and March CPS-based estimates of poverty. Both the overall poverty rate and, perhaps more important, the distribution of poverty across groups may be affected. The Census Bureau has recently begun a research program to investigate the undercoverage problem in greater depth and take steps to reduce it (Shapiro and Bettin, 1992).

Household and Person Nonresponse

Relative to many other surveys, the CPS obtains high response rates. Yet, 4-5 percent fail to respond to the CPS, and another 9 percent of people in otherwise interviewed households fail to respond (Citro, 1991:26). In addition, a considerable number of people, although responding to the basic CPS labor force questionnaire, do not respond to the March income supplement. Nonresponse to the supplement is treated together with other cases of failing to answer one or more specific questions (see below). To adjust for whole household nonresponse to the basic CPS, the Census Bureau increases the weights of responding households; to adjust for person nonresponse, it imputes a complete data record for another person with similar demographic characteristics. These procedures assume that respondents represent the characteristics of nonrespondents; this assumption has not been adequately tested.

Like all household surveys, SIPP experiences household nonresponse, and like all longitudinal surveys, it suffers cumulative sample loss or attrition at each successive interview wave (some households that fail to respond at an interview wave are subsequently brought back into the survey). In addition, it experiences "type Z" nonresponse—the failure to obtain information, either in person or by proxy, for individual members of otherwise cooperating households.

Attrition in SIPP to date has been highest at the first and second interviews—5-8 percent of eligible households at Wave 1 and 4-6 percent of eligible households at Wave 2. Thereafter, the additional loss is only 2-3 percent in each of Waves 3-5 and less than 1 percent in each subsequent wave. By Wave 6 (after 2 years of interviewing), cumulative sample loss is 18-20 percent of eligible households; by Wave 8, it is 21-22 percent (Bowie, 1991). The Panel to Evaluate SIPP estimated that total sample attrition at the end of 12 waves (4 years) might be 25 percent (Citro and Kalton, 1993:102). The attrition experience in SIPP is quite comparable to that in the ISDP (Nelson, Bowie, and Walker, 1987) and the PSID (with the exception that, as noted above, the PSID experienced a larger sample loss at the first two waves).

Attrition reduces the number of cases that are available for analysis—including the number available for longitudinal analysis over all or part of the time span of a panel and the number available for cross-sectional analysis from interview waves—and thereby increases the sampling error of the estimates. More important, the people who drop out may differ from those who remain in the survey. To the extent that adjustments to the weights for survey respondents do not compensate for these differences, estimates from the survey may be biased.

The available evidence does suggest that people who drop out of SIPP differ from those who stay in the survey. Studies of nonresponse from the 1984 SIPP panel show that household noninterview rates after the first wave tended to be higher for renters, for households located in large metropolitan areas, and for households headed by young adults. Individuals who did not complete all of the interview waves, compared with those who did, tended to include more residents of large metropolitan areas, renters, members of racial minorities, children and other relatives of the reference person, people aged 15-24, never-married people, and people with no savings accounts or other assets (Jabine, King, and Petroni, 1990:35-37, Table 5.4). A recent analysis of attrition from the 1990 SIPP panel obtained similar results (Lamas, Tin, and Eargle, 1994). This study found that attrition was more likely to occur among young adults, males, minority groups, never-married people, poor people, and people with lower educational attainment.

In addition, more limited evidence suggests that the current noninterview weighting adjustments do not fully compensate for differential attrition across groups. One evaluation of the procedures to adjust for household non-response at each wave developed two sets of weights for Wave 2 households in the 1984 panel—one set based on all Wave 2 households and one set based just on those Wave 2 households that provided interviews at Wave 6. Comparing Wave 2 estimates from these two samples showed that the latter set produced higher estimates of median income and fewer households with low monthly income than those produced with the former set, evidence that the weights do not adequately adjust for higher attrition rates among low-income households (Petroni and King, 1988). A subsequent study that compared samples from the 1985 panel of all Wave 2 households and those that provided interviews at Wave 6 obtained similar findings (King et al., 1990).

With regard to annual estimates of poverty from SIPP, one study (Lamas, Tin, and Eargle, 1994) found that the inclusion of people with missing waves, using an imputation process, produced somewhat higher poverty rates than the use of complete reporters. Approximately one-sixth of the difference between annual poverty rates in SIPP and the March CPS is apparently due to attrition bias.

It is important to note that the current cross-sectional nonresponse adjust-ments in SIPP make only minimal use of the information that is available from previous waves for many current nonrespondents. Also, in constructing lon-gitudinal files from SIPP panels, the Census Bureau assigns zero weights to original sample members who missed only one or a few waves in addition to those who missed all or most waves. The Census Bureau has recently com-mitted itself to an intensive program of research to improve the weighting adjustments for attrition as part of the decision to move to 4-year panels for SIPP with no overlap (Weinberg and Petroni, 1992).

Item Nonresponse

In addition to household and person nonresponse, there is substantial item nonresponse in the March CPS. The Census Bureau imputes as much as 20 percent of the total income in the CPS. For some income sources, imputation rates are even higher—as much as one-third of nonfarm self-employment income, interest, and dividend payments are imputed (Bureau of the Census, 1989a:Table A-2; Bureau of the Census, 1992b:Table C-1).

SIPP compares favorably with the March CPS on item nonresponse rates: overall, only 11 percent of total regular money income for 1984 was imputed in SIPP, compared with 20 percent in the March CPS. The SIPP and March CPS imputation rates for earnings were 10 percent and 19 percent, respectively; for public and private transfers, 12 percent and 21 percent, respectively; and for property income, 24 percent and 32 percent, respectively (Jabine, King, and Petroni, 1990:Table 10.8; see also Citro and Kalton, 1993:Tables 3-4, 3-5 for comparisons of nonresponse rates for such specific income sources as AFDC and SSI).

The imputation process maximizes the available sample size for analysis from a survey by providing filled-in records for respondents whose records would otherwise have to be discarded if key analytical variables were missing. However, the process can introduce error. No definitive evaluation has been conducted of the imputation procedures used in the March CPS or SIPP; however, available evidence suggests that the procedures are a source of error and could be improved.

The Census Bureau currently applies very complex procedures, which it refers to as statistical matches, to impute values in the March CPS for whole groups of variables, such as income and employment-related items. The records are classified by a number of characteristics, and the record that is the best match is selected as the "donor" to supply the missing values to the record requiring imputation (the "host"). The Census Bureau's statistical matching procedures have, over the years, replaced somewhat less complex "hot-deck" imputations for more and more items. In the hot-deck method, the data records are arrayed by geographic area and processed sequentially, and the reported values are used to update matrices of characteristics. A record with a missing item has the most recently updated value assigned from the appropriate matrix. Hot-deck methods are largely used for imputation in SIPP.

David et al. (1986) compared the Census Bureau's imputations of earnings in the March CPS with a regression-based imputation—using data from the Internal Revenue Service from a 1981 exact-match CPS-IRS file as the measure of truth—and found that the CPS methods performed quite well in reproducing the overall shape of the earnings distribution. However, they and other analysts have determined that the CPS imputations are less successful for small groups, such as minorities and specific occupations (Coder, no date: Lillard, Smith, and Welch, 1986). Coder (1991), in an exact match of the March 1986 CPS with IRS records for married couples with earnings, found that records with imputations for CPS earnings contributed significantly to the overall underestimate of wages and salaries in the CPS in comparison with the IRS tax returns. Thus, while mean CPS earnings in cases with no imputations were 98 percent of mean IRS earnings, mean CPS earnings in cases with imputations were only 89 percent of mean IRS earnings. Also, while 95 percent of cases with no imputations had CPS earnings within 1 decile of IRS earnings, only 66 percent of cases with imputations were in this close agreement.

The available evidence suggests that the SIPP imputation procedures could also be improved. Several studies have focused on the population eligible for assistance programs and have identified problems because the current procedures do not take low income or receipt of program benefits into account in imputing program-related variables. Doyle and Dalrymple (1987) found that the imputation of income in the 1984 SIPP panel for households reporting receipt of food stamps produced a larger proportion of such households with high monthly incomes that would make them ineligible for Food Stamp Program benefits than households that reported both their cash income and food stamps. Allin and Doyle (1990) compared program participants from the 1984 SIPP panel whom they simulated to be eligible for food stamp benefits with participants whom they simulated to be ineligible because of excessive incomes or asset holdings: they found that only 5 percent of the eligible participants but 28 percent of the ineligible participants had some or all income or asset values imputed.

Coder (1992b), in an exact match of the 1990 SIPP panel with IRS records for married couples with earnings, found results similar to the 1986 CPS-IRS exact-match study reported above. Records with imputations for SIPP earnings contributed significantly to the overall underestimate of wages and salaries in the SIPP in comparison with the IRS tax returns. Thus, while mean SIPP earnings in cases with no imputations were 94 percent of mean IRS earnings, mean SIPP earnings in cases with imputations were only 85 percent of mean IRS earnings. Also, while 88 percent of cases with no imputations had SIPP earnings within 1 decile of IRS earnings, only 75 percent of cases with imputations were in this close agreement.

Other Sources of Error

A number of other error sources have been identified in the March CPS and SIPP, particularly with regard to poverty and related income statistics, although no definitive results are available on their effects.

The CPS, like other surveys with a rotation group design, is subject to rotation group bias, in that respondents who are newer to the survey give different responses than do respondents who have been in the survey for a longer period. For example, the unemployment rate estimated for households in the incoming CPS rotation group each month is 7 percent higher than the average for all eight rotation groups (Bailar, 1989:Table 6). There has been no analysis of how rotation group bias might affect poverty and income estimates from the March supplement.

Reporting errors, as distinct from nonresponse, are also a potential problem. Very few record checks that compare survey reports with independent sources (e.g., tax or program records) for the same people have been conducted for the March CPS. Coder (1991) conducted such a record-check study in his 1986 exact-match CPS-IRS analysis. He noted that the net CPS aggregate underestimate of 2-3 percent masked widespread over- and underreporting of amounts and that the imputation procedures did little to correct the bias from nonresponse. Despite these errors, the CPS distribution of earnings was very similar to that derived from the IRS. The most serious error problems were concentrated at the bottom and top of the distribution.

Estimates of poverty and income from the March CPS are affected by the fact that the sample comprises persons present at the March interview who are asked about income in the preceding calendar year. Thus, income from people who died during the year or otherwise left the survey universe is missed entirely (this is not true for SIPP). Also, family composition is measured as of the March following the income reference year, and no information is obtained about intrayear changes in composition. For example, two people found to be married as of March will be classified as a married couple for the entire income reference year and assigned the combined income of both spouses for that year. However, this treatment is misleading, with regard to classification both by family type and by income level, if, in fact, the couple's marriage took place after the start of the income year. The limited available evidence suggests that annual poverty rates in the CPS may be biased upwards to some extent by the mismatch of family composition and income (see Czajka and Citro, 1982; Williams, 1987; see also Lamas, Tin, and Eargle, 1994).

In SIPP, researchers have looked at the equivalent of rotation group bias, namely time-in-sample or conditioning effects. As a panel progresses, respondents may acquire new knowledge that affects their behavior: for example, they may apply for benefits from government assistance programs as a direct consequence of learning about such programs from the survey. They may also gain experience with the questionnaire that leads them to give either less accurate or more accurate answers than in earlier interviews. However, studies conducted with SIPP to date suggest that conditioning effects are scattered and of limited effect (see, e.g., Pennell and Lepkowski, 1992).

Some record-check studies have been conducted with SIPP, including the 1990 SIPP-IRS exact match (Coder, 1992b). Marquis and Moore (1990a, 1990b) carried out a record-check study that matched SIPP records in four states from the first two waves of the 1984 panel with records from eight state and federal programs (AFDC, food stamps, unemployment insurance, worker's compensation, federal civil service retirement, Social Security, SSI, and veterans' pensions and compensation). The results showed negatively biased participation rates for most programs: that is, net underreporting of participation, although there were overreports as well as underreports. For most programs, there appeared to be relatively little bias in reporting of benefit amounts for those who correctly reported their participation. In one state, a large proportion of AFDC recipients incorrectly reported their benefits as general assistance.

One problem identified in SIPP and other longitudinal surveys is the "seam" phenomenon, in which respondents are more likely to report changes (e.g., going off or on a welfare program) between pairs of months that span two interviews (e.g., for SIPP, months 4-5, 8-9, 12-13, etc.) than between pairs of months for which data are collected from the same interview. The seam problem affects most variables for which monthly data are collected in SIPP—often strongly. For example, in the first year of the 1984 SIPP panel, over twice as many nonparticipants reported entering the Social Security program between seam months than nonseam months (Jabine, King, and Petroni, 1990:Table 6.2). The reasons for the occurrence and extent of the seam phenomenon are not well understood, but it clearly results in errors in the timing of transitions in SIPP and the duration of spells of program participation (and perhaps of poverty). It may or may not result in errors in the number of transitions that occur within a given period. For example, in the case of food stamps, total exits and entrances from SIPP are close to the rates derived from food stamp administrative records. In contrast, whether due to the seam effect or other factors, entrance rates from SIPP for SSI are significantly higher than those shown by program records (Jabine, King, and Petroni, 1990:59-60). The Census Bureau has pursued research and testing of alternative questionnaire designs and interviewing procedures that could reduce the seam problem and produce more accurate income reporting overall (see, e.g., Marquis, Moore, and Bogen, 1991). To date, there have been few positive results.

Aggregate Comparisons

Aggregate comparisons of income estimates from SIPP and CPS, like comparisons of internal indicators of data quality, show a mixed picture. On balance, SIPP seems to be doing a somewhat better job of income reporting, but not for all income types. Moreover, it may be that the gains in SIPP are not holding up over time.

Comparisons of 1984 estimates from the 1984 SIPP and March 1985 CPS showed SIPP as a percentage of CPS as follows (Jabine, King, and Petroni, 1990:Table 10.8):

Total money income	100.1
Regular money income	99.9
Earnings	98.2
All other	106.0
Public and private transfers	111.6
Property income	103.1
All other regular money income	37.0
Lump-sum payments	N.A. (not collected in CPS)

SIPP performed better than the March CPS with the notable exception of earnings. (The low ratio for all other regular money income is presumably due to higher levels of reporting of specific income types in SIPP than in the

March CPS.) Census Bureau analysts assume that many SIPP respondents are reporting their net paychecks rather than their gross earnings as requested by the survey.

Coder and Scoon-Rogers (1994) reported comparisons for detailed income sources for 1984 and 1990. These comparisons indicate that some of the gains in income reporting seen in SIPP at the outset of the survey may no longer be occurring. However, they noted that the 1990 SIPP panel may not be comparable to the 1984 panel because it contained an added sample, carried over from the 1989 panel, of households headed by single mothers and minorities. The weighting adjustments for these added cases may be problematic.

As with the review of internal indicators of data quality, it is difficult from the available comparisons of aggregates to draw conclusions about the implications for estimates of poverty and related income statistics. Perhaps the most telling summary indicator available is the fact, noted above, that SIPP poverty estimates are consistently several percentage points below those from the March CPS. Lamas, Tin, and Eargle (1994) found that only about one-sixth of this difference could be explained by attrition bias in SIPP. Another one-sixth of the difference appears due to more accurate measurement of family composition during the income reporting year in SIPP than in the March CPS. The remaining two-thirds difference, it is hypothesized, is explained by more complete reporting of income in SIPP for the lower end of the income distribution. In that regard, respondents to SIPP report more sources of income than respondents to the March CPS; they also report higher amounts for such income sources as Social Security, Railroad Retirement, SSI, unemployment compensation, veterans' payments, and child support payments, all of which are important to the low-income population. However, reporting of AFDC and other cash welfare is currently no more complete in SIPP than in the March CPS (Coder and Scoon-Rogers, 1994:Table 1). Clearly, much more analytical work needs to be done, including work to look at differences in income reporting among population groups within and across the surveys and the development of a complete time series of poverty and related income statistics from SIPP for comparison with the March CPS.

The Interdependence of Time and Money

In the panel's primary focus on the measurement of poverty in the United States, we discuss the rationale for, and the measurement of, a concept of poverty based on the lack of family resources needed to obtain an adequate level of food, clothing, shelter, and a little more. Setting the poverty threshold, we suggest, should be informed by the actual level of expenditure on these commodities by consumer units, with the threshold determined as an appropriate fraction of the median expenditure by a reference family type, with a small additional amount to allow for other expenditures.

The concept of poverty that we contend should be used as the U.S. official poverty measure—economic poverty—is based on having the money or near-money resources needed for consumption. We stress at several points in the volume that this concept of poverty should not be considered the only relevant measure of deprivation. A measure of economic poverty should be supplemented by other measures that might reflect psychological deprivation, exposure to extreme risks of physical harm, illiteracy, lack of adequate medical care, and so forth.

In this appendix we address an issue that is neither as separable from the measure of economic poverty as psychological or even health-related factors are, nor as easily incorporated into an economic measure as the flow of services from owned homes might be: how to treat the valuable resource of time. Because of the unique problems posed by this one issue, we devote this appendix to considering it alone.

"TIME IS MONEY"

The old adage that "time is money" essentially says it all, but unfortunately it does not tell one how to measure the value of time when measuring the available economic resources in a family unit. Nor does it tell one how to take account of the fact that two families with similar economic resources might have vastly different time resources that somehow should be taken into account in determining their material well-being. In this section we first illustrate the dilemma and the seemingly inadequate strategy of just ignoring the value of time when measuring a family's command over resources. Next we show actual expenditure data that reinforce the concern that it is not appropriate simply to count all the dollars of income and ignore all the time resources.

Illustration

To illustrate the issue simply, consider two households. Household A has one adult; household B has two adults; neither has any children. The official (1992) poverty thresholds for these households (averaged by age of the head) are $7,143 and $9,137, respectively. This pair of thresholds implies that household B requires 128 percent as much income as household A to be at comparable poverty thresholds.

With these numbers, we can illustrate the question of time; see Table C-1. Since there are 168 hours in each week, household A has a total of 168 hours available every week, and B has twice that much time, 336 hours, since both adults have 168. Suppose that within each week every person requires 70 hours for sleep, personal hygiene, and eating—8 hours for sleep and 2 hours for personal hygiene and eating. (We use these values only for illustration and profess no expertise about their magnitudes; if the numbers are changed, the same points apply.) Subtracting this 70 hours per week from the total of 168 leaves just under 100 hours per person for discretionary use, that is, for all other activities.

Next, assume that the adults in households A and B each have a wage rate of $3.57. We selected this arbitrary wage rate to yield exactly $7,143 in annual income per adult if that adult worked 40 hours each week for 50 weeks of the year. This wage rate permits the full-time earner in household A to achieve exactly the poverty threshold level of income. Subtracting that 40 hours from the discretionary weekly hours, the adult in that household has now 58 hours available for all remaining activities. But for household B, the two adults only need to be employed a combined total of 51 hours per week to earn the poverty threshold level of income. One of the two might work full time, for 40 hours a week, and the other work part time for about 11 hours a week; or they might both work part time, averaging a little over 25 hours of work per

TABLE C-1   A Comparison of the Value of Time in Two Households

Factors in Valuing Time	Household Composition	
	A: One Adult	B: Two Adults
Official Poverty Threshold, 1992[a]	$7,143	$9,137
Relation of Thresholds	1.00	1.28
Time Allocation, Weekly Hours		
Total	168	336
Personal care (subtract)	−70	−140
Discretionary, net	98	196
Needed to earn poverty		
threshold @$3.57/hour (subtract)	−40	−51
Available, net	58	145
Available per person, net	58	72.5
Valuing the Nonmarket Time		
Hours available per week	58	145
Annual value @$3.57/hour	$10,353	$25,882
Assuming No Scale Economies		
in Nonmarket Time		
Scale	1.00	2.00
Monetary equivalent	$10,353	$20,706
Extra resources for B	—	$5,176
Assuming the Same Scale Economies in		
Nonmarket Time as in Money Usage		
Scale	1.00	1.28
Monetary equivalent	$10,353	$13,252
Extra resources for B	—	$12,630

[a]Weighted averages from Bureau of the Census (1993c:Table A).

week. After subtracting these work hours, household B has 145 hours available for all remaining activities.

If the two households have exactly met their poverty threshold level of income, and all adults have the same (arbitrarily set) hourly wage rate, then the two households are equally well off in terms of economic resources. That is, after all, just what these poverty threshold levels are supposed to achieve. But notice that in household B, the remaining discretionary time is a total of 145 hours or 72.5 hours per person; in household A it is 58 hours. This fact highlights the underlying issue: having set poverty threshold levels of income for households A and B that reflect the economies of scale in living together (putting aside whether the scale economies are correctly measured or not) necessarily results in the larger household's having more discretionary time per adult than the smaller household. Thus, the two households are not equally well off at the poverty thresholds, even though those thresholds were set at levels that were intended to achieve just that condition. After meeting their personal care needs and working enough (at a similar wage rate) to earn the poverty threshold level of income, each person in household B has 72.5 free hours, but the person in household A has only 58 hours. It looks as though the two people in household B are better off than the person in household A.

This particular illustration makes the point simply: if one ignores time in measuring poverty, one overlooks an important resource that can be converted into money. If we had used larger households in the illustration, the point could be made with even larger discrepancies. (Different values for the personal care needs or for the scale economies or for the wage rate in the illustration do not qualitatively change the conclusion.)

Moreover, since time is used in earning the money that meets the poverty thresholds, time is not just an example of a separate and independent resource that has been overlooked or set aside. Unlike many other resources, this resource—time—is generally correlated with the money earned. In many cases, it is traded for money in the labor market. Thus, for many family units, time is systematically and negatively correlated with money: those who have more leisure or home time have less money, and those who spend more time in the labor market earning money have correspondingly less discretionary time for other activities.

To return to the illustrative example above, one can get an estimate of the monetary value of the extra time in household B in comparison with household A (see Table C-1). To do so, one needs to decide two things: what money value to use in measuring the time value of the discretionary time, and what (if any) scale economies to assume in the use of that nonmarket time. For the former, we use the market wage rate of $3.57. (Again, the point made here could be made with many other arbitrarily set nonmarket time valuations.) Regarding scale economies, we use two extreme assumptions to suggest bounds on the point: first, that there are no scale economies in nonmarket time use; second, that the economies of scale are the same as the scale economies in using money.

The 58 discretionary hours available to household A have the value $10,353, and the 145 discretionary hours in household B have the value $25,882. Under the assumption that there are no scale economies in using this nonmarket time, household B would need twice as much time as A to achieve the same per capita outcome, which is $20,706 worth of time, leaving as a residual an extra bit of time in household B that is valued at $5,176. That extra resource—the time valued at $5,176—seems to be inconsistent with viewing the two households as equally well off. Under the assumption that scale economies are the same for nonmarket time as for purchased commodities, household B needs only $13,252 in time value to obtain what household A obtains ($10,353 × 1.28); this implies that household B has an extra bit of time that is valued at $12,630. Again, household B seems to be better off than household A, and that is inconsistent with the goals that were set in establishing poverty thresholds for the two households. These dollar values on the available discretionary time simply quantify the point made earlier: the household with more discretionary time appears to be better off than the other one.

Expenditure Data

The illustrative example depicts the logic that if both time and money have value, and if poverty thresholds are defined on the basis of equivalence in money income only, then no matter how the money equivalents are set, the combined value of the time and money that households have at their disposal is misspecified. If the money alone is correctly calculated, when one looks at the value of time there is an apparent inconsistency.

In this section, we discuss a related aspect of the interdependence of time and money: those families that have more than one adult employed in the job market appear to spend at least some, and perhaps a sizable portion, of the second earner's added income on goods and services that are associated with earning that money. Thus, it is arguable that some portion of those earnings is not in fact a net increase in the family's real income and does not reflect a real increase in command over resources. If this is so, it raises the question of how to adjust for this simple substitution of money for nonmarket time when one measures a family's level of income.

The relevant data on expenditures are not hard to find, but the implications for what should be done to account for the differences are not so easy to find. Lazear and Michael (1980b) compare two sets of households from the 1972-1973 Consumer Expenditure Survey (CEX), both with two adults and no children, one set with one earner and the other with two earners. The before-tax income for these two sets differed by 35 percent (with the two-earner couples having the higher income, of course). In terms of total current consumption, however, the difference was only 17 percent. That is, the two-earner families both faced higher taxes and saved a higher portion of their income, so in terms of spending on goods and services, the difference, on average, was far less than the difference in gross (before-tax) income. More revealing, the two-earner families spent much more than one-earner families on items that can be considered market substitutes for home-produced goods: restaurant expenditures were 55 percent higher, dry cleaning services were 42 percent higher, and women's clothing was 60 percent higher, while expenditures on food at home were actually 15 percent lower. (Rental expenditures by renters were 12 percent higher.)

It appears that much of the income earned by the second earner is spent on making it possible to earn that income. Thus, the net addition to the family's resources is less than the added income, since that income is at least partially offset by less time in the nonmarket activities by that second earner. On the basis of this evidence, Michael (1985:136) argues: "Almost certainly the impact on real income [of the second earner's wage earnings] is a small fraction of the change in money income."

A more recent article by Jacobs, Shipp, and Brown (1989) uses the 1984–1986 CEX data and includes families that have children, so they can observe expenditures on child care, which the Lazear and Michael study did not consider. This study concludes (p. 15): "When a wife becomes a second earner, husband-wife families spend more on work-related and timesaving items such as child care and food away from home." They exploit the quarterly data from the CEX and compare family spending patterns in the second quarter of the survey year to that in the fifth quarter, looking specifically at those families in which the wife began employment between those two times and comparing the changes to a control group in which the wife was not employed throughout the year. The results were inconclusive in this strategy, but when a multivariate regression model was used, controlling for household characteristics, they find (Jacobs, Shipp, and Brown, 1989:21):

> Families in which the wife is employed spend significantly more on food away from home, child care, women's apparel and gasoline and motor oil than do families in which the wife does not work outside the home.

Another recent study by Hanson and Ooms (1991) uses the 1980-1983 CEX data and suggests a further refinement. They conclude that the two-earner families that have relatively low levels of husband's earnings actually expend proportionately more on "work-related expenditures and taxes" (an increment of 69 percent) in comparison with families with middle levels of husband's earnings (an increment of 56 percent) or to families with upper levels of husband's earnings (an increment of only 29 percent). So to disregard work-related expenditures may be particularly problematic for lower income families.

Discussion

All these studies simply show the not-remarkable fact that when a second adult in the family enters the work force and earns income, some of that income is spent buying in the marketplace goods and services other families secure by nonmarket efforts. A skeptic might well ask: "So what? Isn't this also the case for the first earner? If the household had zero earners, wouldn't that household be inclined to do even more nonmarket production—growing its own food, sewing its own clothing, and so forth?" This point is correct, but a poverty threshold implicitly assumes some amount of nonmarket time and some likely amount of labor market effort: thus, a threshold of, say, $15,000 in money income for a family of some particular size and structure has embedded within it some implicit amount of time in the home. But when one begins to compare households of different sizes and structures, one confronts the fact that there is a violation of the implicit assumption that the differences in money somehow also correspond to the differences in available nonmarket time. When it is clear that the nonmarket time in different families is far from proportionate to the money income in those two families, one may become uneasy in treating those families as equally well off.

Consider the extreme example in which one family obtains the threshold level of money from labor market earnings and another family of identical structure and size receives the same income completely from government assistance programs. It is discomforting to characterize these two families as exactly equally well off: the second family has much more nonmarket time available than the working family, and somehow this should be taken into account.

The illustration of households A and B above emphasized that when one looks only at the available money, a family's available total resources, including discretionary time, is almost surely misspecified. The expenditure data from the several CEX studies make the same point in reverse: some of the money earned is used to facilitate the earnings itself, and other of the money earned is used to buy in the marketplace goods and services that are typically produced at home by families with less earnings. Both these observations emphasize the intricately intertwined linkages between money and time. Time is money and to some degree the two are interchangeable: to disregard time is to misspecify the available resources in the family unit. Yet time and money are not fully interchangeable in all cases, of course; there are many uses of money that have no own-time substitute. For instance, no amount of one's own time can heal an abscessed tooth—a dentist is needed and, for that, money (or, at least, barter) is essential.

In an effort to measure economic poverty, it is easiest to just ignore nonmarket time, and treat money as money, but the panel finds this inadequate. In fact, we argue in the text that near-money—food stamps, school lunches, and housing subsidies, for example—should be counted as part of a family's resources in comparing resources with the poverty threshold. In the proposed poverty measure, we convert near-money to money equivalence. If time is near-money, perhaps it, too, should be converted to money in the measurement of a family's resources. Similarly, in the text we argue that some expenditures are necessary to obtain labor market earnings—child care and other work-related expenses, for example—and should be subtracted from earnings in measuring the available money resources. In the proposed poverty measure, we convert gross money into net money available to expend on food, clothing, and shelter, and a little more. If time at home can be used to obtain food or clothing or shelter, perhaps it, too, should be valued in measuring a family's resources to obtain these commodities up to the poverty threshold levels.

If one argues for subtracting expenditures that substitute for time at home doing certain tasks, such as child care, when measuring the relevant level of family income for determining poverty status, then it seems logical to argue that time at home does legitimately enter into the determination of the relevant measure of money income in determining poverty status. If so, the issue becomes what level of nonmarket time is implicitly assumed in setting the poverty threshold levels of money income for a household of one adult, or for a family with two adults and no children, or a family with one child, and so on. To be frank, we do not know how to incorporate time in a feasible and manageable way. Consequently, we do not know how to adjust for more or less time as one measures money resources to compare with those poverty thresholds. We next review two suggestions from the literature.

RESEARCH APPROACHES

Time Poor: A Measurement

Perhaps the best statement of the problem with ignoring time that has an associated suggestion regarding its solution is Vickery (1977), who stressed the importance of time as a resource and suggested a two-dimensional poverty definition. As shown in Figure C-1, Vickery suggested that a poverty threshold should have both a minimum money level, such as M_0 in that figure, and also a minimum time level, such as T_0, and with some tradeoff, as depicted by the curved line segment AB. Households with resources to the left of T_0 would be considered time-poor, and those below M_0 would be considered monetarily poor; those to the right and above M_0, T_0, and AB would be considered not poor. Of course, setting the level T_0 and the tradeoff AB would require judgment, as does setting the minimum income level, M_0. (Vickery had some suggestions about these minimum levels.)

We suggest that a key element in this determination of poverty would be a household's ability to convert time into money—the wage rate of the adult(s) in the unit—which we depict at two levels in lines L and H in the figure. As drawn, the household with the lower wage rate, L, would be considered in poverty; the household with the higher wage rate, H, would not be considered in poverty. Notice that the second household might choose a position along its wage line at which its nonmarket time was in fact below time poverty, but it could as well select a position along its wage line that put its income below money poverty. In neither case would the household be considered in poverty, however, since these choices are discretionary.

Notice that this strategy for defining which households are in poverty places the burden of the definition of poverty heavily on the notion of the wage rate, the best indicator of the potential tradeoff between time and money. To define poverty by the wage rate instead of by the actual income received

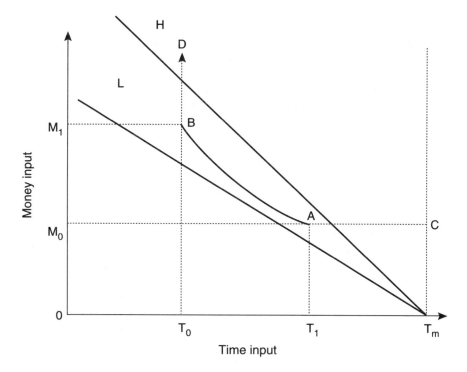

FIGURE C-1 Time and money tradeoffs in the poverty threshold for a household.
SOURCE: Adapted from Vickery (1977).

can, in fact, resolve much of the problem of disregarding time, but it places a very heavy burden on the determination of the relevant, available wage rate for the adults in the household. Even when that wage is determined, there is the issue of whether it is in fact available and, if so, for how many hours. In fact, using a given wage rate as depicted in Figure C-1 assumes that the adult can trade any number of hours for dollars at that wage rate. But the presence of unemployment, of various rigidities in hours of work on certain jobs, and the high rate of job turnover, especially among those who are less skilled, causes one to doubt that assumption. And if that wage is not actually available, this theoretically appealing strategy for measuring poverty would be quite difficult to implement empirically. Considering the complexity of measuring the relevant wage rate for all persons and units and of knowing the constraints on its availability across hours of work and from week to week, we as a panel do not recommend adopting this strategy for measuring poverty. In light of the practical difficulties it raises, we do not consider it a feasible alternative. It is possible that with further research this analytically attractive alternative would become tractable and implementable, but it is not so today.

Calculating Earnings Capacity

The use of the wage rate as the key determinant of the poverty status of a household unit is very similar to the solution to the problem advocated by Haveman in a series of articles (see Garfinkel and Haveman, 1977; Haveman, 1992, 1993; Haveman and Buron, 1991, 1993). The strategy suggested by Haveman and his colleagues is to estimate the earnings capacity of the adults in the household and to use that capacity, for a person employed in a full-time job minus the costs incurred in having that job, as the estimate of income against which a poverty threshold is compared. As Haveman (1992:12) puts it: "Does a family have the skills and capabilities to earn its way out of poverty were it fully to use them?" If so, the suggestion is to define that family as not in poverty; if not, to define that family as in poverty.

This suggestion is quite similar to the suggestion above of relying on the level of the market wage rate (adjusting for the necessary costs of employment) as the measure of poverty status. Haveman has, in fact, implemented his suggestion, using the Current Population Survey (CPS), to estimate the earnings capacity of the families and unrelated individuals in the CPS and then to consider the composition and magnitude of poverty so defined.

There can be philosophical differences about whether it is preferable to measure poverty on the basis of the actual income received or the potential income that might be received if the family unit "played by the rules" and worked for pay as much as some other family does. Once the allocation of time becomes a focus, this distinction between actual and potential earnings is relevant. We as a panel have taken no position on the matter of the preferable measure, because we stress a preemptive issue: estimating the wage potential with the precision necessary to implement this method of measuring official poverty in the United States is not yet feasible. Neither the wage rate that might be earned if a job were available, nor the likelihood of finding a job that offered that wage rate for the number of hours preferred by the individual, is a calculation that can easily be made. Thus, we do not take a position on the matter of the relative attractiveness of using a wage rate definition or an actual income definition of family resources. We urge continued research to address this matter, but do not consider it sufficiently resolved to warrant implementation now.

A few of the issues not yet resolved—which convinced us that earnings capacity is not yet feasible as an alternative to income for determining poverty status—include the following:

(1) Is it preferable to use the actual earnings of those who have full-time earnings or to use an imputed earnings potential for those families as well as for those who have no actual earnings? Imputation is surely necessary for those who do not have actual earnings, but then it is not clear how to link these imputed cases to the many others with full-time or part-time earnings.

(2) Is it preferable to use the actual wage rate for units with part-time employment and scale up their potential earnings to full time or to use an imputed wage rate for them as well?

(3) How does one build into the estimates derived from imputation an appropriate variability based on the error term of the estimation model for those units that require imputation?

(4) How should one estimate the capacity for those who have retired or are elderly and have not had a history of earnings at an earlier age?

Furthermore, if earnings capacity were fully measurable and brought into the measurement of poverty, then other analytic issues would be raised. For example, by introducing leisure time as a commodity that is purchased with the available resources of time and money, there is then a need to take account of the fact that those with a high wage rate face a relatively high price for that commodity. Until it is clear how to estimate the capacity to earn with greater precision and consistency than is now the case, an earnings capacity definition of resources should not be the basis of the poverty measure. Even when enough is known about how to integrate time and money resources in the measurement of poverty, it will also be necessary to consider how that introduction might alter the level that is set as the threshold for poverty. It would not be reasonable to simply add the value of some or all nonmarket time without considering how that modification on the resource side should affect the level of the threshold.

CONCLUSION

There is at present no feasible way to improve the measurement of poverty by incorporating the time allocation of families. We encourage further research that might yield a better solution in the near future, but we see no way adequately to address this perplexing issue now. The earnings capacity estimate of available income, suggested by Haveman and colleagues, and the wage rate usage as suggested above in the context of Vickery's analytic figure, both address the issue, but they are not warranted as a replacement for the current strategy of estimating income directly. Although there are important contributions in the literature regarding how Americans actually spend their nonmarket time (e.g., see Juster and Stafford, 1985; Robinson, 1977; and Walker and Woods, 1976), and analytically how to understand its allocation (e.g., Becker, 1965), we know of no implementable solution to the concern addressed here.

Thus, many concerns about the treatment or nontreatment of time are unresolved. One of these concerns is that some families are probably considered to be impoverished that could spend enough time working for pay to earn enough to get themselves out of poverty but do not do so. At the other end of the spectrum is concern that some families probably devote so much of their limited time and energy to earning money, that despite having income a little above the poverty threshold, they are "time poor" and quite impoverished. Both of these concerns, among others, need to be addressed by further work on the proper method for introducing the value of time into the measurement of poverty.

Assistance Programs for People with Low Incomes

T his appendix describes assistance programs, partly or wholly financed by the federal government, that provided income support, near–cash income support, or other benefits and services to people with low income through 1994. Table D-1 categorizes 70 programs by the type of test they use to determine income eligibility for program benefits. In fiscal 1992 the expenditures of these programs totaled $279 billion. Of these 70 programs,

- 14 of them (20%), which account for 2 percent of the expenditures, use the poverty guidelines (or a multiple of them) as the sole criterion of income eligibility (see Part A of Table D-1);
- 13 of them (19%), which account for 56 percent of the expenditures, accord eligibility to people already participating in another program, such as Aid to Families with Dependent Children (AFDC) and Supplemental Security Income (SSI), and also permit other people to qualify by comparing their incomes to the poverty guidelines (see Part B of Table D-1);[1]

---

[1] In some programs, the comparison is to a multiple of the poverty guidelines if that level is higher than a percentage of state median income or a percentage of the lower living standard income level defined by the U.S. Department of Labor. The lower living standard income levels are published by the department's Employment and Training Administration for 25 metropolitan areas and for metropolitan and nonmetropolitan components of the four census regions, Alaska, and Hawaii. These levels represent the Bureau of Labor Statistics lower level family budget, developed for 1967 on the basis of 1960-1961 consumer expenditure data and last published for 1981, updated for price changes. In 1993, 70 percent of the lower living standard income level for a family of four varied from $14,300 in nonmetropolitan areas of the South to $23,870 in metropolitan areas of Hawaii; in comparison, the federal poverty guideline for a family of four in 1993 was $14,350 (Burke, 1993:Tables 12,14).

TABLE D-1 Expenditures on Government Assistance Programs for Low-Income People, by Type of Income Test, Fiscal 1992

Program[a]	Expenditures[b] (million $)
A. *Programs that link eligibility solely to the federal poverty guidelines*	
Special Supplemental Nutrition Program for Women, Infants, and Children (WIC)	2,600
Maternal and Child Health Services Block Grant	1,059
Child and Adult Care Food Program	624
Community Health Centers	537
Community Services Block Grant	438
Special Programs for Students from Disadvantaged Backgrounds (TRIO Programs)	385
Legal Services	350
Summer Food Service Program for Children	203
Title X Family Planning Services	150
Foster Grandparents	66
Migrant Health Centers	58
Senior Companions	29
Follow Through	9
Special Milk Program (free segment)	2
Total	6,510 (2%)
B. *Programs that link eligibility to the federal poverty guidelines and also to participation in other programs (e.g., AFDC, SSI, or food stamps)*	
Medicaid	118,067
Food Stamps	24,918
School Lunch (free and reduced-price segments)	3,895
Head Start	2,753
Training for Disadvantaged Adults and Youth[c]	1,774
Low-Income Home Energy Assistance Program (LIHEAP)[d]	1,594
Summer Youth Employment and Training Program[c]	1,183
Job Corps[c]	955
School Breakfast (free and reduced-price segments)	782
Senior Community Service Employment Program	395
Weatherization Assistance	174
Commodity Supplemental Food Program (CSFP)	90
Vocational Education Opportunities, Disadvantaged Activities	N.A.
Total	156,580 (56%)
C. *Programs that link eligibility to a percentage of the local area median income defined by the Department of Housing and Urban Development*	
Section 8 Low-Income Housing Assistance	12,307
Low-Rent Public Housing	5,008
Rural Housing Loans (Section 502)	1,468
Child Care and Development Block Grant	825
Section 236 Interest Reduction Payments	652
Rural Rental Housing Loans (Section 515)	573

TABLE D-1   *Continued*

Program[a]	Expenditures[b] (million $)
C.—*continued*	
Rural Rental Assistance Payments (Section 521)	320
Section 101 Rent Supplements	54
Section 235 Homeownership Assistance for Low-Income Families	45
Rural Housing Repair Loans and Grants (Section 504)	24
Rural Housing Preservation Grants (Section 533)	23
Home Investment Partnerships[e]	3
Total	21,302 (8%)
D. *Programs that have their own income eligibility standards (or that link eligibility to participation in another program)*	
Aid to Families with Dependent Children (AFDC)	24,923
Supplemental Security Income (SSI)	22,774
Earned Income Tax Credit (EITC)	9,553
Medical Care for Veterans Without Service-Connected Disability	7,838
Stafford Loans (formerly Guaranteed Student Loans)	5,683
Social Services Block Grant (Title XX)	5,419
Pell Grants	5,374
Foster Care	4,170
Pensions for Needy Veterans, Their Dependents, and Survivors	3,667
Job Opportunities and Basic Skills Program (JOBS) (successor to the Work Incentive Program—WIN)	1,010
Child Care for AFDC Recipients (and ex-recipients)	755
"At Risk" Child Care (to avert AFDC eligibility)	604
College Work-Study Program	595
Supplemental Educational Opportunity Grants (SEOG)	520
Adoption Assistance	402
Emergency Assistance (EA) to Needy Families with Children	268
The Emergency Food Assistance Program (TEFAP)	250
Perkins Loans	156
Assistance to Refugees and Cuban/Haitian Entrants (cash component)	139
State Student Incentive Grant (SSIG) Program	127
Dependency and Indemnity Compensation (DIC) and Death Compensation for Parents of Veterans	68
Fellowships for Graduate and Professional Study	63
Health Professions Student Loans and Scholarships[f]	48
General Assistance to Indians	46
Medical Assistance to Refugees and Cuban/Haitian Entrants	42
Farm Labor Housing Loans (Section 514) and Grants (Section 516)	29
Social Services for Refugees and Cuban/Haitian Entrants	26
Indian Housing Improvement Grants	20
Rural Housing Self-Help Technical Assistance Grants (Section 523) and Rural Housing Site Loans (Sections 523 and 524)[g]	9
Ellender Fellowships	4
Child Development Associate Scholarship Program[h]	1
Total	94,583 (34%)

continued on next page

TABLE D-1 *Continued*

NOTE: The poverty guidelines are issued annually by the U.S. Department of Health and Human Services (HHS). They are developed by smoothing the official poverty thresholds for different size families. For historical reasons, the guidelines are higher than the thresholds for Alaska (by 25%) and Hawaii (by 15%). A few programs use the official thresholds rather than the guidelines.

[a]Programs are listed in decreasing order of fiscal 1992 expenditures.

[b]Expenditures include federal, state, and local outlays for benefits and administrative costs.

[c]These programs also permit eligibility on the basis of 70 percent of the Department of Labor lower living standard income level for specific areas when that level is higher than the poverty guidelines.

[d]This program also permits eligibility on the basis of 60 percent of state median income.

[e]This program links eligibility to 75 percent of state median income for families of the same size.

[f]This program includes a provision to forgive loans to needy students who fail to complete studies, in which need is defined as a percentage of the federal poverty guidelines.

[g]This program also permits eligibility on the basis of a percentage of the local area median income defined by the Department of Housing and Urban Development.

[h]This program accords eligibility to people with incomes below 195 percent of the Department of Labor lower living standard income level.

- 12 of them (17%), which account for 8 percent of expenditures, determine eligibility on the basis of comparing family income to a percentage of the local area median family income defined by the U.S. Department of Housing and Urban Development (HUD), or, in one case, a percentage of state median income for families of the same size (see Part C of Table D-1);[2]
- 31 of them (44%), which account for 34 percent of expenditures, have their own income eligibility standards or accord eligibility to people who qualify for other kinds of assistance (see Part D of Table D-1).[3]

For some of the 31 programs that have their own income eligibility standards, such as AFDC, Foster Care, and Aid to Refugees, the responsibility for determining income eligibility standards rests with the individual states (or localities). For other programs, such as the Earned Income Tax Credit (EITC), the federal portion of SSI, veterans' pensions, and various education grant and loan programs, federal standards apply.

The 14 assistance programs that use the poverty guidelines as the sole

---

[2] Almost all of these programs provide some type of housing assistance to low-income families. HUD prepares estimates of median family income for metropolitan areas and non-metropolitan counties in the United States (Office of Policy Development and Research, 1992b).

[3] One program assigned to this category—the Child Development Associate Scholarship Program—does not, properly speaking, have its own income eligibility standard, but it does not fit any of the other three categories either. It accords eligibility to people with income below 195 percent of the Department of Labor lower living standard income level.

criterion for income eligibility have uniform nationwide eligibility standards (with the exception of Alaska and Hawaii, for which the guidelines are higher than in other states). Ten other programs (e.g., veterans' pensions, EITC) also have uniform standards. The remaining 46 programs have standards that vary by geographic area. Some of these programs, as a sole eligibility criterion or as one of their criteria, explicitly have a comparison of income with a standard that varies by geographic area: either a percentage of the local area median income defined by HUD, a percentage of the Department of Labor lower living standard income level, or a percentage of state median family income. Other programs (e.g., AFDC) have eligibility standards that vary because they are set by the states (or localities). Still other programs (e.g., Head Start, School Lunch) have varying eligibility standards in practice because one of their criteria is participation in another program, such as AFDC, in which individual states or localities set the standards (however, *benefits* do not usually vary by area for these programs).

Below are brief descriptions of all 27 programs that have as at least one of their income eligibility criteria a comparison of income with the poverty guidelines. The descriptions are organized alphabetically within categories of types of benefits: medical, food, education, other services, jobs and training, and energy. The last section of the appendix describes a few of the major cash and near-cash assistance programs that use a test of income eligibility other than the poverty guidelines. Descriptions are included for AFDC, the EITC, housing assistance, SSI, and veterans' pensions. The information in this appendix is derived largely from Burke (1993), supplemented by U.S. House of Representatives (1994).

PROGRAMS THAT TIE ELIGIBILITY TO THE POVERTY GUIDELINES

Medical Programs

Community Health Centers Centers receive grant money to provide primary care services to medically underserved populations, defined on the basis of such factors as the ratio of primary care doctors to population, infant mortality rate, percentage of elderly, and percentage of families with incomes below the poverty level. Families with incomes below 100 percent of poverty are entitled to free services; those with incomes between 100 and 200 percent of poverty are required to make partial payment; and those with higher incomes are required to make full payment for services.

Maternal and Child Health Services Block Grant (Title V) Funds are provided to the states to undertake various activities to improve the health status of mothers and children (e.g., prenatal care, well-child care, dental care, immunization, screening for lead poisoning, etc.). States determine eligibility criteria, but, according to federal law, they are supposed to target mothers and children with low incomes or limited availability of health services. Low income is defined as income below 100 percent of the federal poverty guidelines. States cannot charge low-income people for services under the block grant; they can charge others for services, based on a sliding scale that takes account of family income, resources, and size.

Medicaid   Traditionally, states have been required to provide Medicaid benefits to elderly, blind, and disabled people who receive SSI and to parents and children who receive AFDC. Hence, the income eligibility guidelines for these two programs (see next section) govern Medicaid eligibility for these groups.

There are various exceptions and modifications to the general rule that SSI and AFDC recipients are eligible for Medicaid. For example, states can—and 12 states do—apply the more restrictive criteria that were in effect in 1972 for low-income elderly, blind, and disabled people before the implementation of SSI. Conversely, states must extend Medicaid eligibility to certain groups who do not receive AFDC but who meet AFDC eligibility requirements: examples are first-time pregnant women, members of two-parent families in which the principal earner is unemployed, and people who do not receive a payment because the amount would be less than $10. States must also continue Medicaid coverage for 4-12 months for families that stop receiving AFDC. States must also continue Medicaid coverage for certain groups of people who lose SSI eligibility.

In addition, states may choose to cover the "medically needy," that is, people who are categorically eligible for AFDC or SSI but whose incomes are somewhat above the AFDC or SSI limits. People can be deemed medically needy if their incomes fall below a state-set standard that does not exceed 133 percent of the state's AFDC maximum benefit or if their incomes fall below AFDC or SSI limits after deducting out-of-pocket medical expenses.

Beginning in the mid-1980s, Congress has allowed—and, in some cases, required—states to provide Medicaid benefits to people on the basis of comparing their family incomes with the federal poverty guidelines rather than with AFDC or SSI standards. A growing number of people are becoming eligible on the basis of these income-to-poverty ratios, although the majority of Medicaid beneficiaries are still AFDC or SSI recipients (see, e.g., U.S. House of Representatives, 1994:Table 18-2). At present, states must extend Medicaid benefits to pregnant women and children up to age 6 with family incomes below 133 percent of the federal poverty guidelines. States must also cover all children under age 19 who were born after September 1983 and whose family incomes are below 100 percent of the poverty guidelines. In addition, states may provide coverage to pregnant women and children under age 1 with family incomes between 133 and 185 percent of the poverty guidelines. Finally, states must provide limited coverage (and may provide full coverage) for elderly and disabled people who are eligible for Medicare and whose family incomes are below 100 percent of the poverty guidelines.

Migrant Health Centers   Centers receive grant money to provide services in areas with large numbers of migratory farm workers. Free service is given to people whose principal employment is in agriculture on a seasonal basis and whose family incomes are below 100 percent of the federal poverty guidelines; partial payment, on a sliding scale, is required for people with incomes between 100 and 200 percent of the poverty guidelines.

Title X Family Planning Services   Clinics must provide family planning services to all people who request them. Priority must be given to people from families with low incomes. Services are provided free of charge to people with incomes below 100 percent of the federal poverty guidelines; partial payment is required for people with incomes between 100 and 250 percent of the poverty guidelines.

Food Programs

Child and Adult Care Food Program   Free meals in child and adult day care centers are available to those whose household incomes are not above 130 percent of the federal poverty guidelines. Those whose household incomes are above 130 percent, but not above 185 percent, of the poverty guidelines are eligible for a reduced price meal.

Commodity Supplemental Food Program   Commodities are provided to local projects in 63 areas that offer food packages to low-income mothers, children, and elderly persons. People eligible for food packages include pregnant women, breastfeeding women, postpartum women, infants, and children up to age 6 who qualify for food, health, or welfare benefits under a government program for low-income people. Depending on state requirements, such people may also have to be designated as being at nutritional risk or may have to live in the service area. Also eligible are elderly people with incomes below the federal poverty guidelines.

Food Stamps   Households composed entirely of recipients of AFDC or SSI are automatically eligible for food stamps, so long as they meet food stamp employment-related requirements (e.g., certain nonworking able-bodied adult household members must register for employment and accept a suitable job if offered one). Hence, the income eligibility requirements for these two programs apply (see next section).

Households that are not automatically eligible for food stamps on the basis of receiving AFDC or SSI must meet certain income and asset requirements. Households without elderly or disabled members qualify if they have gross monthly incomes below 130 percent of the poverty guidelines (gross income excludes a few kinds of payments, such as the EITC) or net monthly incomes below 100 percent of the poverty guidelines. Households with an elderly or disabled member need only meet the net income test. Elderly people are defined as those aged 60 or older; disabled people are generally those receiving such government disability benefits as Social Security or SSI disability payments. Countable liquid assets (including a portion of the value of vehicles) cannot exceed $2,000 for households without elderly or disabled members and $3,000 for households with an elderly or disabled member.

Net monthly income for households without elderly or disabled members is gross monthly income minus: a standard deduction that does not vary by household size ($131 a month in fiscal 1994); 20 percent of any earned income (to allow for taxes and work expenses); out-of-pocket dependent care expenses, when necessary for work or training, up to $200 per month for each dependent under age 2 and up to $175 for other dependents; and shelter expenses that exceed 50 percent of counted income after all other deductions up to a legislatively set ceiling ($231 a month as of July 1994).

Net monthly income for households with an elderly or disabled member is gross monthly income minus: the standard, earned income, and dependent care deductions noted above; shelter expenses that exceed 50 percent of counted income after all other deductions, with no ceiling; and out-of-pocket medical care expenditures for the elderly or disabled member that exceed $35 a month.

School Lunch and School Breakfast Programs   For the School Lunch Program, all school children are eligible to receive at least a partly subsidized meal in participating schools and institutions. Children whose gross family incomes are at or below 130 percent of the federal poverty guidelines are eligible for a free lunch and children in households receiving AFDC or food stamps are automatically eligible for a free lunch. Children whose gross family incomes are more than 130 percent but not more than 185 percent of the guidelines are eligible for a reduced-price lunch (not more than 40 cents per meal). Other children pay whatever the full school price is for a lunch, which, however, is less than cost because of the federal subsidy.

The School Breakfast Program operates similarly, except that the subsidy for breakfasts for non-needy children is smaller. The income eligibility guidelines for school breakfasts are the same as for school lunches. Almost all participants in the School Breakfast Program—98 percent—are children who receive free or reduced-price breakfasts; in contrast, 48 percent of participants in the School Lunch Program receive free or reduced-price lunches.

Special Milk Program   Children in participating schools and residential child care institutions whose gross family incomes are at or below 130 percent of the federal poverty guidelines are eligible for free or partially subsidized milk. Participating schools can elect to provide free milk or to require partial payment. The Special Milk Program operates mainly in schools and institutions that do not participate in the School Lunch or School Breakfast Programs.

Special Supplemental Nutrition Program for Women, Infants, and Children (WIC) Supplemental foods are provided to low-income pregnant women, new mothers, nursing mothers, infants, and children up to age 5 who are judged to be at nutritional risk by a local agency. Income limits for WIC are to be no less than those set by states or local agencies for free or reduced-price health care so long as they are no greater than 185 percent and no less than 100 percent of the federal poverty guidelines.

Summer Food Service Program for Children There are no individual income requirements for participation. Eligibility for benefits is tied to the location and type of sponsor operating a program. Eligible programs must operate in areas where at least 50 percent of the children are from families with incomes at or below 185 percent of the federal poverty guidelines.

Education Programs

Follow Through Children from families whose incomes are below 100 percent of the official poverty guidelines are eligible for special educational services in the early elementary grades. At least 60 percent of participants must have participated in Head Start or similar preschool programs with a focus on pupils from low-income families.

Head Start Children from families with incomes below 100 percent of the federal poverty guidelines are eligible for Head Start, as are children from families receiving AFDC or other public assistance. No more than 10 percent of participating children, including handicapped children, can be from nonpoor families.

Special Programs for Students from Disadvantaged Backgrounds These programs (e.g., Upward Bound, Talent Search) are for college students. Eligibility criteria differ somewhat for the various programs, but generally two-thirds of participants must be low-income, first-generation college students. Low income is defined as taxable income below 150 percent of the Census Bureau poverty thresholds.

Vocational Education Opportunities, Disadvantaged Activities (Perkins Act) Vocational education services and activities are available to disadvantaged individuals, including members of economically disadvantaged families, migrants, people with limited English proficiency, and high school dropouts or potential dropouts. States are required to adopt a uniform method to determine who is economically disadvantaged by using one or more of the following tests: annual incomes below 100 percent of the official poverty line, eligibility for free or reduced-price school lunch or food stamps, eligibility for AFDC or other public assistance, receipt of a Pell Grant or comparable state needs-based education assistance, or eligibility for participation in programs under the Job Training Partnership Act.

Other Service Programs

Community Services Block Grant   Beneficiaries of programs funded by the Community Services Block Grant (which include nutrition services, emergency services, and employment services) must have incomes no higher than 100 percent of the federal poverty guidelines, or, at state option, 125 percent of the poverty guidelines.

Legal Services   The eligibility level for Legal Services is set by individual programs, but incomes may not exceed 125 percent of the federal poverty guidelines unless specifically authorized by the Legal Services Corporation. However, there are exceptions to the income limits in specified circumstances: for example, services can be provided to people with incomes between 125 and 187.5 percent of the federal poverty guidelines if they have exceptional medical care expenses, child care or other work-related expenses, certain debts or expenses associated with age or disability, or meet other criteria. Individual programs are also required to establish "specific and reasonable" limits each year on assets that income-eligible people may hold, taking into account the special needs of elderly, institutionalized, and handicapped people.

Jobs and Training Programs

Foster Grandparents   People who are at least 60 years of age, no longer in the regular work force, and of low income are eligible for a stipend plus transportation and meal costs. The low-income test is met for people with family incomes below 125 percent of the federal poverty guidelines or below 100 percent of the guidelines plus any SSI supplement that is provided by the state, whichever figure is higher.

Job Corps   Economically disadvantaged youths aged 14 through 21 who live in a disorienting environment are eligible to receive basic education, vocational skills training, counseling, work experience, and health services. The definition of "economically disadvantaged" (which applies to all programs authorized by the Job Training Partnership Act) includes recipients of AFDC or other cash welfare; recipients of food stamps; people with countable family incomes below 100 percent of the federal poverty guidelines or below 70 percent of the lower living standard income level, whichever is higher; foster children whose care is supported by the government; and handicapped adults whose own incomes meet the program's limit but whose families' incomes exceed it. The definition of countable income excludes unemployment compensation, child support, and welfare payments.

Senior Community Service Employment Program   People aged 55 and over with low incomes are eligible for part-time community service jobs for which their wages are subsidized by the federal government. People meet the income eligibility criteria if their countable incomes are less than 125 percent of the federal poverty guidelines or if they are receiving regular cash welfare. Countable income is gross income minus welfare payments, disability payments, unemployment benefits, trade adjustment benefits, capital gains, certain veterans' payments, and one-time unearned income payments or unearned income payments of fixed duration. There is an extra $500 deduction for reenrollees.

Senior Companions   Volunteers at least 60 years of age, no longer in the regular work force, and of low income are eligible for a stipend plus transportation and meal costs. The definition of low income is the same as in the Foster Grandparents Program.

Summer Youth Employment and Training Program   Education, training, and summer jobs are available for economically disadvantaged youths aged 16-21 who are unemployed, underemployed, or in school, and, at local option, economically disadvantaged youths aged 14-15. The definition of economically disadvantaged is the same as in the Job Corps.

Training for Disadvantaged Adults and Youth   This program of education, training, and supportive services must have 90 percent of its participants who are economically disadvantaged. The definition of economically disadvantaged is the same as in the Job Corps.

Energy Programs

Low-Income Home Energy Assistance Program (LIHEAP)   LIHEAP is designed to help low-income households meet their energy-related expenses, including home heating or cooling bills, weatherization, and energy-related emergencies. The federal government makes block grants to the states, which have considerable discretion in regard to determining eligibility and benefits. States can elect to make LIHEAP payments to households that receive benefits from AFDC, SSI, or the Veterans' Administration. They can also provide benefits to households with incomes of less than 150 percent of the federal poverty guidelines or 60 percent of the state's median income, whichever is greater. The income ceiling for eligibility cannot be less than 110 percent of the poverty guidelines.

States must ensure that the largest benefits go to households with the lowest income and highest energy costs relative to their incomes, taking account of family size. LIHEAP benefits cannot be counted as income for purposes of determining eligibility or benefits for any other federal or state assistance program. In fiscal 1992, average benefits for heating assistance ranged widely, presumably as a function of climate conditions as well as state choices regarding eligibility and benefit levels, from $39 in Texas to $459 in Massachusetts.

Weatherization Assistance   Weatherization aid is available to families receiving AFDC, SSI, or state assistance program benefits or whose family incomes are below 125 percent of the federal poverty guidelines.

SELECTED PROGRAMS WITH THEIR OWN INCOME ELIGIBILITY STANDARDS

Aid to Families with Dependent Children   AFDC is a state-administered program with funding provided by both the states and the federal government through a matching provision. The program was established by the Social Security Act of 1935. In order to qualify for federal funding, a state must establish a standard of need that defines in monetary amounts the basic needs the state wishes to recognize as appropriate for an assistance standard of living; however, neither the components of the standard nor the methods for setting the standard are prescribed by federal law or regulation. Each state must apply this standard uniformly and statewide in determining financial eligibility for assistance, although it may vary the standard to account for family size or composition, area cost-of-living differentials, or other factors.

Although states are required to establish need standards, they may adopt lower payment standards for benefits: they may set a maximum payment that is below the need standard; they may pay a percentage of the difference between a family's income and the need standard; or they may pay a percentage of the need standard.

Recently, a number of states have lowered their payment standards to satisfy budget constraints and to try to induce recipients to adopt preferred behaviors. As examples, some states no longer provide an additional benefit for an additional child, or they condition benefit amounts on such actions as recipients' obtaining immunization shots for their children. (See Wiseman, 1993, for a list of these kinds of changes in payment standards for which states had waivers from the federal government approved or pending in 1992.)

Over the years, amendments to the law, court decisions, and federal regulations have formally reaffirmed the states' autonomy in setting AFDC benefit levels. In particular, the 1967 amendments to the Social Security Act affirmed the right of states to set payment maximums and to apply "ratable reductions" in order to set benefits lower than their standards of need. The

1967 amendments included a provision to require states to update their need standards to reflect cost-of-living increases since the standards were adopted; however, states were not required to pay benefits consistent with these increases. No such requirement to adjust need standards for inflation has been legislated since 1967.

Although the states have very wide latitude in setting their need and payment standards, federal regulations have always been more specific about the resource side of the equation for determining AFDC eligibility and benefits (see U.S. House of Representatives, 1994:327-329; Solomon and Neisner, 1993). Currently, to receive AFDC payments, a family must pass two income tests. First, a family's gross monthly income cannot be higher than a certain percentage of the state's need standard. This provision was first adopted in 1981, with the limit initially set at 150 percent and raised to 185 percent in 1984. Second, a family's net or countable monthly income must not exceed 100 percent of the need standard or 100 percent of the payment standard in the many states in which the payment standard is below the need standard.

Families must also meet an asset test. Federal regulations currently limit assets or "countable resources" to $1,000 per family, excluding a home and car (provided the equity value of the car does not exceed $1,500). States must also exclude burial plots from countable resources and may exclude such essential items for daily living as clothing and furniture (U.S. House of Representatives, 1994:331). Finally, families must meet various other state and federal requirements (e.g., provisions for work, education, or training).

The definition of countable income for AFDC is gross income minus various exclusions. Currently, states must deduct from gross income the following unearned income components: the first $50 of monthly child support receipts; certain Department of Education grants and loans to college students; the value of Department of Agriculture donated foods; benefits from child nutrition programs; and payments to participants in Volunteers in Service to America (VISTA), some payments to certain Indian tribes, and Agent Orange settlement payments. In addition, states must deduct from gross income the following earned income components: a standard work expense deduction of $90 per month and actual child care expenses up to a ceiling of $175 per month per child ($200 for a child under age 2 and less for part-time work). For AFDC recipients who obtain employment subsequent to enrollment, the states must deduct an additional $30 of earnings per month for the first 12 months and an additional one-third of remaining earnings for the first 4 months. The states must also ignore any benefits from the EITC. Finally, although states have the authority to count food stamp benefits as income for purposes of determining AFDC benefits, no state currently does so. Rather, the process works the other way: AFDC benefits are counted as income for purposes of determining food stamp benefits.

In January 1994 the AFDC need standards for the 50 states and Washington, D.C., showed considerable variation, from $1,648 per month in New Hampshire to $320 per month in Indiana, with a median value of $574 (and a coefficient of variation of 41%). The maximum AFDC benefit showed similar variation from $923 per month in Alaska to $120 in Mississippi, with a median value of $366 (and a coefficient of variation of 40%).[4] The maximum combined AFDC and food stamp benefit showed less variation, from $1,208 in Alaska to $415 in Mississippi, with a median value of $658 (and a coefficient of variation of 22%); see Table 8-1. In relation to the poverty thresholds, in January 1994 the median state AFDC need standard was 60 percent of the poverty threshold for a family of three, and the median state AFDC maximum payment was 38 percent of that threshold (see Table 8-3).

Earned Income Tax Credit   The EITC was enacted in 1975 to provide tax relief to low-income working families and improve incentives to work. It is refundable, thereby serving as a kind of negative income tax. The EITC was recently expanded to increase the basic benefit for families with more than one child and to provide an EITC for childless workers. For tax year 1994 the maximum EITC credit is 26.3 percent of earnings of $7,750 for a family with one qualifying child and 30 percent of earnings of $8,425 for a family with two or more qualifying children. To qualify, a child must be related to and live with the taxpayer(s) more than 6 months of the year and must be under age 19 (or 24 if a full-time student) or be permanently and totally disabled. For families with higher adjusted gross incomes (from $11,000 up to a ceiling of $23,750 (one child) or $25,300 (two or more children) for tax year 1994), the amount of the credit is reduced fractionally for each added dollar of income. The maximum credit for childless workers is 7.65 percent of earnings of $4,000, and it phases out at adjusted gross income of $9,000. There is no geographic variation in the EITC (as is true of all provisions of the federal income tax). EITC benefits cannot be counted as income for determining eligibility or benefits for AFDC, Medicaid, SSI, food stamps, or low-income housing programs.

Section 8 Low-Income Housing Assistance and Low-Rent Public Housing The Section 8 program provides rent subsidies to low-income families and single people, defined as those with incomes at or below 80 percent of the area median (adjusted for family size) as determined by the Department of Housing and Urban Development. A large proportion of subsidies is supposed to go to "very low income" households—those with incomes below 50 percent of the area median.

Countable annual income is defined as gross annual income (which excludes a few sources, such as earnings of children, foster care payments, educa-

---

[4] All dollar amounts are for a three-person AFDC unit, consisting of a caretaker and two children.

tional scholarships, and lump sums) minus the following: $480 for each family member (other than the head or spouse) who is under 18, older and disabled, or a full-time student; $400 for an elderly family member; medical expenses of more than 3 percent of gross income for an elderly family member; and child care and handicapped assistance expenses necessary for a family member to work or further his or her education.[5] For families with net family assets above $5,000 (including the net cash value of real property, savings, stocks, bonds, and other forms of investment but excluding furniture and automobiles), the greater of the following is included in countable income: actual income from all net family assets or a percentage of their value based on the current passbook savings rate.

Section 8 families pay a rent equal to 30 percent of their countable income or 10 percent of gross income, whichever is higher, and the federal government makes up the difference.

The low-rent public housing program operates in the same manner as the Section 8 program, but the benefit is a rent subsidy for a unit in a public housing project rather than a rent subsidy for a unit of the recipient's choosing.

Supplemental Security Income   The SSI program provides monthly cash benefits to needy aged, blind, and disabled people. SSI began operating in 1974, replacing the former federal-state programs for old-age assistance, aid to the blind, and aid to the permanently disabled. About 40 percent of SSI recipients are over age 65; the remainder are disabled. Children can qualify for benefits on the basis of disability, and children can also benefit indirectly because they live in a household with one or more SSI recipients.

SSI is unique among current assistance programs in that it provides a nationwide federal benefit (indexed each year for inflation) that is supplemented by most states. State supplementation is required for people who received benefits under one of the former federal-state programs that were more generous than the federal SSI benefits, although relatively few SSI beneficiaries receive supplementation for this reason. States can also choose to supplement the federal benefit for other beneficiaries in their state, and only seven states do not currently provide some form of supplementation. In the aggregate, 44 percent of SSI beneficiaries receive some type of state supplement (U.S. House of Representatives, 1994:222-223).

To be eligible for SSI benefits, aged, blind, or disabled people must have countable monthly incomes that do not exceed the federal benefit standard plus the applicable state supplementation. Countable income is gross income minus: $20 of unearned income (not counting such means-tested income as

---

[5] Legislation in 1990 liberalized the deductions allowed from gross income by increasing the dependent allowance from $480 to $550 per dependent; allowing a deduction of 10 percent of earned income; and extending the medical expense deduction to nonelderly families. However, these liberalizations were only to take effect if approved in an appropriations measure, which, to date, has not occurred.

veterans' pensions or government-provided in-kind assistance) and the first $65 of earned income plus one-half of remaining earnings. Blind recipients are also allowed to deduct reasonable work expenses, and disabled recipients are also allowed to deduct work and living expenses caused by their disabilities. SSI recipients must apply for other benefits, such as Social Security, for which they are eligible. Also, if a recipient is living in another person's household and receiving support and maintenance from that person, that support is valued as income to the recipient in the amount of one-third of the federal benefit standard. The income of an ineligible spouse or parent also figures into the recipient's income. Finally, SSI recipients cannot have countable assets that exceed $2,000 for individuals or $3,000 for married couples.

As of January 1994 the maximum federal SSI benefit for a single individual living in his or her own home was 77 percent of the corresponding official 1993 poverty threshold; for couples, the maximum benefit was 92 percent of the corresponding threshold. State SSI supplements vary, although not as widely as AFDC payment levels. In looking at only those states (about half) that supplement the federal benefit for single aged people, the median combined federal-state benefit in those states was 83 percent of the official 1993 poverty threshold, with a range from 77 to 142 percent. The addition of food stamps raised the median benefit in these states to 95 percent of the poverty threshold, with a range from 92 to 156 percent (U.S. House of Representatives, 1994:Tables 6-1, 6-7, 6-8).

Pensions for Needy Veterans, Their Dependents, and Survivors   The federal government provides pensions to veterans who served honorably for at least 90 days (including at least 1 day of wartime service), who are totally and permanently disabled for reasons not related to their military service, and who have incomes below the prescribed limits. (Veterans disabled during military service are eligible for disability compensation payments, for which there is no income test.) Survivors of veterans who die from a nonservice cause who meet the income test are also eligible for pensions.

There are different definitions of countable income for veterans who established pension eligibility at different times. For those entitled after January 1979, virtually all of their income is counted with the exception of public or private cash welfare aid. In addition, veterans must meet an asset test, in which a determination is made of whether their property (excluding a home and personal effects) is of sufficient value that it could be converted to provide income support.

Maximum pension amounts (paid to those with no countable income) are about the same as the official poverty thresholds for veterans with no more than two dependents. For widows and widowers and for veterans with three or more dependents, the maximum pension amounts are 60–80 percent of the corresponding poverty thresholds.

References and Bibliography

Aaron, Henry J.
  1985 Comment: The evaluation of Census Bureau procedures for the measurement
        of noncash benefits and the incidence of poverty. Pp. 57-62 in *Proceedings of the
        Bureau of the Census Conference on the Measurement of Noncash Benefits*. Washing-
        ton, D.C.: U.S. Department of Commerce.
Adams, Terry K., and Greg J. Duncan
  1988 The Persistence of Urban Poverty and Its Demographic and Behavioral Corre-
        lates. Survey Research Center, Institute for Social Research, University of
        Michigan.
Adler, N.E., T. Boyce, M.A. Chesney, S. Cohen, S. Folkman, R.L. Kahn, and
S.L. Syme
  1994 Socioeconomic status and health: The challenge of the gradient. *American
        Psychologist* 49(1):5-14.
Advisory Council on Public Welfare
  1966 *Having the Power, We Have the Duty*. Report to the Secretary of Health, Educa-
        tion, and Welfare. Washington, D.C.: U.S. Department of Health, Education,
        and Welfare.
Agency for Health Care Policy and Research
  1992 *Private Health Insurance Premiums in 1987: Policyholders Under Age 65*. National
        Medical Expenditure Survey Data Summary 5, AHCPR Publication No. 92-
        0061. Prepared by J. Vistnes. Washington, D.C.: U.S. Department of Health
        and Human Services.
Allin, Susan, and Pat Doyle
  1990 *Analysis of the Quality of SIPP as It Pertains to the Food Stamp Program*. Final
        Report to the Food and Nutrition Service, U.S. Department of Agriculture.
        Washington, D.C.: Mathematica Policy Research, Inc.
American Chamber of Commerce Researchers Association
  1992 *ACCRA Cost of Living Index: Comparative Data for 300 Urban Areas, Third*

Quarter 1992. Vol. 25, No. 3. Louisville, Ky.: American Chamber of Commerce Researchers Assocation.

An, Chong-Bum, Robert Haveman, and Barbara Wolfe
   1991   *Teen Out-of-Wedlock Births and Welfare Receipt: The Role of Childhood Events and Economic Circumstances.* Discussion Paper 944-91, Institute for Research on Poverty. Madison: University of Wisconsin.

Appelbaum, Diana Karter
   1977   The level of the poverty line: A historical survey. *Social Service Review* 51(3)(September):514-523.

Ashworth, Karl, Martha Hill, and Robert Walker
   1992   A New Approach to Poverty Dynamics. Paper prepared for the American Statistical Association winter meeting, Ft. Lauderdale, Fla. Centre for Research in Social Policy, Loughborough University of Technology, United Kingdom, and Survey Research Center, University of Michigan.

Assistant Secretary for Planning and Evaluation
   1978   *Summary Report: Seattle-Denver Income Maintenance Experiment—Mid-Experimental Labor Supply Results and a Generalization to the National Population.* Office of Income Security Policy. Washington, D.C.: U.S. Department of Health, Education, and Welfare.
   1983   *Overview of the Seattle-Denver Income Maintenance Experiment Final Report.* Office of Income Security Policy. Washington, D.C.: U.S. Department of Health and Human Services.

Atkinson, Anthony B.
   1985   How Should We Measure Poverty? Some Conceptual Issues. Discussion Paper No. 82. Prepared for the Symposium on Statistics for the Measurement of Poverty organized on behalf of the European Community by the University of Frankfurt and the Deutsches Institut für Wirtschaftsforschung, Berlin. Economic and Social Research Council Programme on Taxation, Incentives and the Distribution of Income, London School of Economics, England. [Reprinted in part in Atkinson, 1989:7-24]
   1989   *Poverty and Social Security.* Hemel Hempstead, Eng.: Harvester-Wheatsheaf.

Atkinson, A.B., and J. Micklewright
   1992   *Economic Transformation in Eastern Europe and the Distribution of Income.* Cambridge, Eng.: Cambridge University Press.

Bailar, Barbara A.
   1989   The design of panel surveys. In D. Kasprzyk, G. Duncan, G. Kalton, and M.P. Singh, eds., *Panel Surveys.* New York: J.W. Wiley and Sons, Inc.

Bailis, Lawrence, ed.
   1987   Annotated Bibliography of Research on Welfare Dependence of the Non-Elderly and Its Links to Welfare Policy and Programs. Prepared for the Office of the Assistant Secretary for Planning and Evaluation, U.S. Department of Health and Human Services. Center for Human Resources, Heller Graduate School, Brandeis University, Waltham, Mass.

Barreiros, Lidia
   1989   Poverty Measurement: A European Perspective. Contributed paper to the Seminar on Poverty Statistics in the European Community, Noordwijk. Statistical Office of the European Communities [Eurostat], Luxembourg.

1992   How to measure poverty in Europe?   The methodological experience of the
       European Statistical Office. Pp. 281–306 in *Poverty Measurement for Economies in
       Transition in Eastern European Countries*. Warsaw: Polish Statistical Association
       and Polish Central Statistical Office.

Baydar, Nazli, Jeanne Brooks-Gunn, and Frank F. Furstenburg, Jr.
1993   Early warning signs of functional illiteracy: Predictors in childhood and adoles-
       cence. *Child Development* 64(3):815–829.

Becker, Gary S.
1965   A theory of the allocation of time. *Economic Journal* 75:493–517.

Becketti, Sean, William Gould, Lee Lillard, and Finis Welch
1988   The PSID after fourteen years: An evaluation. *Journal of Labor Economics*
       6(4):472–492.

Betson, David
1990   *Alternative Estimates of the Cost of Children from the 1980-1986 Consumer Expendi-
       ture Survey*. Office of the Assistant Secretary for Planning and Evaluation. Wash-
       ington, D.C.: U.S. Department of Health and Human Services.
1995   Technical Documentation for the Analysis of Alternative Poverty Measures with
       the March 1993 Current Population Survey. Paper prepared for the Panel on
       Poverty and Family Assistance, Committee on National Statistics, National Re-
       search Council. Department of Economics, University of Notre Dame.

Betson, David, and Robert Michael
1993   A Recommendation for the Construction of Equivalence Scales. Unpublished
       memorandum prepared for the Panel on Poverty and Family Assistance, Com-
       mittee on National Statistics, National Research Council. Department of Eco-
       nomics, University of Notre Dame.

Blackley, D., J. Follain, and H. Lee
1986   An evaluation of hedonic price indexes for thirty-four large SMSAs. *Journal of
       the American Real Estate and Urban Economics Association* 14(2):179–205.

Blakorby, Charles, and David Donaldson
1980   Ethical indices for the measurement of poverty. *American Economic Review*
       48(4):1053–1060.

Blank, Rebecca M.
1988   The effect of welfare and wage levels on the location decisions of female-headed
       households. *Journal of Urban Economics* 24:186–211.
1989   The effect of medical need and Medicaid on AFDC participation. *Journal of
       Human Resources* 24(1):54–87.

Blinder, Alan S.
1985   Comment: Measuring income—What kind should be in? Pp. 28–31 in *Proceed-
       ings of the Bureau of the Census Conference on the Measurement of Noncash Benefits*.
       Washington, D.C.: U.S. Department of Commerce.

Bloomquist, G., M. Berger, and J. Hoehn
1988   New estimates of quality of life in urban areas. *American Economic Review*
       78(March):89–107.

Boggess, W. Scott
1993   Family Structure, Economic Status, and High School Completion. Paper pre-
       pared for the American Statistical Association winter meeting, Ft. Lauderdale,
       Fla. Population Studies Center, University of Michigan.

Boldin, Paul, and John Burghardt
  1989   *Analysis of Household Expenditures in Relation to the Food Stamp Program Benefit Structure.* Prepared for the Food and Nutrition Service, U.S. Department of Agriculture. Washington, D.C.: Mathematica Policy Research, Inc.
Bosworth, Barry, Gary Burtless, and John Sabelhaus
  1991   The decline in saving: Evidence from household surveys. *Brookings Papers on Economic Activity* 1991(1):183-256.
Bowie, Chester E.
  1991   SIPP Household Sample Loss: 1984-1990 Panels. Unpublished memorandum. Bureau of the Census, U.S. Department of Commerce, Washington, D.C.
Bradbury, Bruce
  1989   Family size equivalence scales and survey evaluations of income and well-being. *Journal of Social Policy* 18(3)(July):383-408.
Bradshaw, Jonathan
  1991   *Seeking a Behavioural Representation of Modest but Adequate Levels of Living.* Working Paper No. 13. Family Budget Unit, Department of Social Policy and Social Work. Heslington, Eng.: University of York.
  1993   *Budget Standards for the United Kingdom.* Aldershot, Eng.: Avebury.
Brooks-Gunn, Jeanne
  1990   Promoting healthy development in young children: What educational interventions work? Pp. 125-145 in D.E. Rodgers and E. Ginzberg, eds., *Improving the Life Chances of Children at Risk.* Boulder, Colo.: Westview Press.
Brooks-Gunn, Jeanne, Greg J. Duncan, Pamela Kato Lebanov, and Naomi Sealand
  1993   Do neighborhoods influence child and adolescent development? *American Journal of Sociology* 99(2):353-395.
Brooks-Gunn, Jeanne, Guang Guo, and Frank F. Furstenberg, Jr.
  1993   Who drops out of and who continues beyond high school? A 20-year follow-up of black urban youth. *Journal of Research on Adolescence* 3(3):271-294.
Browning, Edgar K.
  1985   Comment: The evaluation of Census Bureau procedures for the measurement of noncash benefits and the incidence of poverty. Pp. 63-67 in *Proceedings of the Bureau of the Census Conference on the Measurement of Noncash Benefits.* Washington, D.C.: U.S. Department of Commerce.
Browning, Martin
  1992   Children and household economic behavior. *Journal of Economic Literature* 30(3): 1434-1475.
Browning, Martin, and Costas Meghir
  1991   The effects of male and female labor supply on commodity demands. *Econometrica* 59(4):925-951.
Brush, Lorelei R.
  1987a Child Care Used by Working Women in the AFDC Population: An Analysis of the SIPP Data Base. Prepared for the Office of the Assistant Secretary for Planning and Evaluation, U.S. Department of Health and Human Services. Analysis, Research and Training, McLean, Va.
  1987b Usage of Different Kinds of Child Care: An Analysis of the SIPP Data Base. Prepared for the Office of the Assistant Secretary for Planning and Evaluation,

U.S. Department of Health and Human Services. Analysis, Research and Training, McLean, Va.

Buhmann, Brigitte, Lee Rainwater, Guenther Schmaus, and Timothy M. Smeeding
  1988   Equivalence scales, well-being, inequality, and poverty: Sensitivity estimates across ten countries using the Luxembourg Income Study (LIS) database. *The Review of Income and Wealth* 34(2):115-142.

Bumpass, Larry, and James A. Sweet
  1989   National estimates of cohabitation. *Demography* 26(4):615-625.

Bureau of the Census
  1967   *1960 Census of Population, Subject Reports, Socioeconomic Status.* PC(2)-5C. Washington, D.C.: U.S. Department of Commerce.
  1969   *Poverty in the United States: 1959-1968.* Current Population Reports, Consumer Income, Series P-60, No. 68. Washington, D.C.: U.S. Department of Commerce.
  1973   *The Current Population Survey: A Report of Methodology.* Technical Paper No. 7. Washington, D.C.: U.S. Department of Commerce.
  1975   *Historical Statistics of the United States, Colonial Times to 1970, Bicentennial Edition, Part 1.* Washington, D.C.: U.S. Department of Commerce.
  1978a   *The Current Population Survey: Design and Methodology.* Technical Paper 40. Washington, D.C.: U.S. Department of Commerce.
  1978b   *1972-1973 U.S. Consumer Expenditure Survey: A Preliminary Evaluation.* Technical Paper No. 45. Washington, D.C.: U.S. Department of Commerce.
  1982   *Money Income of Households, Families, and Persons in the United States: 1980.* Current Population Reports, Consumer Income, Series P-60, No. 132. Washington, D.C.: U.S. Department of Commerce.
  1985   *Income Nonresponses: March 1983 CPS.* Technical Paper No. 54. Washington, D.C.: U.S. Department of Commerce.
  1986   *Estimates of Poverty Including the Value of Noncash Benefits: 1985.* Technical Paper No. 56. Washington, D.C.: U.S. Department of Commerce.
  1988a   *Estimates of Poverty Including the Value of Noncash Benefits: 1987.* Technical Paper No. 58. Washington, D.C.: U.S. Department of Commerce.
  1988b   *Measuring the Effect of Benefits and Taxes on Income and Poverty: 1986.* Current Population Reports, Consumer Income, Series P-60, No. 164-RD-1. Washington, D.C.: U.S. Department of Commerce.
  1989a   *Money Income of Households, Families, and Persons in the United States: 1987.* Current Population Reports, Consumer Income, Series P-60, No. 162. Washington, D.C.: U.S. Department of Commerce.
  1989b   *Transitions in Income and Poverty Status: 1984-85.* Current Population Reports, Household Economic Studies, Series P-70, No. 15-RD-1. Washington, D.C.: U.S. Department of Commerce.
  1991   *The American Housing Survey for the United States in 1991.* Current Housing Reports, Series H150/91. Washington, D.C.: U.S. Department of Commerce.
  1992a   *Measuring the Effect of Benefits and Taxes on Income and Poverty: 1979 to 1991.* Current Population Reports, Consumer Income, Series P-60, No. 182-RD. Washington, D.C.: U.S. Department of Commerce.
  1992b   *Money Income of Households, Families, and Persons in the United States: 1991.*

Current Population Reports, Consumer Income, Series P-60, No. 180. Washington, D.C.: U.S. Department of Commerce.

1992c *Poverty in the United States: 1991.* Current Population Reports, Consumer Income, Series P-60, No. 181. Washington, D.C.: U.S. Department of Commerce.

1992d *Statistical Abstract of the United States 1992.* 112th Edition. Washington, D.C.: U.S. Department of Commerce.

1993a *Measuring the Effect of Benefits and Taxes on Income and Poverty: 1992.* Current Population Reports, Consumer Income, Series P-60, No. 186-RD. Washington, D.C.: U.S. Department of Commerce.

1993b *Money Income of Households, Families, and Persons in the United States: 1992.* Current Population Reports, Consumer Income, Series P-60, No. 184. Washington, D.C.: U.S. Department of Commerce.

1993c *Poverty in the United States: 1992.* Current Population Reports, Consumer Income, Series P-60, No. 185. Washington, D.C.: U.S. Department of Commerce.

1993d *Statistical Abstract of the United States 1993.* 113th Edition. Washington, D.C.: U.S. Department of Commerce.

1995 *Income, Poverty, and Valuation of Noncash Benefits: 1993.* Current Population Reports, Consumer Income, Series P-60, No. 188. Washington, D.C.: U.S. Department of Commerce.

no Report on the SIPP 1984 Panel Wave 6 Annual Roundup and Tax Data.
date(a) Unpublished memorandum. U.S. Department of Commerce, Washington, D.C.

no Size of Family—Families by Total Money Income in 1989, by State.
date(b) Unpublished tabulations from the 1990 census. U.S. Department of Commerce, Washington, D.C.

Bureau of Labor Statistics
1969 *Three Standards of Living for an Urban Family of Four Persons, Spring 1967.* Bulletin No. 1570-5. Washington, D.C.: U.S. Department of Labor.

1982 Autumn 1981 Urban Family Budgets and Comparative Indexes for Selected Urban Areas. USDL 82-139. U.S. Department of Labor, Washington, D.C.

no Consumer expenditures and income. Chapter 18 in *BLS Handbook of Methods.*
date Bulletin 2285. Washington, D.C.: U.S. Department of Labor.

Burke, Vee
1993 *Cash and Noncash Benefits for Persons with Limited Income: Eligibility Rules, Recipient and Expenditure Data, FY 1990-92.* Congressional Research Report for Congress No. 93-832 EPW, Congressional Research Service. Washington, D.C.: U.S. Government Printing Office.

Burtless, Gary
1986 In-Kind Transfers and the Trend in Poverty. The Brookings Institution, Washington, D.C.

Callan, Tim, Brian Nolan, and Christopher T. Whelan
1992 Resources, deprivation, and the measurement of poverty. Pp. 99-134 in *Poverty Measurement for Economies in Transition in Eastern European Countries.* Warsaw: Polish Statistical Association and Polish Central Statistical Office.

Center on Social Welfare Policy and Law
  1988   Analysis of 1988 Benefit Levels in the Program of Aid to Families with Depen-
          dent Children. Washington, D.C.
Chapman, David W., Leroy Bailey, and Daniel Kasprzyk
  1986   Nonresponse adjustment procedures at the U.S. Bureau of the Census. *Survey
          Methodology* 12(2):161-180.
Chernick, Howard, and Andrew Reschovsky
  1986   The Taxation of the Poor: Impacts of Federal Tax Reform Proposals. Draft
          report. Department of Economics, Hunter College.
Chiswick, Barry R.
  1985   The evaluation of Census Bureau procedures for the measurement of noncash
          benefits and the incidence of poverty. Pp. 36-56 in *Proceedings of the Bureau of the
          Census Conference on the Measurement of Noncash Benefits.* Washington, D.C.:
          U.S. Department of Commerce.
Citro, Constance F.
  1991   Databases for microsimulation: A comparison of the March CPS and SIPP. Pp.
          11-61 in Constance F. Citro and Eric A. Hanushek, eds., *Improving Information
          for Social Policy Decisions: The Uses of Microsimulation Modeling, Vol. II, Technical
          Papers.* Panel to Evaluate Microsimulation Models for Social Welfare Programs,
          Committee on National Statistics, National Research Council. Washington,
          D.C.: National Academy Press.
Citro, Constance F., and Michael L. Cohen, eds.
  1985   *The Bicentennial Census: New Directions for Methodology in 1990.* Panel on De-
          cennial Census Methodology, Committee on National Statistics, National Re-
          search Council. Washington, D.C.: National Academy Press.
Citro, Constance F., and Eric A. Hanushek, eds.
  1991   *Improving Information for Social Policy Decisions: The Uses of Microsimulation Model-
          ing.* 2 vols. Panel to Evaluate Microsimulation Models for Social Welfare
          Programs, Committee on National Statistics, National Research Council. Wash-
          ington, D.C.: National Academy Press.
Citro, Constance F., and Graham Kalton, eds.
  1993   *The Future of the Survey of Income and Program Participation.* Panel to Evaluate the
          Survey of Income and Program Participation, Committee on National Statistics,
          National Research Council. Washington, D.C.: National Academy Press.
Clark, Rebecca L.
  1988   Out-Migration Among Welfare Recipients. Paper presented at the Population
          Association of America annual meeting, New Orleans, La. Population Studies
          and Training Center and Department of Sociology, Brown University.
  1990   Does Welfare Affect Migration? Unpublished paper. The Urban Institute,
          Washington, D.C.
  1992   Do They Leave the Safety Net? The Effect of Level of State Welfare Payments
          on the Outmigration of Low-Income Mothers. Paper prepared for the Popula-
          tion Association of America annual meeting, Denver, Colo. The Urban Insti-
          tute, Washington, D.C.
Clark, Stephen, Richard Hemming, and David Ulph
  1981   On indices for the measurement of poverty. *The Economic Journal* 91:515-526.

Clubb, Jerome M., Peter A. Granda, and Erik W. Austin
  1991   Understanding Living Conditions: The Cost of Living Surveys in the U.S.,
          1888-1937. Paper prepared for the Joint Statistical Meetings, Atlanta, Ga.
          Inter-University Consortium for Political and Social Research, University of
          Michigan.
Coder, John
  1991   Exploring Nonsampling Errors in the Wage and Salary Income Data from the
          March Current Population Survey. Paper prepared for the Allied Social Sci-
          ences Association/Society of Government Economists meeting, Washington,
          D.C. Bureau of the Census, U.S. Department of Commerce, Washington,
          D.C.
  1992a   Measurement Errors in the Income Data from the March CPS. Background
          materials prepared for the Panel on Poverty and Family Assistance, Committee
          on National Statistics, National Research Council. Bureau of the Census, U.S.
          Department of Commerce, Washington, D.C.
  1992b   Using administrative record information to evaluate the quality of the income
          data collected in the Survey of Income and Program Participation. In *Proceedings
          of Statistics Canada Symposium 92—Design and Analysis of Longitudinal Surveys.*
          Ottawa: Statistics Canada.
  no   The Current Population Survey Earnings Imputation System: An Explanation
  date   and Evaluation. Bureau of the Census, U.S. Department of Commerce, Wash-
          ington, D.C.
Coder, John, and Lydia Scoon-Rogers
  1994   Evaluating the Quality of Income Data Collected in the Annual Supplement to
          the March Current Population Survey and the Survey of Income and Program
          Participation. Bureau of the Census, U.S. Department of Commerce, Washing-
          ton, D.C.
Cohany, Sharon R., Anne E. Polivka, and Jennifer M. Rothgeb
  1994   Revisions in the Current Population Survey effective January 1994. *Employment
          and Earnings* 41(2)(February):13-37.
Colasanto, Diane, Arie Kapteyn, and Jacques van der Gaag
  1984   Two subjective definitions of poverty: Results from the Wisconsin Basic Needs
          Study. *Journal of Human Resources* 28(1):127-138.
Committee on National Statistics
  1989   *The Survey of Income and Program Participation: An Interim Assessment.* National
          Research Council. Washington, D.C.: National Academy Press.
Conference on Economic Progress
  1959   *The Federal Budget and "The General Welfare"—We Can Afford to Serve Our Hu-
          man Needs.* Washington, D.C.: Conference on Economic Progress.
Congressional Budget Office
  1977a   *Poverty Status of Families Under Alternative Definitions of Income.* Prepared by John
          Korbel. Washington, D.C.: U.S. Government Printing Office.
  1977b   *Welfare Reform: Issues, Objectives, and Approaches.* Prepared by John Korbel and
          William Hoagland. Washington, D.C.: U.S. Government Printing Office.
  1987   *The Changing Distribution of Federal Taxes: 1975-1990.* Prepared by Richard
          Kasten and Frank Sammartino. Washington, D.C.: U.S. Government Printing
          Office.

1989a *Fiscal Federalism and the Partnership Act of 1987.* Prepared by Janice Peskin. Washington, D.C.: U.S. Government Printing Office.
1989b *Work and Welfare: The Family Support Act of 1988.* Staff Working Paper by Janice Peskin, Julia Isaacs, and Alan Fairbank. Washington, D.C.: U.S. Government Printing Office.

Congressional Research Service
1991 *Cash and Noncash Benefits for Persons with Limited Income: Eligibility Rules, Recipient and Expenditure Data, FY 1988-90.* Compiled by Vee Burke, Education and Public Welfare Division. Washington, D.C.: U.S. Government Printing Office.

Corbett, Thomas
1993 Child poverty and welfare reform: Progress or paralysis? *Focus* 15(1):1-17. [Institute for Research on Poverty, University of Wisconsin-Madison]

Council of Economic Advisers
1992 *Economic Report of the President.* Washington, D.C.: U.S. Government Printing Office.

Curtin, Richard T., F. Thomas Juster, and James N. Morgan
1989 Survey estimates of wealth: An assessment of quality. Pp. 473-552 [including comments by Eugene Smolensky] in Robert E. Lipsey and Helen Stone Tice, eds., *The Measurement of Saving, Investment, and Wealth.* Chicago: University of Chicago Press.

Cutler, David M., and Lawrence F. Katz
1991 Macroeconomic performance and the disadvantaged. *Brookings Papers on Economic Activity* 1991(2):1-74.
1992 Rising inequality? Changes in the distribution of income and consumption in the 1980s. *American Economic Review* 82(2)(May):546-551.

Czajka, John L., and Constance F. Citro
1982 Analysis of household income and poverty statistics under alternative measures of household and family composition. In *Proceedings of the Social Statistics Section.* Washington, D.C.: American Statistical Association.

Danziger, Sheldon, Robert Haveman, and Robert Plotnick
1981 How income transfers affect work, savings, and the income distribution: A critical review. *Journal of Economic Literature* 19(3):975-1028.

Danziger, Sheldon, George Jakubson, Saul Schwartz, and Eugene Smolensky
1982 Work and welfare as determinants of female poverty and household headship. *Quarterly Journal of Economics* 97(3):519-534.

Danziger, Sheldon, Jacques van der Gaag, Michael K. Taussig, and Eugene Smolensky
1984 The direct measurement of welfare levels: How much does it cost to make ends meet? *Review of Economics and Statistics* 66(3):500-505.

David, Martin, and John Fitzgerald
1987 Measuring Poverty and Crises: A Comparison of Annual and Subannual Accounting Periods Using the Survey of Income and Program Participation. Institute for Research on Poverty, University of Wisconsin-Madison.

David, Martin, Roderick J.A. Little, Michael E. Samuhel, and Robert K. Triest
1986 Alternative methods for CPS income imputation. *Journal of the American Statistical Association* 81(393):28-41.

Davidson, Gestur, and Ira Moscovice
  1989   Health insurance and welfare reentry. *HSR: Health Services Research* 24(5)(December):599-614.
Dear, Ronald B.
  1982   No more poverty in America? A critique of Martin Anderson's theory of welfare. *Children and Youth Services Review* 4(1-2):5-34.
Deaton, Angus, and John Muellbauer
  1980   *Economics and Consumer Behavior.* Cambridge, Eng.: Cambridge University Press.
  1986   On measuring child costs: With applications to poor countries. *Journal of Political Economy* 94(August):720-744.
de Neufville, Judith I.
  1975   *Social Indicators and Public Policy.* New York: Elsevier Scientific Publishing Company.
de Vos, Klaas, and Thesia I. Garner
  1991   An evaluation of subjective poverty definitions: Comparing results from the U.S. and the Netherlands. *The Review of Income and Wealth* 37(3)(September):267-285.
Donaldson, David, and John A. Weymark
  1986   Properties of fixed-population poverty indices. *International Economic Review* 27:667-88.
Doyle, Pat, Karen Beauregard, and Enrique Lamas
  1993   Health Benefits and Poverty: An Analysis on the National Medical Expenditure Survey. Center for Intramural Research, Agency for Health Care Policy and Research, U.S. Department of Health and Human Services, Washington, D.C.
Doyle, Pat, and Robert Dalrymple
  1987   The impact of imputation procedures on distributional characteristics of the low income population. Pp. 483-508 in *Proceedings of the Bureau of the Census Third Annual Research Conference.* Washington, D.C.: U.S. Department of Commerce.
Dublin, Louis I., and Alfred J. Lotka
  1946   *The Money Value of a Man.* 2nd edition. New York: Ronald Press.
Duncan, Greg J.
  1989   Panel Studies of Poverty: Prospects and Problems. Survey Research Center, University of Michigan.
  1992   Talking Points for a Discussion of the Temporal Aspects of Poverty. Unpublished memorandum for the Panel on Poverty and Family Assistance, Committee on National Statistics, National Research Council. Survey Research Center, University of Michigan.
Duncan, Greg J., Bjorn Gustafsson, Richard Hauser, Gunther Schmauss, Hans Messinger, Ruud Muffels, Brian Nolan, and Jean-Claude Ray
  1993   Poverty dynamics in eight countries. *Journal of Population Economics.* 6(3)(August):215-234.
Duncan, Greg J., and Martha S. Hill
  1991   Panel Study of Income Dynamics: Research uses and recent innovations. *ICPSR Bulletin* (February):1-4.

Duncan, Greg J., and Saul D. Hoffman
  1990 Welfare benefits, economic opportunities, and out-of-wedlock births among black teenage girls. *Demography* 27(4):519-535.
Duncan, Greg J., F. Thomas Juster, and James N. Morgan
  1984 The role of panel studies in a world of scarce resources. Pp. 302-328 in Seymour Sudman and Mary A. Spaeth, eds., *The Collection and Analysis of Economic and Consumer Behavior Data: In Memory of Robert Ferber*. Bureau of Economic and Business Research. Champaign: University of Illinois.
Duncan, Greg J., and Willard Rodgers
  1991 Has children's poverty become more persistent? *American Sociological Review* 56(4)(August):538-550.
Duncan, Greg J., Timothy M. Smeeding, and Willard Rodgers
  1992 Why Is the Middle Class Shrinking? Paper presented to the Association for Public Policy Analysis and Management Research Conference, October. Survey Research Center, University of Michigan.
Eargle, Judith
  1990 *Household Wealth and Asset Ownership: 1988*. Current Population Reports, Household Economic Studies, Series P-70, No. 22. Bureau of the Census. Washington, D.C.: U.S. Department of Commerce.
Economic Research Service
  1976 Analytical support for cost-of-living differentials in the poverty threshold. Technical Paper XV. *The Measure of Poverty*. Washington, D.C.: U.S. Department of Health, Education, and Welfare.
Edmonston, Barry, and Charles Schultze, eds.
  1995 *Modernizing the U.S. Census*. Panel on Census Requirements in the Year 2000 and Beyond, Committee on National Statistics, National Research Council. Washington, D.C.: National Academy Press.
Egbuono, L., and B. Starfield
  1982 Child health and social status. *Pediatrics* 69(5):550-557.
Eisen, M., C.A. Donald, J.E. Ware, and R.H. Brook
  1980 *Conceptualization and Measurement of Health for Children in the Health Insurance Study*. R-2313-HEW. Santa Monica, Calif.: The Rand Corporation.
Ellwood, David T.
  1987 *Understanding Dependency: Choices, Confidence, or Culture?* Prepared for the Office of the Assistant Secretary for Planning and Evaluation, U.S. Department of Health and Human Services. Center for Human Resources, Heller Graduate School. Waltham, Mass: Brandeis University.
Ellwood, David, and Mary Jo Bane
  1985 The impact of AFDC on family structure and living arrangements. In R. Erenberg, ed., *Research in Labor Economics, Vol. 7*. Greenwich, Conn: JAI Press.
Ellwood, David T., and Lawrence H. Summers
  1985 Measuring income: What kind should be in? Pp. 8-27 in *Proceedings of the Bureau of the Census Conference on the Measurement of Noncash Benefits*. Washington, D.C.: U.S. Department of Commerce.
Engel, Ernst
  1895 Die lebenskosten belgischer arbeiter-familien früher und jetzt. *International Statistical Institute Bulletin* 9:1-74.

Engel, Rafael J.
   1989   Economic vulnerability of the transitory poor elderly. In *Proceedings of the Social Statistics Section*. Alexandria, Va.: American Statistical Association.
Eurostat
   1990   Inequality and Poverty in Europe (1980-1985). *Rapid Reports*, Population and Social Conditions, No. 7.
Expert Committee on Family Budget Revisions (Watts Committee)
   1980   *New American Family Budget Standards*. Madison: Institute for Research on Poverty, University of Wisconsin; New York: Center for the Social Sciences, Columbia University.
Falk, Gene, and Joe Richardson
   1985   *Families with Children: Selected Characteristics of Benefit Recipients from the Survey of Income and Program Participation (SIPP)*. Report No. 85-220-EPW. Congressional Research Service. Washington, D.C.: U.S. Government Printing Office.
Family Budget Unit
   1990   *The Work of the Family Budget Unit*. Working Paper No. 1. Department of Social Policy and Social Work. Heslington, Eng.: University of York.
Fay, Robert E.
   1989   An analysis of within-household undercoverage in the Current Population Survey. Pp. 156-175 in *Proceedings of the Bureau of the Census Fifth Annual Research Conference*. Washington, D.C.: U.S. Department of Commerce.
Fay, Robert, Jeffrey S. Passel, and Gregory J. Robinson
   1988   *The Coverage of the Population in the 1980 Census*. 1980 Census of Population and Housing Evaluation Research Report No. PHC80-E4. Bureau of the Census. Washington, D.C.: U.S. Department of Commerce.
Fein, David
   1989   The Social Sources of Census Omission: Racial and Ethnic Differences in Omission Rates in Recent U.S. Censuses. Dissertation submitted to Sociology Department, Princeton University.
Fendler, Carol, and Mollie Orshansky
   1979   Improving the poverty definition. Pp. 640-645 in *Proceedings of the Social Statistics Section*. Washington, D.C.: American Statistical Association.
Findlay, Jeanette, and Robert E. Wright
   1992   Gender, Poverty and Intra-Household Distribution of Resources. Luxembourg Income Study, Working Paper No. 83. Department of Political Economy, University of Glasgow, Scotland.
Fisher, Gordon M.
   1985   Estimates of the Poverty Population Under the Current Official Definition for Years Before 1959: Initial Results. Draft (October). U.S. Department of Health and Human Services, Washington, D.C.
   1992a The development and history of the poverty thresholds. *Social Security Bulletin* 55(4)(Winter):3-14.
   1992b The Development of the Orshansky Poverty Thresholds and Their Subsequent History as the Official U.S. Poverty Measure. Draft (May). U.S. Department of Health and Human Services, Washington, D.C.
   1992c Poverty guidelines for 1992. *Social Security Bulletin* 55(1)(Spring):43-46.

1993 From Hunter to Orshansky: An Overview of (Unofficial) Poverty Lines in the United States from 1904 to 1965. Paper presented at the Association for Public Policy Analysis and Management Research Conference, October. U.S. Department of Health and Human Services, Washington, D.C

1994 Is There Such a Thing as an Absolute Poverty Line Over Time? Evidence from the United States, Britain, Canada, and Australia. Paper presented at the Association for Public Policy Analysis and Management Research Conference, October. U.S. Department of Health and Human Services, Washington, D.C.

Fitzgerald, Hiram E., Barry M. Lester, and Barry Zuckerman, eds.

1995 *Children of Poverty: Research, Health Care, and Policy Issues.* New York: Garland.

Flik, Robert J., and Bernard M.A. van Praag

1991 Subjective poverty line definitions. *De Economist* 139(3):311-330.

Food and Nutrition Service

1984 *The Effects of Legislative Changes in 1981 and 1982 on Food Stamp Program Benefits.* Interim Report to Congress. Office of Analysis and Evaluation. Washington, D.C.: U.S. Department of Agriculture.

1988a Background Information on Eligibility for the WIC Program. U.S. Department of Agriculture, Washington, D.C.

1988b *Characteristics of the National School Lunch and School Breakfast Program Participants.* Office of Analysis and Evaluation. Washington, D.C.: U.S. Department of Agriculture.

1988c *Food Stamp Program Participation Rates Among the Poverty Population, 1980-1987.* Prepared by Carole Trippe and Harold Beebout, Mathematica Policy Research, Inc., Washington, D.C. Office of Analysis and Evaluation. Washington, D.C.: U.S. Department of Agriculture.

1989 *Food Stamp Analytic Studies—The Dynamics of Food Stamp Program Participation.* Prepared by Nancy R. Burstein and Mary G. Visher, Abt Associates, Inc., Cambridge, Mass. Office of Analysis and Evaluation. Washington, D.C.: U.S. Department of Agriculture.

1991 *Eligibility Guidance for School Meals Manual.* U.S. Department of Agriculture, Washington, D.C.

Foster, James

1984 On economic poverty: A survey of aggregate measures. In R.L. Basmann and George F. Rhodes, Jr., eds., *Advances in Econometrics, Vol. 3.* London: JAI Press Inc.

Foster, James, Joel Greer, and Erik Thorbecke

1984 A class of decomposable poverty measures. *Econometrica* 52:761-766.

Fraker, Thomas, and Robert Moffitt

1985 *The Effects of Food Stamp Benefits on the Market Labor of Female Heads of Households.* Final Report to the Food and Nutrition Service, U.S. Department of Agriculture. Washington, D.C.: Mathematica Policy Research, Inc.

1988 The effect of food stamps on labor supply: A bivariate selection model. *Journal of Public Economics* 35:25-56.

1989 *The Effect of Food Stamps on the Labor Supply of Unmarried Adults Without Dependent Children.* Final Report to the Food and Nutrition Service, U.S. Department of Agriculture. Washington, D.C.: Mathematica Policy Research, Inc.

Fraker, Thomas, Robert Moffitt, and Douglas Wolf
  1985   Effective tax rates and guarantees in the AFDC program, 1967-1982. *Journal of Human Resources* 20(2):251-263.
Friedman, Milton
  1957   *A Theory of the Consumption Function.* Princeton, N.J.: Princeton University Press.
Friedman, Rose D.
  1965   *Poverty: Definition and Perspective.* Washington, D.C.: American Enterprise Institute.
Fuchs, Victor R.
  1965   Toward a theory of poverty. Pp. 71-91 in Task Force on Economic Growth and Opportunity, *The Concept of Poverty.* Washington, D.C.: Chamber of Commerce of the United States.
Gabe, Thomas, and Sharon Stephan
  1988   *Child Day Care: Patterns of Use Among Families with Preschool Children.* Education and Public Welfare Division, Congressional Research Service. Washington, D.C.: U.S. Government Printing Office.
Garfinkel, Irwin, and Robert Haveman.
  1977   *Earnings Capacity, Poverty and Inequality.* New York: Academic Press.
Gieseman, Raymond
  1987   The Consumer Expenditure Survey: Quality control by comparative analysis. *Monthly Labor Review* 110(March):8-14.
Gillingham, Robert
  1975   Place to place rent comparisons. *Annals of Economic and Social Measurement* 4(1):153-173.
  1981   Estimating inter-city differences in the price of housing services: Further evidence. *Urban Studies* 18:365-369.
Goedhart, Theo, Victor Halberstadt, Arie Kapteyn, and Bernard M.S. van Praag
  1977   The poverty line: Concept and measurement. *Journal of Human Resources* 12(4):503-520.
Goodreau, Karen, Howard Oberheu, and Denton Vaughan
  1984   An assessment of the quality of survey reports of income from the Aid to Families with Dependent Children (AFDC) program. *Journal of Business and Economic Statistics* 2(2):179-186.
Gottschalk, Peter
  1992   The intergenerational transmission of welfare participation: Facts and possible causes. *Journal of Policy Analysis and Management* 11(2):254-272.
Grall, Timothy S.
  1994   *Households at Risk: Their Housing Situation.* Current Housing Reports, Series H121/94-2. Bureau of the Census. Washington, D.C.: U.S. Department of Commerce.
Gramlich, Edward, and Deborah Laren
  1984   Migration and income redistribution responsibilities. *Journal of Human Resources* 19(4):489-511.
Green, Gordon
  1983   Underreporting of Income in Household Surveys. Bureau of the Census, U.S. Department of Commerce, Washington, D.C.

Greenlees, J.
   1982   An empirical evaluation of the CPI Home Purchase Index, 1973-1978. *Journal of the American Real Estate and Urban Economics Association* 10:1-24.
Greger, Janet
   1985   *A Review of The Thrifty Food Plan and Its Use in the Food Stamp Program.* Report prepared for the Subcommittee on Domestic Marketing, Consumer Relations, and Nutrition, Committee on Agriculture, U.S. House of Representatives. Washington, D.C.: U.S. Government Printing Office.
Groeneveld, Lyle, Michael Hannan, and Nancy Tuma
   1983   Income and marital events: Review of previous research. In *Final Report of the Seattle-Denver Income Maintenance Experiments.* Menlo Park, Calif.: SRI International.
Gueron, Judith M.
   1987   *Reforming Welfare with Work.* Occasional Paper 2. Project on Social Welfare and the American Future. New York: Ford Foundation.
Haber, Sheldon E.
   1988   Valuing In-Kind Benefits and the Measurement of Poverty and Income. Department of Economics, George Washington University.
   1989a   The Fungible Value of Government and Employer Provided In-Kind Health Benefits. Department of Economics, George Washington University.
   1989b   Recipient Value and Market Value: How They Measure Up in Counting the Poor. Department of Economics, George Washington University.
Hafner-Eaton, C.
   1993   Physician utilization disparities between the uninsured and insured: Comparisons of the chronically ill, acutely ill, and well nonelderly populations. *Journal of the American Medical Association* 269(6):787-792.
Hagenaars, Aldi
   1986   *The Perception of Poverty.* Amsterdam: North Holland Publishing Company.
   1987   A class of poverty indices. *International Economic Review* 28:583-607.
Hagenaars, Aldi, and Klaas de Vos
   1988   The definition and measurement of poverty. *Journal of Human Resources* 23(2): 211-221.
Hagenaars, Aldi, and Bernard M.S. van Praag
   1985   A synthesis of poverty line definitions. *The Review of Income and Wealth* 31:139-154.
Hahn, Beth A.
   1994   Health care utilization: The effect of extending insurance to adults on Medicaid or uninsured. *Medical Care* 32(3):227-239.
Hahn, B., and D. Lefkowitz
   1992   *Annual Expenses and Sources of Payment for Health Care Services.* National Medical Expenditure Survey Research Findings 14, AHCPR Publication No. 93-00007. Agency for Health Care Policy and Research. Washington, D.C.: U.S. Department of Health and Human Services.
Hanson, Sandra L., and Theodora Ooms
   1991   The economic costs and rewards of two-earner, two parent families. *Journal of Marriage and the Family* 53(August):622-634.

Hauver, James H., John A. Goodman, and Marc A. Grainer
    1981   The federal poverty thresholds: Appearance and reality. *Journal of Consumer Research* 8(June):1-10.
Haveman, Robert
    1992   Who Are the Nation's "Truly Poor"?: Problems and Pitfalls in Defining and Measuring Poverty. Draft. Institute for Research on Poverty, University of Wisconsin-Madison.
    1993   Who are the nation's "truly poor"?: Problems and pitfalls in (re)defining and measuring poverty. *The Brookings Review* 11(1)(Winter):24-27.
Haveman, Robert, and Larry F. Buron
    1991   *Who Are the Truly Poor? Patterns of Official and Net Earnings Capacity Poverty, 1973-1988.* Discussion Paper 956-91, Institute for Research on Poverty. Madison: University of Wisconsin.
    1993   Escaping poverty through work: The problem of low earnings capacity in the United States, 1973-1988. *The Review of Income and Wealth.*
Haveman, Robert, and Barbara Wolfe
    1993   Intergenerational Determinants of the Education Level of Young Adults. Paper prepared for the American Statistical Association winter meeting, Ft. Lauderdale, Fla. University of Wisconsin-Madison.
Haveman, Robert, Barbara Wolfe, and James Spaulding
    1991   Childhood events and circumstances influencing high school completion. *Demography* 29(1):133-157.
Hayghe, Howard V., and Suzanne M. Bianchi
    1993   Changes in the Labor Force Role of Married Mothers. Paper presented at the American Statistical Association winter meeting, Ft. Lauderdale, Fla. Bureau of Labor Statistics, U.S. Department of Labor, and Bureau of the Census, U.S. Department of Commerce, Washington, D.C.
Hernandez, Donald
    1993   *America's Children: Resources from Family, Government, and the Economy.* New York: Russell Sage Foundation.
Hill, Martha S.
    1992   *The Panel Study of Income Dynamics: A User's Guide.* Part of the series, *Guides to Major Social Science Data Bases.* Newbury Park, Calif.: Sage Publications, Inc.
Hoffman, Saul, and Greg Duncan
    1988   A comparison of choice-based multinomial and nested logit models: The family structure and welfare use decisions of divorced or separated women. *Journal of Human Resources* 23(4):550-562.
Hopkins, Kevin R.
    1987   *Welfare Dependency—Behavior, Culture, and Public Policy.* Prepared for the Office of the Assistant Secretary for Planning and Evaluation, U.S. Department of Health and Human Services. Alexandria, Va.: Hudson Institute.
Hoppe, Robert A.
    1988   Two Types of Poverty, Two Types of Policy. Paper presented at "Towards Rural Development Policy for the 1990s: Enhancing Income and Employment Opportunities," symposium sponsored by the Congressional Research Service for the Joint Economic Committee. Economic Research Service, U.S. Department of Agriculture, Washington, D.C.

Hurd, Michael D.
  1990 Research on the elderly: Economic status, retirement, and consumption and savings. *Journal of Economic Literature* 28(June):565-637.
Huston, Aletha C., ed.
  1991 *Children in Poverty: Child Development and Public Policy.* New York: Cambridge University Press.
Huston, Aletha C., Vonnie McLoyd, and Cynthia Garcia Coll
  1994 Children and poverty: Issues in contemporary research. *Child Development* (Special Issue: Children and Poverty) 65(2):275-282.
Hutchens, Robert, George Jakubson, and Saul Schwartz
  1989 AFDC and the formation of subfamilies. *Journal of Human Resources* 24(4):599-628.
Interagency Forum on Aging-Related Statistics
  1990 *Income Data for the Elderly: Guidelines.* Income Working Group. Washington, D.C.: Interagency Forum on Aging-Related Statistics.
Jabine, Thomas B., Karen E. King, and Rita J. Petroni
  1990 *Survey of Income and Program Participation: Quality Profile.* Bureau of the Census. Washington, D.C.: U.S. Department of Commerce.
Jacobs, Eva, and Stephanie Shipp
  1990 A history of the U.S. Consumer Expenditure Survey: 1935 to 1988. In *Proceedings of the Social Statistics Section.* Alexandria, Va.: American Statistical Association.
Jacobs, Eva, Stephanie Shipp, and Gregory Brown
  1989 Families of working wives spending more on services and nondurables. *Monthly Labor Review* (February):15-23.
Jenkins, Stephen P.
  1991 Poverty measurement and the within-household distribution: Agenda for action. *Journal of Social Policy* 20(4):457-483.
Johnson, David S., and Thesia I. Garner
  1993 Estimating unique equivalence scales. Pp. 420-427 in *Proceedings of the Social Statistics Section.* Alexandria, Va.: American Statistical Association.
Johnson, Paul, and Steven Webb
  1992 Official statistics on poverty in the United Kingdom. Pp. 135-154 in *Poverty Measurement for Economies in Transition in Eastern European Countries.* Warsaw: Polish Statistical Association and Polish Central Statistical Office.
Jorgenson, Dale W., and Daniel T. Slesnick
  1987 Aggregate consumer behavior and household equivalence scales. *Journal of Business and Economic Statistics* 5(2):219-232.
Juster, F. Thomas, and Kathleen A. Kuester
  1991 Differences in the measurement of wealth, wealth inequality and wealth composition obtained from alternative U.S. wealth surveys. *The Review of Income and Wealth* 37(1):33-62.
Juster, F. Thomas, and Frank P. Stafford
  1985 *Time, Goods, and Well-Being.* Survey Research Center. Ann Arbor: University of Michigan.
Juster, F. Thomas, and Richard Suzman
  1993 *The Health and Retirement Study: An Overview.* Health and Retirement Study

Working Paper Series, Core Paper No. 94-1001. Institute for Social Research
and National Institute on Aging. Ann Arbor: University of Michigan; Washington, D.C.: U.S. Department of Health and Human Services.

Kakwani, Nanak
  1980   On a class of poverty measures. *Econometrica* 48:437-446.

Kalton, Graham, Daniel Kasprzyk, and David B. McMillen
  1989   Nonsampling errors in panel surveys. Pp. 249-270 in D. Kasprzyk, G. Duncan,
         G. Kalton, and M.P. Singh, eds., *Panel Surveys*. New York: J.W. Wiley and
         Sons, Inc.

Kapteyn, Arie
  1977   A Theory of Preference Formation. Dissertation submitted to Leyden Univer-
         sity, The Netherlands.

Kerr, R., and B. Peterkin
  1975   *The Effect of Household Size on the Cost of Diets That Are Nutritionally Equivalent.*
         CFE(Adm.)325. Consumer and Food Economics Institute. Washington, D.C.:
         U.S. Department of Agriculture.

Kiernan, K.E., and V. Estaugh.
  1993   *Cohabitation: Extra-Marital Childbearing and Social Policy.* Occasional Paper 17.
         London, Eng.: Family Policy Studies Center.

Kilpatrick, Robert W.
  1973   The income elasticity of the poverty line. *Review of Economics and Statistics*
         55(3)(August):327-332.

King, Jill
  1976   The consumer price index. Technical Paper V. *The Measure of Poverty*. Wash-
         ington, D.C.: U.S. Department of Health, Education, and Welfare.

King, Karen E., S. Patricia Chou, Maryann K. McCormick, and Rita J. Petroni
  1990   Investigations of the SIPP's cross-sectional noninterview adjustment method and
         variables. In *Proceedings of the Survey Research Methods Section*. Alexandria, Va.:
         American Statistical Association.

Klerman, Lorraine
  1991   The health of poor children: Problems and programs. Pp. 136-157 in Aletha C.
         Huston, ed., *Children in Poverty: Child Development and Public Policy.* New York:
         Cambridge University Press.

Kokoski, Mary F.
  1991   New research on interarea consumer price differences. *Monthly Labor Review*
         (July):31-34.

Kokoski, Mary, Patrick Cardiff, and Brent Moulton
  1992   Interarea Price Indices for Consumer Goods and Services: An Hedonic Ap-
         proach Using CPI Data. Preliminary draft. Bureau of Labor Statistics, Wash-
         ington, D.C.
  1994   *Interarea Price Indices for Consumer Goods and Services: An Hedonic Approach Using
         CPI Data.* BLS Working Paper No. 256, Bureau of Labor Statistics. Washing-
         ton, D.C.: U.S. Department of Labor.

Korbin, Jill E., ed.
  1992   Special issue: The impact of poverty on children. *American Behavioral Scientist*
         35(3).

Kundu, A., and T.E. Smith
   1983   An impossibility theorem on poverty indices. *International Economic Review* 24(June):423-434.
Lamas, Enrique, Jan Tin, and Judith Eargle
   1994   The Effect of Attrition on Income and Poverty Estimates from the Survey of Income and Program Participation (SIPP). Paper presented at the Conference on Attrition in Longitudinal Surveys. Bureau of the Census, U.S. Department of Commerce, Washington, D.C.
Larin, Kathryn A., with Kathryn H. Porter
   1992   *Enough to Live On: Setting an Appropriate AFDC Need Standard.* Washington, D.C.: Center on Budget and Policy Priorities.
Laumann, E.O., J.H. Gagnon, R.T. Michael, and S. Michaels
   1994   *The Social Organization of Sexuality.* Chicago: University of Chicago Press.
Lazear, Edward, and Robert Michael
   1980a Family size and the distribution of real per capita income. *American Economic Review* 70(1):91-107.
   1980b Real income equivalence among one-earner and two-earner families. *American Economic Review* 70(2)(May):203-208.
   1988   *Allocation of Income Within the Household.* Chicago: University of Chicago Press.
Lefkowitz, D., and A. Monheit
   1991   *Health Insurance, Use of Health Services, and Health Care Expenditures.* National Medical Expenditure Survey Research Findings 12, AHCPR Publication No. 92-0017. Agency for Health Care Policy and Research. Washington, D.C.: U.S. Department of Health and Human Services.
Lepkowski, James M.
   1989   Treatment of wave nonresponse in panel surveys. Pp. 348-374 in D. Kasprzyk, G. Duncan, G. Kalton, and M.P. Singh, eds., *Panel Surveys.* New York: J.W. Wiley and Sons, Inc.
Lepkowski, James M., Graham Kalton, and Daniel Kasprzyk
   1990   Measurement Errors in Panel Surveys. Paper prepared for the International Conference on Measurement Errors in Surveys, Tucson, Ariz. Institute for Social Research, University of Michigan.
Lerman, Robert I., and Donald L. Lerman
   1989   Income sources and income inequality: Measurements from three U.S. income surveys. *Journal of Economic and Social Measurement* 15(2):167-189.
Lerman, Robert I., and Shlomo Yitzhaki
   1989   The Time Dimension in Poverty and Inequality. Draft paper prepared for the Office of the Assistant Secretary for Planning and Evaluation, U.S. Department of Health and Human Services. Brandeis University and Hebrew University, Israel.
Levine, Daniel B., and Linda Ingram, eds.
   1988   *Income and Poverty Statistics: Problems of Concept and Measurement. Report of a Workshop.* Committee on National Statistics, National Research Council. Washington, D.C.: National Academy Press.
Lewis, Gordon H., and Richard C. Michel, eds.
   1990   *Microsimulation Techniques for Tax and Transfer Analysis.* Washington, D.C.: The Urban Institute Press.

Lillard, Lee A., James P. Smith, and Finis Welch
  1986   What do we really know about wages? The importance of nonreporting and census imputation. *Journal of Political Economy* 94(31):489-506.
Lillard, Lee A., and R.J. Willis
  1978   Dynamic aspects of earning mobility. *Econometrics* 46(5):985-1012.
Lindert, Peter H.
  1978   *Fertility and Scarcity in America.* Princeton: Princeton University Press.
Lundberg, Shelly, and Robert Plotnick
  1990   Adolescent premarital childbearing: Do opportunity costs matter? Paper prepared for the May 1990 Population Association of America conference, Toronto, Canada.
Mack, Joanna, and Stewart Lansley
  1985   *Poor Britain.* London, Eng.: George Allen & Unwin, Ltd.
Mahoney, Bette, Milo B. Sunderhauf, and Murray S. Weitzman
  1973   Consolidated Report of Subcommittee Chairmen: Review of Poverty Statistics. Unpublished memorandum to Paul Krueger. U.S. Office of Management and Budget, Washington, D.C.
Maritato, Nancy
  1992   Subjective Measures of Poverty. Unpublished paper prepared for the Panel on Poverty and Family Assistance, Committee on National Statistics, National Research Council. Office of the Assistant Secretary for Planning and Evaluation, U.S. Department of Health and Human Services.
Marquis, Kent H., and Jeffrey C. Moore
  1990a Measurement errors in SIPP program reports. Pp. 721-745 in *Proceedings of the Bureau of the Census Sixth Annual Research Conference.* Washington, D.C.: U.S. Department of Commerce.
  1990b SIPP Record Check Final Report. Draft. Bureau of the Census, U.S. Department of Commerce, Washington, D.C.
Marquis, Kent H., Jeffrey C. Moore, and Karen E. Bogen
  1991   A Cognitive Approach to Redesigning Measurement in the Survey of Income and Program Participation. Draft background paper prepared for the American Statistical Association/Survey Research Methods Section Working Group on Technical Aspects of SIPP. Bureau of the Census, U.S. Department of Commerce, Washington, D.C.
Mayer, Susan, and Christopher Jencks
  1993   Recent trends in economic inequality in the United States: Income vs. expenditures vs. material well-being. In Dimitri Papadimitriou and Edward Wolff, eds., *Poverty and Prosperity in the USA in the Late Twentieth Century.* London, Eng.: Macmillan.
McCormick, M.C., J. Baker, J. Brooks-Gunn, J. Turner, J. Workman-Daniels, and G. Peckham
  1991   Cohort reconstruction: Which infants can be restudied at school age? *Pediatric and Perinatal Epidemiology* 5:410-422.
Michael, Robert T.
  1985   Consequences of the rise in female labor force participation rates: Questions and probes. *Journal of Labor Economics* 3(No. 1, Pt. 2):S117-S146.

Michael, Robert T., and Edward P. Lazear
  1986   Estimating the personal distribution of income with adjustment for within-fam-
         ily variation. *Journal of Labor Economics* 4:S216-S244.
Michalos, Alex C.
  1989   Discrepancies between perceived income needs and actual incomes. *Social Indi-
         cators Research* 21(3)(June):293-296.
Michel, Richard C., and Frank S. Levy
  1991   Family income: Slower growth and less equity. *Forum for Applied Research and
         Public Policy* (Summer):40-49.
Millar, Jane, and Caroline Glendinning
  1989   Survey article: Gender and poverty. *Journal of Social Policy* 18(3):363-381.
Modigliani, Franco, and Richard Brumberg
  1954   Utility analysis and the consumption function: An interpretation of cross-sec-
         tion data. In K. Kurihara, ed., *Post-Keynesian Economics*. New Brunswick:
         Rutgers University Press.
Moffitt, Robert
  1992   Incentive effects of the U.S. welfare system: A review. *Journal of Economic
         Literature* 30(March):1-61.
Moffitt, Robert, and Barbara Wolfe
  1990   *The Effect of the Medicaid Program on Welfare Participation and Labor Supply*. Dis-
         cussion Paper No. 909-90, Institute for Research on Poverty. Madison: Uni-
         versity of Wisconsin.
Monheit, Alan C., and Claudia L. Schur
  1988   The dynamics of health insurance loss: A tale of two cohorts. *Inquiry*
         25(Fall):315-327.
Moon, Marilyn
  1977   *The Measurement of Economic Welfare: Its Application to the Aged Poor*. New York:
         Academic Press.
  1993   Incorporating Health Issues in the Measurement of Poverty. Unpublished paper
         prepared for the Panel on Poverty and Family Assistance, Committee on Na-
         tional Statistics, National Research Council. The Urban Institute, Washington,
         D.C.
Morissette, Rene, and Susan Poulin
  1991   Income Satisfaction Supplement: Summary of Four Survey Years. Labour and
         Household Surveys Analysis Division, Statistics Canada, Ottawa, Canada.
Moulton, Brent R.
  1992   Interarea Indexes of the Cost of Shelter Using Hedonic Quality and Adjustment
         Techniques. Bureau of Labor Statistics, U.S. Department of Labor, Washing-
         ton, D.C.
Muth, Richard
  1971   The derived demand for urban residential land. *Urban Studies* 8:243-254.
National Opinion Research Center
  no   The National Data Program for the Social Sciences [description of the General
  date   Social Survey]. Chicago, Ill.
Nelson, Charles T., and Gordon W. Green, Jr.
  1986   Estimating after-tax income of households, using the March Current Population

Survey. Pp. 27-36 in *Proceedings of the Business and Economic Statistics Section.* Washington, D.C.: American Statistical Association.

Nelson, Dawn D., Chet Bowie, and Annetta Walker
  1987 *Survey of Income and Program Participation (SIPP) Sample Loss and the Efforts to Reduce It.* SIPP Working Paper No. 8709. Bureau of the Census. Washington, D.C.: U.S. Department of Commerce.

Nelson, Julie
  1993 Household equivalence scales: Theory versus policy? *Journal of Labor Economics* 11(3):471-493.

Nelson, Kathryn P., and F. Stevens Redburn
  1994 Rethinking Priority Needs for Rental Assistance: Limitations of "Worst Case Needs." Paper prepared for the American Real Estate and Urban Economics Association midyear meeting. U.S. Department of Housing and Urban Development, Washington, D.C.

Neter, John, and Joseph Waksberg
  1965 *Response Errors in Collection of Expenditures Data by Household Interview: An Experimental Study.* Technical Paper No. 11. Bureau of the Census. Washington, D.C.: U.S. Department of Commerce.

Newhouse, Joseph P., and The Insurance Experiment Group
  1993 *Free for All? Lessons from the RAND Health Insurance Experiment.* Cambridge, Mass.: Harvard University Press.

Nicholson, J.L.
  1976 Appraisal of different methods of estimating equivalence scales and their results. *The Review of Income and Wealth* 22:1-18.

O'Connell, Martin, and Amara Bachu
  1990 *Who's Minding the Kids? Child Care Arrangements: Winter, 1986-87.* Current Population Reports, Household Economic Studies, Series P-70, No. 20. Bureau of the Census. Washington, D.C.: U.S. Department of Commerce.

Office of Policy Development and Research
  1992a Fair Market Rents for the Section 8 Housing Assistance Payments Program. U.S. Department of Housing and Urban Development, Washington, D.C.
  1992b FY 1992 Income Limits Briefing Material. U.S. Department of Housing and Urban Development, Washington, D.C.

Office of Technology Assessment
  1992 *Does Health Insurance Make a Difference?—Background Paper.* OTA-BP-H-99. Washington, D.C.: U.S. Government Printing Office.
  1994 *Understanding Estimates of National Health Expenditures Under Health Reform.* OTA-H-594. Washington, D.C.: U.S. Government Printing Office.

O'Hare, William
  1990 What does it take to get along? *American Demographics* 12(5)(May):36-39.
  1991 Review of Literature on Post-Censal Estimates of State and Sub-State Poverty. Urban Research Institute, University of Louisville.

O'Hare, William, Taynia Mann, Kathryn Porter, and Robert Greenstein
  1990 *Real Life Poverty in America: Where the American Public Would Set the Poverty Line.* Washington, D.C.: Center on Budget and Policy Priorities and Families USA Foundation.

O'Higgins, Michael, and Stephen Jenkins
  1990   Poverty in the EC: Estimates for 1975, 1980, and 1985. Pp. 187-212 in
         Rudolph Teekens and Bernard M.S. van Praag, eds., *Analysing Poverty in the
         European Community: Policy Issues, Research Options, and Data Sources.* Luxem-
         bourg: Office of Official Publications of the European Communities.
Oldfield, Nina
  1992   *Using Budget Standards to Estimate the Cost of Children.* Working Paper No. 15.
         Family Budget Unit, Department of Social Policy and Social Work. Heslington,
         Eng.: University of York.
O'Neill, June
  1985   Comment: The statistical measurement of poverty. Pp. 96-98 in *Proceedings of
         the Bureau of the Census Conference on the Measurement of Noncash Benefits.* Wash-
         ington, D.C.: U.S. Department of Commerce.
Organization for Economic Cooperation and Development
  1982   *The OECD List of Social Indicators.* Paris: Organization for Economic Coopera-
         tion and Development.
Orshansky, Mollie
  1963   Children of the poor. *Social Security Bulletin* 26(7)(July):3-13.
  1965a Counting the poor: another look at the poverty profile. *Social Security Bulletin*
         28(1)(January):3-29.
  1965b Who's who among the poor: a demographic view of poverty. *Social Security
         Bulletin* 28(7)(July):3-32.
  1966a More about the poor in 1964. *Social Security Bulletin* 29(5)(May):3-38.
  1966b The poor in city and suburb, 1964. *Social Security Bulletin* 29(12)(December):22-
         37.
  1966c Recounting the poor—a five-year review. *Social Security Bulletin* 29(4)(April):20-
         37.
  1968a Demography and ecology of poverty. Pp. 1-29 in *Proceedings of a Conference on
         Research in Poverty.* Washington, D.C.: Bureau of Social Science Research, Inc.
  1968b The shape of poverty in 1966. *Social Security Bulletin* 31(3)(March):3-32.
  1969   How poverty is measured. *Monthly Labor Review* 92(2)(February):37-41.
  1976   Documentation of background information and rationale for current poverty
         matrix. Technical Paper I (reprints Orshansky *Social Security Bulletin* articles).
         The Measure of Poverty. Washington, D.C.: U.S. Department of Health, Educa-
         tion, and Welfare.
  1986   Statement. Pp. 116-124 in U.S. House of Representatives, *Census Bureau Mea-
         surement of Noncash Benefits: Hearings Before the Subcommittee on Census and Popu-
         lation of the Committee on Post Office and Civil Service.* Serial No. 99-51. Wash-
         ington, D.C.: U.S. Government Printing Office.
Orshansky, Mollie, Harold W. Watts, Bradley R. Schiller, and John J. Korbel
  1978   Measuring poverty: a debate. *Public Welfare* 36(2):46-55.
Paglin, Morton
  1980   *Poverty and Transfers In-Kind: A Re-Evaluation of Poverty in the United States.*
         Stanford: Hoover Institution Press, Stanford University.
Pahl, Jan
  1989   *Money and Marriage.* London, Eng.: Macmillan.

Parker, L., S. Greer, and B. Zuckerman
    1988   Double "jeopardy": The impact of poverty on early child development. *The Pediatric Clinics of North America* 35:1227-1240.
Pearl, Robert B.
    1968   *Methodology of Consumer Expenditures Surveys.* Working Paper No. 27. Bureau of the Census. Washington, D.C.: U.S. Department of Commerce.
    1979   *Reevaluation of the 1972-73 U.S. Consumer Expenditure Survey.* Technical Paper No. 46. Bureau of the Census. Washington, D.C.: U.S. Department of Commerce.
Pechman, Joseph A.
    1985   *Who Paid the Taxes, 1966-1985?* Washington, D.C.: The Brookings Institution.
Pennell, Steven G., and James M. Lepkowski
    1992   Panel Conditioning Effects in the Survey of Income and Program Participation. Paper prepared for the American Statistical Association annual meeting. Survey Research Center, University of Michigan.
Peterkin, Betty, Andrea Blum, Richard Kerr, and Linda Cleveland
    1983   The Thrifty Food Plan, 1983. CNO(Adm.)365. Consumer Nutrition Division, Human Nutrition Information Service, U.S. Department of Agriculture, Washington, D.C.
Peterson, Paul E., and Mark C. Rom
    1989   American federalism, welfare policy and residential choices. *American Political Science Review* 83(3):711-728.
    1990   *Welfare Magnets—A New Case for a National Standard.* Washington, D.C.: The Brookings Institution.
Petroni, Rita J., and Karen E. King
    1988   Evaluation of the Survey of Income and Program Participation's cross-sectional noninterview adjustment methods. Pp. 342-347 in *Proceedings of the Survey Research Methods Section.* Alexandria, Va.: American Statistical Association.
Phipps, Shelley A.
    1993   Measuring poverty among Canadian households: Sensitivity to choice of measure and scale. *Journal of Human Resources* 28(1):162-184.
Plotnick, Robert D.
    1989   How much poverty is reduced by state income transfers? *Monthly Labor Review* 112(7)(July):21-26.
    1990   Welfare and out-of-wedlock childbearing: Evidence from the 1980s. *Journal of Marriage and the Family* 52(August):735-746.
Plotnick, Robert D., and Richard F. Winters
    1985   A politico-economic theory of redistribution. *American Political Science Review* 79(2):458-73.
Pollak, Robert, and Terrence J. Wales
    1979   Welfare comparisons and equivalence scales. *American Economic Review* 69 (March):216-21.
Poulin, Susan
    1988   An Application of Analytic Techniques to Canadian Income Satisfaction Data. Staff report. Labor and Household Surveys Analysis Division, Statistics Canada, Ottawa.

President's Commission on Income Maintenance Programs
  1969   Poverty Amid Plenty—The American Paradox. Washington, D.C.: U.S. Government Printing Office.
Quinn, Joseph F., Richard V. Burkhauser, and Daniel A. Myers
  1990   Passing the Torch: The Influence of Economic Incentives on Work and Retirement. Kalamazoo, Mich.: W.E. Upjohn Institute for Employment Research.
Rabin, R.L.
  1970   Implementation of the cost-of-living adjustment for AFDC recipients: A case study of welfare administration. University of Pennsylvania Law Review 118(8): 1143-1166.
Radbill, Larry M., and Kathleen Short
  1992   Extended Measures of Well-Being: Selected Data from the 1984 Survey of Income and Program Participation. Current Population Reports, Household Economic Studies, Series P-70, No. 26. Bureau of the Census. Washington, D.C.: U.S. Department of Commerce.
Rainwater, Lee
  1974   What Money Buys: Inequality and the Social Meanings of Income. New York: Basic Books, Inc.
  1990   Poverty and Equivalence as Social Constructions. Luxembourg Income Study, Working Paper No. 55. Harvard University.
  1992   Poverty in American Eyes. Luxembourg Income Study, Working Paper No. 80. Harvard University.
Ramey, C.T., D.M. Bryant, B.H. Wasik, J.J. Sparling, K.H. Fendt, and L.M. LaVange
  1992   The Infant Health and Development Program for low birth weight premature infants: Progam elements, family participation, and child intelligence. Pediatrics 3(March):454-465.
Ravallion, Martin
  1992   Poverty Comparisons: A Guide to Concepts and Methods. Living Standards Measurement Study, Working Paper No. 88. Washington, D.C.: The World Bank.
Ravallion, Martin, Gaurav Datt, and Dominique van de Walle
  1991   Quantifying absolute poverty in the developing world. The Review of Income and Wealth 37(4):345-361.
Rawlings, Steve W.
  1993   Household and Family Characteristics: March 1992. Current Population Reports, Series P-20, No. 467. Bureau of the Census. Washington, D.C.: U.S. Department of Commerce.
Rees, Albert
  1985   Comment: Measuring income—What kind should be in? Pp. 32-35 in Proceedings of the Bureau of the Census Conference on the Measurement of Noncash Benefits. Washington, D.C.: U.S. Department of Commerce.
Renwick, Trudi J.
  1993a   Budget-based poverty measurement: 1992 basic needs budgets for American families. Pp. 573-582 in Proceedings of the Social Statistics Section. Alexandria, Va.: American Statistical Association.
  1993b   Budget-Based Poverty Thresholds and Equivalence Scales. Paper prepared for the American Statistical Association winter meeting, Ft. Lauderdale, Fla. Skidmore College.

Renwick, Trudi J., and Barbara R. Bergmann
  1993   A budget-based definition of poverty with an application to single-parent fami-
         lies. *Journal of Human Resources* 28(1):1–24.
Roback, J.
  1982   Wages, rents, and the quality of life. *Journal of Political Economy* 90(Decem-
         ber):1257–1278.
Robinson, Gregory J.
  1990   Preliminary Estimates of the United States Resident Population on April 1,
         1990, Based on Demographic Analysis. Paper presented to the Census Advisory
         Committee of the American Statistical Association and the Census Advisory
         Committee on Population Statistics. Bureau of the Census, U.S. Department of
         Commerce, Washington, D.C.
Robinson, John P.
  1977   *How Americans Use Time: A Social-Psychological Analysis of Everyday Behavior.*
         New York: Praeger Publishers.
Rodgers, Joan R., and John L. Rodgers
  1991   Measuring the intensity of poverty among subpopulations. *Journal of Human
         Resources* 26(2):338–361.
  1993   Chronic poverty in the United States. *Journal of Human Resources* 28(1):25–54.
Rosen, H. S.
  1978   Estimating inter-city differences in the price of housing services. *Urban Studies*
         15:351–355.
  1979   Wage-based indexes of urban quality of life. In Peter Mieszkowski and Mahlon
         Straszheim, eds., *Current Issues in Urban Economics*. Baltimore, Md.: Johns
         Hopkins University Press.
Rothbarth, E.
  1943   Notes on a method of determining equivalent incomes for families of different
         composition. Appendix 4 in C. Madge, ed., *War-Time Pattern of Saving and
         Spending*. Cambridge, Eng.: Cambridge University Press.
Ruggles, Patricia
  1988a Accounting Period Impacts on the Measured Duration of Poverty Spells. The
         Urban Institute, Washington, D.C.
  1988b *Short Term Fluctuations in Income and Their Relationship to the Characteristics of the
         Low Income Population: New Data from SIPP*. SIPP Working Paper No. 8802.
         Bureau of the Census. Washington, D.C.: U.S. Department of Commerce.
  1990   *Drawing the Line—Alternative Poverty Measures and Their Implications for Public
         Policy*. Washington, D.C.: The Urban Institute Press.
Ruggles, Patricia, and Roberton Williams
  1987   *Transitions In and Out of Poverty: New Data from the Survey of Income and Program
         Participation*. SIPP Working Paper No. 8716. Bureau of the Census. Washing-
         ton, D.C.: U.S. Department of Commerce.
  1989   Longitudinal measures of poverty: Accounting for income and assets over time.
         The Review of Income and Wealth 35(3):225–244.
Rust, John, and Christopher Phelan
  1993   How Social Security and Medicare Affect Retirement Behavior in a World of
         Incomplete Markets. Monograph prepared for Workshop on Pensions and Pub-
         lic Finance in an Aging Society, Rotterdam. University of Wisconsin-Madison.

Rutter, Michael
   1989   Child psychiatric disorders in ICD-10. *Journal of Child Psychology & Psychiatry & Allied Disciplines* 30(4)(July):499-513.
Saluter, Arlene F.
   1992   *Marital Status and Living Arrangements: March 1992.* Currrent Population Reports, Series P-20, No. 468. Bureau of the Census. Washington, D.C.: U.S. Department of Commerce.
Sawhill, Isabel V.
   1988   Poverty in the U.S.: Why is it so persistent? *Journal of Economic Literature* 26(September):1073-1119.
Schirm, Allen L., Gary D. Swearingen, and Cara S. Hendricks
   1992   *Development and Evaluation of Alternative State Estimates of Poverty, Food Stamp Program Eligibility, and Food Stamp Program Participation.* Report to the Food and Nutrition Service, U.S. Department of Agriculture. Washington, D.C.: Mathematica Policy Research, Inc.
Schwarz, John E., and Thomas J. Volgy
   1992   *The Forgotten Americans.* New York: W.W. Norton & Company.
Sen, Amartya
   1976   Poverty: An ordinal approach to measurement. *Econometrica* 44:219-31.
   1983   Poor, relatively speaking. *Oxford Economic Papers* 35:153-169.
   1985   A sociological approach to the measurement of poverty: A reply to Professor Peter Townsend. *Oxford Economic Papers* 37(4):669-676.
   1987   *The Standard of Living.* Tanner Lectures, Clare Hall, Cambridge, 1985. Cambridge Eng.: Cambridge University Press.
   1992   *Inequality Reexamined.* Cambridge, Mass.: Harvard University Press.
Seneca, J.J., and M.K. Taussig
   1971   Family equivalence scales and personal income tax exemptions for children. *Review of Economics and Statistics* 53:253-262.
Shapiro, Gary, and Paul Bettin
   1992   Coverage in Household Surveys. Paper presented to the Census Advisory Committee of the American Statistical Association and the Census Advisory Committee on Population Statistics. Bureau of the Census, U.S. Department of Commerce, Washington, D.C.
Shapiro, Gary, Gregg Diffendal, and David Cantor
   1993   Survey undercoverage: Major causes and new estimates of magnitude. Pp. 638-663 in *Proceedings of the Bureau of the Census 1993 Annual Research Conference.* Washington, D.C.: U.S. Department of Commerce.
Shapiro, Gary M., and Donna Kostanich
   1988   High response error and poor coverage are severely hurting the value of household survey data. Pp. 443-448 in *Proceedings of the Survey Research Methods Section.* Washington, D.C.: American Statistical Association.
Sherwood, Mark
   1975   Family budgets and geographic differences in price levels. *Monthly Labor Review* (April):8-15.
   1977   Bureau of Labor Statistics (BLS) Family Budgets Program. Technical Paper IV. *The Measure of Poverty.* Washington, D.C.: U.S. Department of Health, Education, and Welfare.

Short, Kathleen, and Martina Shea
  1991   *Transitions in Income and Poverty Status: 1987-88.* Current Population Reports, Household Economic Studies, Series P-70, No. 24. Bureau of the Census. Washington, D.C.: U.S. Department of Commerce.
Silberstein, Adriana R.
  1989   Recall effects in the U.S. Consumer Expenditure Survey. *Journal of Official Statistics* 5(2):125-142.
Slesnick, Daniel T.
  1991a Gaining Ground: Poverty in the Postwar United States. Revised July 1991. Department of Economics, University of Texas.
  1991b The standard of living in the United States. *The Review of Income and Wealth* 37(4):363-386.
Smeeding, Timothy M.
  1982   *Alternative Methods for Valuing Selected In-Kind Transfer Benefits and Measuring Their Effect on Poverty.* Technical Paper No. 50. Bureau of the Census. Washington, D.C.: U. S. Department of Commerce.
  1988   Valuation of Noncash Benefits and Their Effect on Poverty: What Needs to Be Done and Why? Statement before the Subcommittee on Census and Population, Committee on Post Office and Civil Service, U.S. House of Representatives, March 22. Vanderbilt University.
Smeeding, Timothy M., and Barbara Boyle Torrey
  1988   Poor children in rich countries. *Science* 242(11 November):873-877.
Smith, Adam
  1776   *Wealth of Nations.* Modern Library Edition, 1993. New York: Random House, Inc.
Smith, James D.
  1987   Measuring the informal economy. *Annals of the American Academy of Political and Social Science* 493(September):83-99.
Smolensky, Eugene
  1985   Comment: The statistical measurement of poverty. Pp. 99-103 in *Proceedings of the Bureau of the Census Conference on the Measurement of Noncash Benefits.* Washington, D.C.: U.S. Department of Commerce.
Solomon, Carmen D.
  1991   *Aid to Families with Dependent Children (AFDC): Need Standards, Payment Standards, and Maximum Benefits.* Congressional Research Service Report for Congress 91-849-EPW. Washington, D.C.: U.S. Government Printing Office.
Solomon, Carmen D., and Jennifer A. Neisner
  1993   *Aid to Families with Dependent Children (AFDC): Need Standards, Payment Standards, and Maximum Benefits.* Congressional Research Service Report for Congress 93-63-EPW. Washington, D.C.: U.S. Government Printing Office.
Sorenson, Elaine
  1993   Noncustodial Fathers: Can They Afford to Pay More Child Support? The Urban Institute, Washington, D.C.
Spillman, B.C.
  1992   The impact of being uninsured on utilization of basic health care. *Inquiry* 29:457-466.

Statistics Canada
 1991 *Income Distributions by Size in Canada—1990.* Household Surveys Division. Ottawa: Statistics Canada.
 1992 *Income After Tax, Distributions by Size in Canada—1990.* Household Surveys Division. Ottawa: Statistics Canada.
Steffick, Diane
 1993 Housing Subsidies. Unpublished memorandum, The Urban Institute, Washington, D.C.
Stein, R.E., S.L. Gortmaker, E.C. Perrin, J.M. Perrin, I.B. Pless, D.K. Walker, and M. Weitzman
 1987 Severity of illness: Concepts and measurements. *The Lancet* 2:1506-1509.
Stephenson, Stanley, Jr.
 1977 Relative measure of poverty. Technical Paper XIV. *The Measure of Poverty.* Washington, D.C.: U.S. Department of Health, Education, and Welfare.
Survey Research Center
 1989 *A Panel Study of Income Dynamics—Procedures and Tape Codes, 1987 Interviewing Year.* Institute for Social Research. Ann Arbor: University of Michigan.
Takayama, Noriyuki
 1979 Poverty, income inequality and their measures: Professor Sen's axiomatic approach reconsidered. *Econometrica* 47:747-759.
Taylor, Amy K., and Jessica S. Banthin
 1994 *Out-of-Pocket Expenditures for Personal Health Services: Changes in 1977 and 1988.* National Medical Expenditure Survey Research Findings 21, AHCPR Publication No. 94-0065. Agency for Health Care Policy and Research. Washington, D.C.: U.S. Department of Health and Human Services.
Thibodeau, T.
 1989 Housing price indexes from the 1974-1983 SIMSA Annual Housing Surveys. *Journal of the American Real Estate and Urban Economics Association* 1(1):100-117.
Thon, Dominique
 1979 On measuring poverty. *The Review of Income and Wealth* 25:429-39.
Thornton, Arland
 1988 Cohabitation and marriage in the 1980s. *Demography* 25(4)(November):497-508.
Townsend, Peter
 1954 Measuring poverty. *British Journal of Sociology* 5(2)(June):130-137.
 1962 The meaning of poverty. *British Journal of Sociology* 13(3)(September):210-227.
 1979 *Poverty in the United Kingdom: A Survey of Household Resources and Standards of Living.* Harmondsworth, Eng.: Penguin Books.
 1985 A sociological approach to the measurement of poverty—A rejoinder to Professor Amartya Sen. *Oxford Economic Papers* 37:659-668.
 1992 *The International Analysis of Poverty.* Hemel Hempstead, Eng.: Harvester-Wheatsheaf
Townsend, Peter, and David Gordon
 1991 What is enough? New evidence on poverty allowing the definition of a minimum benefit. Pp. 35-69 in Michael Adler, Colin Bell, Jochen Clasen, and Adrian Sinfield, eds., *The Sociology of Social Security.* Edinburgh: Edinburgh University Press.

Tsakloglou, Panos
    1990   A Comparison of Poverty Rate Estimates Using Expenditure and Income Data.
            Luxembourg Income Study, Working Paper No. 71. Luxembourg: Statistical
            Office of the European Communities.
Tucker, Clyde, Gil Haugh, Sylvia Johnson-Herring, Sharon Krieger, and Karen Vigliano
    no   The Impact of Political and Economic Conditions on Refusal Rates
    date   to the Current Population Survey and the Consumer Expenditure Surveys.
            Bureau of Labor Statistics, U.S. Department of Labor, Washington, D.C.
Urban Systems Research & Engineering, Inc. (USR&E)
    1980   *AFDC Standards of Need: An Evaluation of Current Practices, Alternative Approaches,*
            and Policy Options. Prepared for the Social Security Administration, U.S. De-
            partment of Health and Human Services. Cambridge, Mass.: Urban Systems
            Research & Engineering, Inc.
U.S. Department of Health, Education, and Welfare
    1976   *The Measure of Poverty.* A report to Congress as mandated by the Education
            Amendments of 1974. Includes 17 technical appendices. Washington, D.C.:
            U.S. Government Printing Office.
U.S. General Accounting Office
    1985a   *An Evaluation of the 1981 AFDC Changes: Final Report.* GAO/PEMD-85-4.
            Washington, D.C.: U.S. Government Printing Office.
    1985b   *Federal Benefit Programs: A Profile.* GAO/HRD-86-14. Washington, D.C.:
            U.S. Government Printing Office.
    1986a   *An Evaluation of the Census Bureau's Measurement Conference.* GAO/PEMD-86-
            8BR. Washington, D.C.: U.S. Government Printing Office.
    1986b   *Noncash Benefits: Initial Results Show Valuation Methods Differentially Affect the*
            Poor. GAO/PEMD-87-7BR. Washington, D.C.: U.S. Government Printing
            Office.
    1987a   *Noncash Benefits: Methodological Review of Experimental Valuation Methods Indicates*
            Many Problems Remain. GAO/PEMD-87-23. Washington, D.C.: U.S. Gov-
            ernment Printing Office.
    1987b   *Welfare—Income and Relative Poverty Status of AFDC Families.* GAO/HRD-88-
            9. Washington, D.C.: U.S. Government Printing Office.
    1988   *Evaluation of Poverty Indicators.* GAO/T-PEMD-88-1. Washington, D.C.: U.S.
            Government Printing Office.
    1992   *Unemployed Parents—An Evaluation of the Effects of Welfare Benefits on Family Sta-*
            bility. GAO/PEMD-92-19BR. Washington, D.C.: U.S. Government Printing
            Office.
U.S. House of Representatives
    1985   *Children in Poverty.* Committee on Ways and Means. Washington, D.C.: U.S.
            Government Printing Office.
    1990   *Overview of Entitlement Programs: 1990 Green Book.* Background material and
            data on programs within the jurisdiction of the Committee on Ways and Means.
            Washington, D.C.: U.S. Government Printing Office.
    1991   *Overview of Entitlement Programs: 1991 Green Book.* Background material and
            data on programs within the jurisdiction of the Committee on Ways and Means.
            Washington, D.C.: U.S. Government Printing Office.
    1992   *Overview of Entitlement Programs: 1992 Green Book.* Background material and

data on programs within the jurisdiction of the Committee on Ways and Means. Washington, D.C.: U.S. Government Printing Office.

1993 *Overview of Entitlement Programs: 1993 Green Book.* Background material and data on programs within the jurisdiction of the Committee on Ways and Means. Washington, D.C.: U.S. Government Printing Office.

1994 *Overview of Entitlement Programs: 1994 Green Book.* Background material and data on programs within the jurisdiction of the Committee on Ways and Means. Washington, D.C.: U.S. Government Printing Office.

U.S. Office of Economic Opportunity

1965 *National Anti-Poverty Plan and 1967 Budget Request.* Washington, D.C.: U.S. Office of Economic Opportunity.

1966 *National Anti-Poverty Plan—FY 1968-FY 1972.* Washington, D.C.: U.S. Office of Economic Opportunity.

U.S. Senate

1986 *Work and Welfare.* Committee on Labor and Human Resources and Committee on Finance. Washington, D.C.: U.S. Government Printing Office.

van den Bosch, Karel

1992 Comparing Longitudinal Poverty Across Countries: Results from Five EC-Countries and Some Methodological Explorations. Paper prepared for the International Social Science Methodology Conference at Trento, Italy. Centre of Social Policy, University of Antwerp, The Netherlands.

van der Gaag, Jacques

1981 *On Measuring the Cost of Children.* Discussion Paper 663-81, Institute for Research on Poverty. Madison: University of Wisconsin.

van Praag, Bernard M.S.

1968 *Individual Welfare Functions and Consumer Behavior.* Amsterdam: North Holland Publishing Company.

van Praag, B.M.S., S. Dubnoff, and N. van der Saar

1988 On the measurement and explanation of standards with respect to income, age, and education. *Journal of Economic Psychology* 9:481-498.

van Praag, Bernard M.S., Theo Goedhart, and Arie Kapteyn

1980 The poverty line: A pilot survey in Europe. *Review of Economics and Statistics* 62:461-465.

Vaughan, Denton R.

1985 Using subjective assessments of income to estimate family equivalence scales: A report on work in progress. Pp. 31-44 in *Survey of Income and Program Participation and Related Longitudinal Surveys: 1984.* Selected papers given at the 1984 annual meeting of the American Statistical Association, Philadelphia, Pa. Bureau of the Census. Washington, D.C.: U.S. Department of Commerce.

1989 *Reflections on the Income Estimates from the Initial Panel of the Survey of Income and Program Participation (SIPP).* ORS Working Paper Series, No. 39. Office of Research and Statistics, Social Security Administration. Washington, D.C.: U.S. Department of Health and Human Services.

1993 Exploring the use of the public's views to set income poverty thresholds and adjust them over time. *Social Security Bulletin* 56(2)(Summer):22-46.

Veit-Wilson, John

1994 *Dignity not Poverty: A Minimum Income Standard for the UK.* Commission on

Social Justice Issue Paper 6.   London, Eng.:   Institute for Public Policy Research.

Vickery, Clair
1977   The time-poor: A new look at poverty. *Journal of Human Resources* 12(1):27-48.

Walker, K.E., and M.E. Woods
1976   *Time Use: A Measure of Household Production of Family Goods and Services.* Washington D.C.:   American Home Economics Association.

Ward, Michael P.
1985   The statistical measurement of poverty.   Pp. 68-95 in *Proceedings of the Bureau of the Census Conference on the Measurement of Noncash Benefits.* Washington, D.C.: U.S. Department of Commerce.

Watts, Harold W.
1967   The iso-prop index: An approach to the determination of differential poverty income thresholds. *Journal of Human Resources* 2(1):3-18.

1968   An economic definition of poverty.   Pp. 316-329 in Daniel P. Moynihan, ed., *On Understanding Poverty: Perspectives from the Social Sciences.* New York: Basic Books.

1980   Special panel suggests changes in BLS Family Budget Program. *Monthly Labor Review* 103(12)(December):3-10.

1986   Have our measures of poverty become poorer?   *Focus* 9(2)(Summer):18-23. [Institute for Research on Poverty, University Wisconsin-Madison]

1993   A Review of Alternative Budget-Based Expenditure Norms.   Unpublished paper prepared for the Panel on Poverty and Family Assistance, Committee on National Statistics, National Research Council.   Columbia University.

Weinberg, Daniel H.
1987   Filling the "poverty gap," 1979-1984. *Journal of Human Resources* 22(4):563-573.

1989   Poverty Dynamics and the Poverty Gap, 1984-1986.   Office of the Assistant Secretary for Planning and Evaluation, U.S. Department of Health and Human Services, Washington, D.C.

1990   Income Inequality and Measures of Well-Being: The Next Decade.   Paper prepared for the Joint Statistical Meetings, Anaheim, Calif. Bureau of the Census, U.S. Department of Commerce, Washington, D.C.

Weinberg, Daniel H., and Enrique J. Lamas
1992   The history and current issues of U.S. poverty measurement.   Pp. 173-199 in *Poverty Measurement for Economies in Transition in Eastern European Countries.* Warsaw: Polish Statistical Association and Polish Central Statistical Office.

1993   Some experimental results on alternative poverty measures.   Pp. 549-555 in *Proceedings of the Social Statistics Section.*   Alexandria, Va.:   American Statistical Association.

Weinberg, Daniel H., and Rita J. Petroni
1992   *The Survey of Income and Program Participation in the 1990s.*   SIPP Working Paper No. 9206.   Bureau of the Census.   Washington, D.C.:   U.S. Department of Commerce.

Weisbrod, Burton A., and W. Lee Hansen
1968   An income-net worth approach to measuring economic welfare. *American Economic Review* 58(5)(December):1315-1329.

Welniak, Edward J., Jr.
  1990 Effects of the March Current Population Survey's new processing system on estimates of income and poverty. In *Proceedings of the Business and Economic Statistics Section*. Alexandria, Va.: American Statistical Association.
Welniak, Edward J., and John F. Coder
  1980 A measure of the bias in the March CPS earnings imputation system. Pp. 421-425 in *Proceedings of the Survey Research Methods Section*. Washington, D.C.: American Statistical Association.
Whiteford, Peter, and Leslie Hicks
  1992 *The Cost of Lone Parents: Evidence from Budget Standards*. Working Paper No. 16. Family Budget Unit, Department of Social Policy and Social Work. Heslington, Eng.: University of York.
Will, B. Phyllis
  1986 Poverty: That Intangible Which Evades Definition or Measurement. Working paper, Statistics Canada, Ottawa.
Williams, Roberton
  1986 Poverty rates and program participation in the SIPP and the CPS. In *Proceedings of the Social Statistics Section*. Alexandria, Va.: American Statistical Association.
  1987 *Measuring Poverty with the SIPP and the CPS*. SIPP Working Paper No. 8723. Bureau of the Census. Washington, D.C.: U.S. Department of Commerce.
Willis, R.J., and R.T. Michael
  1994 Innovation in family formation: Evidence on cohabitation in the United States. Pp. 10-45 in J. Ermisch and K. Ogawa, eds., *The Family, the Market and the State in Aging Societies*. Cambridge, Eng.: Oxford University Press.
Winkler, A.
  1989 The Incentive Effects of Medicaid on Women's Labor Supply. University of Missouri, St. Louis, Mo.
Wise, David A.
  1992 *Topics in the Economics of Aging*. Chicago: The University of Chicago Press.
Wiseman, Michael
  1993 Welfare reform in the states: The Bush legacy. *Focus* 15(1):1-17. [Institute for Research on Poverty, University of Wisconsin-Madison]
Wolfe, Barbara L., and Steven Hill
  1992 *The Health, Earnings Capacity, and Poverty of Single-Mother Families*. Discussion Paper 964-92, Institute for Research on Poverty. Madison: University of Wisconsin.
Wolfe, Barbara, and Robert Moffitt
  1991 A new index to value in-kind benefits. *The Review of Income and Wealth* 37(4): 387-408.
Wolfson, M.C., and J.M. Evans
  1989 *Statistics Canada's Low Income Cut-Offs: Methodological Concerns and Possibilities— A Discussion Paper*. Research Paper Series. Analytical Studies Branch. Ottawa: Statistics Canada.
Ycas, Martynas A., and Charles A. Lininger
  1983 The Income Survey Development Program: Design features and initial findings. Pp. 25-31 in Martin H. David, ed., *Technical, Conceptual, and Administrative*

Lessons of the Income Survey Development Program (ISDP): Papers Presented at a Conference. New York: Social Science Research Council.

Young, Michael
   1952   Distribution of income within the family. British Journal of Sociology 3(4)December:305-321.

Young, Nathan C.
   1991   Longitudinal Analysis of Food Stamp Recipiency in the SIPP: Using Seam Contrasts to Evaluate Measurement Error Bias. Prepared for the Bureau of the Census, U.S. Department of Commerce. Washington, D.C.: The Urban Institute.

Yu, Autumn C. S.
   1992   Low Cost Budget Standards for Three Household Types. Working Paper No. 17. Family Budget Unit, Department of Social Policy and Social Work. Heslington, Eng.: University of York.

Zill, Nicholas, Kristin A. Moore, Ellen Wolpow Smith, Thomas Stief, and Mary Jo Coiro
   1991   The Life Circumstances and Development of Children in Welfare Families: A Profile Based on National Survey Data. Washington, D.C.: Child Trends, Inc.

Biographical Sketches of Panel Members and Staff

ROBERT T. MICHAEL (*Chair*) is the Eliakim Hastings Moore Distinguished Service professor in the Harris School at the University of Chicago. He was founding dean of the Harris School and served as director of the National Opinion Research Center from 1984 through 1989. Previously, he taught in the education department at the University of Chicago and in the economics departments at Stanford University and the University of California at Los Angeles. His research interests are in the economics of the family, including studies of marriage and divorce, the allocation of income within the family, parental investments in children, and adult sexual behavior. He has conducted several national surveys of behavior pertaining to children, schooling, and partnering. At the National Research Council, he chaired the Panel on Pay Equity, and he serves on the Board on Children and Families of the National Research Council/Institute of Medicine. He is a fellow of the American Association for the Advancement of Science. He received a B.A. degree from Ohio Wesleyan University and a Ph.D. degree in economics from Columbia University.

ANTHONY B. ATKINSON is warden of Nuffield College, Oxford. Previously he was professor of political economy at the University of Cambridge and professor of economics at the London School of Economics. His research is in the field of public economics and income distribution. He received a B.A. degree from the University of Cambridge. He is a fellow of the Econometric Society (president, 1988), a fellow of the British Academy, and an honorary member of the American Economic Association. He also served as president of the International Economic Association. He is joint editor of the *Journal of Public Economics*.

DAVID M. BETSON is the director of the Hesburgh Program in Public Service and an associate professor of economics at the University of Notre Dame. He was previously a research associate at the Institute for Research on Poverty at the University of Wisconsin and a staff economist at the Department of Health, Education, and Welfare. His research has dealt with the impact of tax and transfer programs on the economy and the distribution of income. At the National Research Council he served on the Panel to Evaluate Microsimulation Models for Social Welfare Programs of the Committee on National Statistics. He received a B.A. degree from Kalamazoo College and a Ph.D. degree from the University of Wisconsin at Madison.

REBECCA M. BLANK is a professor of economics at Northwestern University and a faculty research associate with the National Bureau of Economic Research. She is also a member of the research faculty at Northwestern University's Center for Urban Affairs and Policy Research, and she serves as codirector of its Urban Poverty Program, an interdisciplinary research and graduate training program. Prior to coming to Northwestern, she taught at Princeton University and served as a senior staff economist with the Council of Economic Advisers. Her research focuses on the interaction among the economy, government antipoverty programs, and the behavior and well-being of low-income families. She recently received the David Kershaw award, given biannually to the young scholar whose work has had the most impact on policy. She has a B.S. degree from the University of Minnesota and a Ph.D. in economics from the Massachusetts Institute of Technology.

LAWRENCE D. BOBO is professor of sociology and director of the Center for Research on Race, Politics, and Society at University of California at Los Angeles. His research interests include racial attitudes and relations, social psychology, public opinion, and political behavior. He has served on the Board of Overseers for the General Social Survey of the National Opinion Research Center, and he has been active in the work of the American Association for Public Opinion Research. At the National Research Council, he served as a senior research associate for the Committee on the Status of Black Americans. He has served on the editorial boards of *Public Opinion Quarterly* and *Social Psychology Quarterly* and is currently on the editorial board of the *American Sociological Review.* He is coauthor of the award-winning book *Racial Attitudes in America* (Harvard University Press). He received a B.A. degree from Loyola Marymount University and M.A. and Ph.D. degrees from the University of Michigan.

JEANNE BROOKS-GUNN is Virginia and Leonard Marx professor in child development and professor of pediatrics at the College of Physicians and Surgeons, Columbia University. She also directs the Center for Young Children and Families at Teachers College and the Adolescent Study Program at Teachers College and the St. Luke-Roosevelt Hospital Center of Columbia University. A developmental psychologist, she received an Ed.M. degree from Harvard University and a Ph.D. degree from the University of Pennsylvania. Her specialty is policy-oriented research focusing on familial influences on children's development—achievement, psychological well-being, school and behavioral problems—and intervention efforts aimed at ameliorating the developmental delays seen in poor and at-risk children.

CONSTANCE F. CITRO (*Study Director*) is a member of the staff of the Committee on National Statistics. She is a former vice president and deputy director of Mathematica Policy Research, Inc., and was an American Statistical Association/National Science Foundation (NSF) research fellow at the Bureau of the Census. For the Committee on National Statistics, she has served or is currently serving as study director for the Panel on Retirement Income Modeling, the Panel to Evaluate the Survey of Income and Program Participation, the Panel to Evaluate Microsimulation Models for Social Welfare Programs, the Panel to Study the NSF Scientific and Technical Personnel Data System, and the Panel on Decennial Census Methodology. Her research has focused on the usefulness and accessibility of large, complex microdata files, as well as analysis related to income measurement and demographic change. She is a fellow of the American Statistical Association. She received a B.A. degree from the University of Rochester and M.A. and Ph.D. degrees in political science from Yale University.

JOHN F. COGAN is a senior fellow at the Hoover Institution and teaches in the Public Policy Program at Stanford University. Previously, he was an associate economist at the Rand Corporation. He has spent considerable time in pubic service beginning in 1981: as assistant secretary for policy in the U.S. Department of Labor and, subsequently, as associate director for economics and government, associate director for human resources, and deputy director at the U.S. Office of Management and Budget. He also served as a member of the U.S. Bipartisan Commission on Comprehensive Health Care (Pepper Commission) and the Social Security "Notch" Commission. He is now pursuing research in the areas of the U.S. budget and fiscal policy, income distribution, and the role of the congressional budget process and its impact on fiscal policy. He received A.B. and Ph.D. degrees in economics from the University of California at Los Angeles.

SHELDON H. DANZIGER is professor of social work and public policy, faculty associate in population studies, and director of the Research and Training Program on Poverty, the Underclass, and Public Policy at the University of Michigan. He received a B.A. degree from Columbia University and a Ph.D. degree in economics from the Massachusetts Institute of Technology.

He was previously on the faculty of the School of Social Work and the Institute for Research on Poverty at the University of Wisconsin, and he was director of the Institute for Research on Poverty. His research focuses on trends in poverty and inequality and the effects of economic and demographic changes and government social programs on disadvantaged groups. He is the coeditor of several volumes, most recently *Confronting Poverty: Prescriptions for Change* (Harvard University Press, 1994). He was a member of the Committee on Research on the Urban Underclass, Social Science Research Council; the Committee on Child Development Research and Public Policy, National Research Council; and the Panel on Employment, Income and Occupations, Committee on the Status of Black Americans, National Research Council.

ANGUS S. DEATON is William Church Osborn professor of public affairs and professor of economics and international affairs at the Woodrow Wilson School of Princeton University. He has previously held appointments at the University of Bristol and Cambridge University in England. He has been a long-time consultant for the World Bank, working on transportation, welfare measurement, price reform, and saving. He is author or coauthor of three books and many journal articles on demand analysis, theoretical and applied econometrics, saving, public finance, and development. His most recent work is on the microeconomics and macroeconomics of saving behavior and on the many issues surrounding the behavior of the prices of primary commodities. In 1978 he was the first recipient of the Frisch Medal of the Econometric Society. He is a fellow of the Econometric Society and was editor of *Econometrica,* and he is a fellow of the American Academy of Arts and Sciences. At the National Research Council, he has served as a member of the Committee on National Statistics.

JUDITH M. GUERON is president of the Manpower Demonstration Research Corporation (MDRC), a nonprofit research organization whose mission is to design and evaluate promising education and employment-related programs aimed at improving the well-being of disadvantaged adults and youth. MDRC has studied more than three dozen, mostly large-scale social policy initiatives; its agenda includes demonstrations or evaluations of school-to-work educational initiatives, teen parent interventions, and efforts to improve child support enforcement and reduce child poverty. The author of many publications, including (with Edward Pauly) *From Welfare to Work* (Russell Sage Foundation, 1991), she also frequently testifies and speaks on the results and implications of MDRC's research, as well as on welfare reform and social policy more broadly. She has served on advisory panels to the U.S. Department of Labor, and she has served on several study committees at the National Research Council. She received a B.A. degree from Radcliffe College and M.A. and Ph.D. degrees in economics from Harvard University.

ROBERT M. HAUSER is Vilas research professor of sociology and formerly served as director of the Institute for Research on Poverty at the University of Wisconsin-Madison, where he has been on the faculty since 1969. He has also held a faculty appointment at Brown University and visiting appointments at the Institute for Advanced Study in Vienna and at the University of Bergen. He received a B.A. degree from the University of Chicago and a Ph.D. degree from the University of Michigan. His publications related to education and social inequality include five books and numerous articles. His current research interests include trends in educational progression and social mobility in the United States among racial and ethnic groups, the effects of families on social and economic inequality, and changes in socioeconomic standing, health, and well-being across the life course. He has won the Paul F. Lazarsfeld award in research methods from the American Sociological Association, and he is a member of the National Academy of Sciences. At the National Research Council, he currently serves on the Commission on Behavioral and Social Sciences and Education and on the Committee on National Statistics. He is a fellow of the American Association for the Advancement of Science, the American Statistical Association, and the American Academy of Arts and Sciences.

NANCY L. MARITATO served as a research associate with the Committee on National Statistics for this and other studies and is now working as an economist in the Office of the Assistant Secretary for Planning and Evaluation at the U.S. Department of Health and Human Services. She received B.A. and M.A. degrees in economics from the University of Wisconsin, where she is currently working on a Ph.D. degree in economics. She was previously a research assistant at the Institute for Research on Poverty at the University of Wisconsin and a junior staff economist with the President's Council of Economic Advisers. Her interests lie in poverty and welfare policy analysis.

ELAINE REARDON served as a research associate for the panel. She recently received a Ph.D. degree from the Harris Graduate School of Public Policy Studies at the University of Chicago. She is now at the Milken Institute for Job and Capital Formation, where her research topics include demand-side factors in black economic progress since 1940; dual-earner households and risk; and the determinants of and policies regarding self-employment.

FRANKLIN D. WILSON is professor of sociology and Afro-American studies and director of the Center for Demography and Ecology at the University of Wisconsin-Madison, where he has taught since 1973. He spent the 1991-1992 academic year in residence at the Bureau of the Census as an American Statistical Association/National Science Foundation/Census Bureau fellow.

He received a B.A. degree from Miles College and M.A. and Ph.D. degrees from Washington State University. As a demographer, he specializes in population distribution and redistribution. His written work has covered such topics as internal migration and urbanization, residential differentiation and geographic mobility within metropolitan areas, and ethnic differences in social and economic well-being. He is currently coprincipal investigator of a project to study the labor market experiences of ethnic populations since 1983, using the 1984 through 1987 panels of the Survey of Income and Program Participation.

Index

see also Consumption and spending patterns; Economic deprivation and well-being; Expert budgets and standards

State-administered programs
eligibility standards, 436, 437, 443
SSI supplementation, 447-448
see also Aid to Families with Dependent Children (AFDC); Aid to Refugees; Foster Care program; Low-Income Home Energy Assistance Program (LIHEAP); Maternal and Child Health Services Block Grant (Title V); Medicaid; Vocational Education Opportunities

Statistical defensibility, 3, 4, 38-39, 40
Statistical Policy Office (OMB), 4, 5, 44
Statistics *see* Data quality; Poverty statistics; Time series and trend data
Statistics Canada, 127, 128, 180n. *See also* Low income cut-offs (LICOs)
Subjective thresholds, 6, 34-35, 47, 50, 51, 54, 134-140, 141, 142
scaling, 174-175
Subsidized housing *see* Rent subsidies
Summer Food Service Program for Children, 441
Summer Youth Employment and Training Program, 443
Supplemental Security Income (SSI)
accounting period, 294
eligibility, 436, 447-448
and participation in other programs, 433, 438, 439, 442, 443, 444
Survey of Consumer Finances, 409n
Survey of Economic Opportunity (SEO), 397, 398
Survey of Income and Program Participation (SIPP), 13, 86, 205, 283-288, 295, 391, 400-402
compared with March Current Population Survey, 278-280, 398, 403, 406-420
data coverage and content, 81-83, 223, 284, 401-402, 404-405, 406-411
data quality, 11, 403-404, 406-410, 411-420

poverty estimates, 11, 81, 214, 278-290, 296, 297-298, 403, 406, 411, 415, 420
sample size and design, 12, 82-83, 205n, 281, 400-401, 404, 409-410, 412
use in setting poverty measure, 11, 12, 40, 82, 83, 278-280, 281-282
Surveys *see* American Housing Survey; Consumer Expenditure Survey; Current Population Survey; Gallup Poll; Income Survey Development Program; March income supplement (March CPS); Panel Study of Income Dynamics; Public opinion polls; Survey of Income and Program Participation

T

Taxes, 25, 29-30, 45, 122, 207, 402
in Consumer Expenditure Survey, 395, 404
data quality, 407
and family resource definition, 2, 4, 5, 37, 40, 69-70, 97, 102, 205, 237-240, 267
in March Current Population Survey, 406-407
in Panel Study of Income Dynamics, 399, 404
policy changes, 3, 28-29
in Survey of Income and Program Participation, 239-240, 404, 407
Telephones, 22, 36, 100
Thresholds *see* Poverty thresholds
Thrifty Food Plan, 33, 111, 114, 116, 122, 149, 168. *See also* Minimum diet (USDA plans)
Time periods
annual accounting period, 13, 72, 85-86, 293-295, 333
long-term measures, 13, 86, 294, 295, 298-301
short-term measures, 13, 72, 85-86, 215, 294, 295-298
Time resources, 399, 421-432
and earnings potential, 430-431